The International Lib

PROBLEMS OF PERSO

Founded by C. K. Ogden

The International Library of Psychology

INDIVIDUAL DIFFERENCES
In 21 Volumes

I	The Practice and Theory of Individual Psychology	*Adler*
II	The Neurotic Constitution	*Adler*
III	Duality	*Bradley*
IV	Problems of Personality	*Campbell et al*
V	An Introduction to Individual Psychology	*Dreikurs*
VI	The Psychology of Alfred Adler and the Development of the Child	*Ganz*
VII	Personality	*Gordon*
VIII	The Art of Interrogation	*Hamilton*
IX	Appraising Personality	*Harrower*
X	Physique and Character	*Kretschmer*
XI	The Psychology of Men of Genius	*Kretschmer*
XII	Handreading	*Laffan*
XIII	On Shame and the Search for Identity	*Lynd*
XIV	A B C of Adler's Psychology	*Mairet*
XV	Alfred Adler: Problems of Neurosis	*Mairet*
XVI	Principles of Experimental Psychology	*Piéron*
XVII	The Psychology of Character	*Roback*
XVIII	The Hands of Children	*Spier*
XIX	The Nature of Intelligence	*Thurstone*
XX	Alfred Adler: The Pattern of Life	*Wolfe*
XXI	The Psychology of Intelligence and Will	*Wyatt*

PROBLEMS OF PERSONALITY

Studies Presented to Dr Morton Prince, Pioneer in American Psychopathology

Edited by
C MACFIE CAMPBELL, H S LANGFELD,
WM MCDOUGALL, A A ROBACK AND
E W TAYLOR

Preface by A A Roback

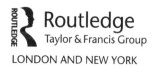

LONDON AND NEW YORK

First published in 1925 by
Kegan Paul, Trench, Trubner & Co., Ltd.
2 Park Square, Milton Park, Abingdon, Oxfordshire OX14 4RN
711 Third Avenue, New York, NY 10017

First issued in paperback 2014

Routledge is an imprint of the Taylor and Francis Group, an informa business

British Library Cataloguing in Publication Data
A CIP catalogue record for this book
is available from the British Library

Problems of Personality
ISBN 978-0415-21054-6
Individual Differences: 21 Volumes
ISBN 0415-21130-1
The International Library of Psychology: 204 Volumes
ISBN 0415-19132-7

ISBN 13: 978-1-138-88251-5 (pbk)
ISBN 13: 978-0-415-21054-6 (hbk)

CONTENTS

PAGE

PREFACE xi

PART ONE

GENERAL ESSAYS

CHAPTER

I. THE EVOLUTION OF INTELLIGENCE AND THE
THRALDOM OF CATCH-PHRASES. G. ELLIOT
SMITH, M.A., LITT.D., M.D., D.SC., F.R.C.P.,
F.R.S., Professor of Anatomy, University of
London 1

II. ABNORMAL PSYCHOLOGY AND SOCIAL PSYCHOLOGY.
ERNEST JONES, M.D., President of The
International Psycho-Analytical Association,
Editor of the *International Journal of Psycho-
Analysis;* formerly Professor of Psychiatry,
University of Toronto ... ... · 13

III. NOTES ON SUGGESTION, EMPATHY, AND BAD
THINKING IN MEDICINE. WILLIAM A. WHITE,
M.D., Superintendent at St. Elizabeth's
Hospital, Washington, D.C. ; Co-editor of the
Psychoanalytic Review and the *Nervous and
Mental Disease Monograph Series;* President,
American Psychiatric Association ; Professor
of Nervous and Mental Diseases, Georgetown
University, and George Washington University ;
and Lecturer on Psychiatry, U.S. Army and
U.S. Navy Medical Schools 27

CONTENTS

PART TWO

STUDIES IN PSYCHOLOGY

CHAPTER   PAGE

IV. DOES THE WILL EXPRESS THE ENTIRE PERSONALITY? ED. CLAPARÈDE, M.D., Professor of Psychology at the University of Geneva 37

V. AN EXPERIENCE DURING DANGER AND THE WIDER FUNCTIONS OF EMOTION. GEORGE M. STRATTON, M.A., PH.D., Professor of Psychology, University of California 45

VI. ON RECENT CONTRIBUTIONS TO THE STUDY OF THE PERSONALITY. C. MACFIE CAMPBELL, M.A., B.Sc., M.R.C.P., M.D., Professor of Psychiatry, Harvard University; Director, Boston Psychopathic Hospital 63

VII. CHARACTER AND INHIBITION. A. A. ROBACK, A.M., PH.D., National Research Council and Harvard University 77

PART THREE

STUDIES IN ABNORMAL PSYCHOLOGY AND PSYCHOPATHOLOGY

VIII. ON MEMORIES WHICH ARE TOO REAL. PIERRE JANET, M.D., LITT.D., Professor of Psychology, Collège de France 139

IX. SOME MEDICO-LEGAL EXPERIENCES, WITH COMMENTS AND REFLECTIONS. CHARLES K. MILLS, M.D., PH.D., LL.D., Professor Emeritus of Neurology, University of Pennsylvania 151

X. SOME MEDICAL ASPECTS OF WITCHCRAFT. E. W. TAYLOR, A.M., M.D.; James Jackson Putnam Professor of Neurology, Harvard Medical School 165

CHAPTER PAGE

XI. Divisions of the Self and Co-Consciousness. T. W. Mitchell, M.D., Editor of *The British Journal of Medical Psychology*; formerly President of the (British) Society for Psychical Research 189

XII. The Handwriting in Nervous Diseases, with Special Reference to the Signatures of William Shakespeare. Charles L. Dana, A.M., M.D., Ll.D., Professor of Nervous Diseases, Cornell University Medical College; Consulting Neurologist to Bellevue Hospital, The Neurological Institute; ex-President of the New York Academy of Medicine 205

XIII. The Static and Kinetic Representations of the Efferent Nervous System in the Psycho-Motor Sphere. J. Ramsay Hunt, M.D., Clinical Professor of Neurology, Columbia University 217

XIV. The Development of Psychopathology as a Branch of Science. Bernard Hart, M.D., Fellow of University College, London; Physician in Psychological Medicine, University College Hospital, London; Lecturer in Psychiatry, University College Hospital Medical School 229

XV. The Subconscious, the Unconscious, and the Co-Conscious. Knight Dunlap, A.M., Ph.D., Professor of Experimental Psychology, Johns Hopkins University 243

XVI. The Association of Psycho-Neurosis with Mental Deficiency. Charles S. Myers, C.B.E., M.A., M.D., D.Sc., F.R.S., Director, National Institute of Industrial Psychology; formerly University Reader in Experimental Psychology, Cambridge 255

PART FOUR

PSYCHOANALYSIS

(*Pro and Con*)

CHAPTER   PAGE

XVII.   PROFESSOR FREUD'S GROUP PSYCHOLOGY AND
        HIS   THEORY   OF   SUGGESTION.   WM.
        MCDOUGALL, M.B., D.Sc., F.R.S., Professor
        of Psychology, Harvard University 267

XVIII. PSYCHOLOGICAL TYPES. C. G. JUNG, M.D., LL.D.,
        formerly of the University of Zürich 287

XIX.   SUGGESTION   AND   PERSONALITY.   WILLIAM
        BROWN, M.D., D.Sc., M.R.C.P., Wilde Reader
        in Mental Philosophy in the University of
        Oxford ; Honorary Consulting Psychologist
        and Lecturer on Medical Psychology, Bethlehem
        Royal Hospital, London ; Lecturer on Psycho-
        therapy, King's College Hospital   303

XX.   THE   UNCONSCIOUS   IN   PSYCHOANALYSIS—A
        CRITICISM. HENRY HERBERT GODDARD, A.M.,
        PH.D., Professor of Abnormal Psychology,
        Ohio State University ; formerly Director of
        Psychological   Research,   Vineland   Training
        School   311

XXI.   UNCONSCIOUS DYNAMICS AND HUMAN BEHAVIOUR :
        A GLIMPSE AT SOME INTER-RELATIONSHIPS OF
        STRUCTURE   AND   FUNCTION.   SMITH   ELY
        JELLIFFE, M.D., PH.D., Managing Editor of
        the *Journal of Nervous and Mental Disease* ;
        Co-editor of *The Psychoanalytic Review*, and
        *Nervous   and   Mental   Disease   Monograph
        Series*   331

XXII.   THE   METAMORPHOSIS   OF   DREAMS.   JOHN   T.
        MACCURDY, M.D., M.A., Lecturer in Psycho-
        pathology, Cambridge University   351

PART FIVE

MISCELLANEOUS PAPERS

Æsthetics

CHAPTER   PAGE

XXIII. CONFLICT AND ADJUSTMENT IN ART. HERBERT
SIDNEY LANGFELD, Ph.D., Professor of Psy-
chology and Director of the Psychological
Laboratory, Princeton University 371

Neurology

XXIV. PRINCE'S "NEUROGRAM" CONCEPT IN ITS
HISTORICAL POSITION. LYDIARD H. HORTON 385

THE STATIC AND KINETIC REPRESENTATION OF
THE EFFERENT NERVOUS SYSTEM IN THE
PSYCHO-MOTOR SPHERE. J. RAMSAY HUNT,
M.D., Clinical Professor of Neurology,
Columbia University ...   *see Paper* XIII

Social Psychology

PROFESSOR FREUD'S GROUP PSYCHOLOGY AND
HIS THEORY OF SUGGESTION. WM.
MCDOUGALL, M.B., D.Sc., F.R.S., Professor of
Psychology, Harvard University *see Paper* XVII

ABNORMAL PSYCHOLOGY AND SOCIAL PSYCHOLOGY.
ERNEST JONES, M.D., President of The
International Psycho-Analytical Association ;
Editor of the *International Journal of Psycho-
Analysis* ; formerly Professor of Psychiatry,
University of Toronto ...   *see Paper* II

Anthropological Psychology

THE EVOLUTION OF INTELLIGENCE AND THE
THRALDOM OF CATCH-PHRASES. G. ELLIOT
SMITH, M.A., Litt.D., M.D., D.Sc., F.R.C.P.,
F.R.S., Professor of Anatomy, University of
London ...   .   *see Paper* I

BIBLIOGRAPHY OF DR MORTON PRINCE'S WRITINGS ... 419

INDEX 427

PREFACE

The practice of bringing out commemorative volumes is viewed with some slight disfavour in this country, though in Germany the *Festschrift* constitutes to this day an expression of deep homage to a man who has reached a landmark in life and has attained high distinction in his chosen field. National temperamental differences are probably at the bottom of this divergence in regard to the publication of such books, but the reason which seems to carry the greatest weight with dissenters hinges about the miscellaneous character of the material almost invariably published in a commemorative volume. This disadvantage is practically inevitable from the very nature of the case ; for the former pupils of a man cannot be expected all to concentrate in one field ; and at the same time it would scarcely be desirable for a contributor to a *Festschrift* to deal with a subject in which he is no longer adept, even if he has not fully lost interest in it.

In the case of the present volume, there is a further complication in that Dr Prince, as will be seen from a glance at the bibliography of his writings, has not maintained any one single intellectual interest throughout life. His earlier years he has devoted partly to philosophy but mainly to purely medical studies. Thence he advanced to neurology and later to psychopathology and abnormal psychology, in which field he has acquired his fame, largely in connection with his multiple-personality researches.

It might consequently have been supposed that the present publication would suffer from the evil referred to above even to a greater extent than is usually the case, inasmuch as the unwitting cause of the volume has been keeping up such varied activities, even in the sphere of intellectual endeavour. Yet the independently-originated collective impulse of the various writers who have been invited to participate in this festive occasion has made it possible to unite the collection of papers under the title of *Problems of Personality*—a subject which well defines the field in which Dr Prince has made his deepest mark as an original observer. It is only by approaching the problem of personality from various angles, from the psychological, the psychiatric, the neurological, the anthropological and other aspects, it is only by studying it not only *per se*, but in its variegated manifestations : in handwriting, in art, genetically through the different stages of evolution, in a social environment, etc., that we can hope to catch a glimpse of this ever-elusive entity which has become a sort of modern thing-in-itself, with all the distinction and limitations of the celebrated Kantian concept. Despite, therefore, the apparent disparity of the studies, especially as gathered from the somewhat artificial classification, there is in each one, though in varying quantities, some material converging in the direction of Dr Prince's chief work.

It is, perhaps, well to mention the fact that the Morton Prince commemorative volume differs from other similar publications in that its collaborators and editors are not pupils of his, but associates to whom Dr Prince has endeared himself by his scientific contributions, as well as by his personal qualities. To point out his merit as a pioneer in psychopathology would be quite unnecessary here, but since his unique position as a mediator between two or more branches of science is often lost sight of, let it be remembered that it was Dr Prince who, at any rate in the United States, supplied the bridge between abnormal psychology and what is ordinarily called general psychology. Through the establishment of the *Journal of Abnormal Psychology* and the publication of symposia he was able to bring about an exchange of views which otherwise would have remained inarticulate ; and, furthermore, through his travels and extra-academic accomplishments he has succeeded in promoting the cause of psychology in distant countries and of American psychology in particular, by effecting a *rapprochement*, more or less international in its scope, among the various workers in psychology, psychopathology and allied fields.

This circumstance would at least partially explain the international character of this volume, which includes contributions from France, Switzerland, and England. That nearly one-half of the collaborators should be British is also more than a coincidence, just as the invitation recently extended to Dr Prince to lecture at the Universities of Oxford, Cambridge, London, and Edinburgh, cannot be regarded as merely fortuitous. As for American universities, the following seats of learning are represented in contributions to this volume : California, Columbia, Cornell, Harvard, Johns Hopkins, Ohio State, Pennsylvania, and Princeton.

There is one other feature to note, *viz.*, that a substantial part of *Problems of Personality* is devoted to a discussion of psychoanalysis in one phase or another. Aside from the fact that Part Four of this volume may be regarded as a symposium on this highly important and widely discussed topic, attention may be directed to the size of the psychoanalytic representation in *Problems of Personality*, which suggests several reflections. In the first place, considering that Dr Prince is rather critical to the new movement in psychopathology, the tribute, coming as it does from theoretically hostile quarters, speaks for itself. But on the other hand, it may be remarked that psychoanalysis must be well situated, if a volume presented to an adversary of the doctrine happens to harbour some of its chief exponents. From these divergent points of view we should conclude, however, that in reality no such hostility exists in intellectual pursuits, as some people are willing to believe ; and it is through such very media as commemorative volumes, naturally brought out only on appropriate occasions and in meritorious cases, that the amenities of science can lead to the further understanding and ultimate solution of generally bothersome problems. In this connection, Dr Prince's merit lies not only in his original contributions, but in bringing his findings into accord with the body of accepted facts, and thus ensuring a clarity of presentation which few specialists even care to acquire. It is through such a careful orientation that Dr Prince has done much to break down the barriers which divided the several schools in his field of science ; and by his generous appreciation of the work of others he has been instrumental in bringing to a focus, under the purview of psychology, a number of divergent views which otherwise might have remained detached and scattered.

A. A. ROBACK,
Secretary of the Board of Editors,

Cambridge, Mass.

THE EVOLUTION OF INTELLIGENCE AND THE THRALDOM OF CATCH-PHRASES

BY

G. ELLIOT SMITH, M.A., Litt.D., M.D., D.Sc., F.R.C.P., F.R.S.

Professor of Anatomy, University of London

THE EVOLUTION OF INTELLIGENCE AND THE THRALDOM OF CATCH-PHRASES

BY

G. ELLIOT SMITH

ALTHOUGH I cannot claim to be either a psychologist or a medical practitioner, my work has always been sufficiently near the fringe of these fields of activity to have enabled me to appreciate the value of Dr Morton Prince's contributions to knowledge and practice. Hence I welcome the opportunity of offering my tribute. But if I have not cultivated the actual field of psychology, I have been able from the immediate *hinterland* of neurology and anthropology, to look into the psychologist's domains, and have detected what seem in this distant vision to be untilled patches well worth cultivating. In these notes I shall call attention to some of these opportunities for useful work.

The chief aim of my work in biology and physical anthropology has been the effort to elucidate the nature of the factors that made possible the emergence of those distinctive qualities of mind which constitute the fundamental distinction between man and all other living creatures ; and on the ethnological or cultural side to discover what light the study of custom and belief sheds upon the use man makes of the great aptitudes which the acquisition of his distinctive type of brain has conferred upon him. In other words, I have been trying to integrate the results of the study of the evolution of the human brain with those revealed by ancient manifestations of human thought and invention, and to use these two departments of historical enquiry to throw some light upon the interpretation of the behaviour of mankind at the present time.

The chief fact that has emerged from this line of investigation has been the demonstration of the fundamental importance in man's ancestors of the cultivation of visual guidance, and especially of the influence of the acquisition of stereoscopic vision, in stimulating the expansion and the distinctive line of evolution of the cerebral cortex, which prepared the way for the emergence of human qualities of mind.

B 3

I have recently summarised the general results of these researches (*Nature*, September 22nd, 1923) and can repeat the statement here.

The Evolution of the Human Brain

Intensive research in comparative anatomy and embryology and discoveries in palæontology have made it possible for us to reconstruct man's pedigree with a confidence that hitherto would not have been justifiable. Using this scheme as a foundation, we can determine precisely what structural changes, especially in the brain, were effected at each stage of the progress of the Primates toward man's estate ; and in the light of the information afforded by physiology and clinical medicine we are able in some measure to interpret the meaning of each of the stages in the attainment of the distinctively human attributes of mind.

In an address delivered at the Dundee meeting of the British Association in 1912, and elsewhere on several occasions since then, I have discussed this problem ; but I make no apology for returning to its consideration again. For, as I have said already, it is the fundamental question in the study of man ; and recent research has cleared up many difficult points since I last wrote on the subject.

Even before the beginning of the Tertiary period the trend had already been determined for that particular line of brain development, the continuation of which eventually led to the emergence of man's distinctive attributes. Moreover, man, as I said in 1912, is " the ultimate product of that line of ancestry which was never compelled to turn aside and adopt protective specialisations, either of structure or mode of life, which would be fatal to its plasticity and power of further development."

Vision the Foundation of Man's Mental Powers

The first step was taken when in a very primitive and unspecialised arboreal mammal, such as the Spectral Tarsier(*Tarsius*) of Borneo and Java, vision became the dominant sense, by which its movements were guided and its behaviour so largely determined. One of the immediate results of the enhancement of the importance of vision was to awaken the animal's curiosity concerning the things it saw around it. Hence it was prompted to handle them, and its hands were guided by visual control in doing so. This brought about not merely increased skill in movement, but also the cultivation of the tactile and kinæsthetic senses, and the building up of an empirical knowledge of the world around it by a correlation of the information obtained experimentally by vision, touch and movement. The acquisition of greater skill affected not merely the hands but also the cerebral mechanisms that regulate all movements ; and one of the ways in which this was expressed was in the attainment of a wider range and an increased precision of the conjugate movements of the eyes, and especially of a more accurate control of convergence. This did not occur, however, until the flattening of the face (reduction of the snout) allowed the eyes to come to the front of the head and look forward so that the visual fields overlapped. Moreover, a very complicated mechanism had to be developed in the brain before these delicate associated movements of the eyes could be effected. The building-up of the instrument for regulating these eye-movements was the fundamental factor in the evolution of man's ancestors, which opened the way for the wider vision and the power of looking forward that are so pre-eminently distinctive of the human intellect. Our common speech is permeated with the symbolism that proclaims the influence of vision in our intellectual life.

The first stage in this process seems to have been the expansion of the prefrontal cortex and the acquisition of the power of voluntarily extending the range of conjugate movements of the eyes and focussing them upon any object. Then came the laborious process of building up in the mid-brain the instrument for effecting these complex adjustments automatically,* so that the animal was then able to fix its gaze upon an object and to concentrate its attention upon the thing seen rather than upon the muscular act incidental to the process of seeing it. This represents the germ of the distinctively human type of attention and of mental concentration in general. But the power of automatically moving the eyes with such accuracy that the images of an object upon the two retinæ could be focussed with precision upon exactly corresponding spots made possible the acquisition of stereoscopic vision, the ability to appreciate the form, size, solidity, and exact position in space of objects. It also prepared the way for the development in each retina of a particularly sensitive spot, the macula lutea, which enabled the animal to appreciate the texture,

* John I. Hunter, " The Oculomotor Nucleus in Tarsius and Nycticebus." *Brain*, 1923.

colour, and other details of objects seen with much more precision than before. Hence probably for the first time in the history of living creatures an animal acquired the power of " seeing," in the sense that we associate with that verb. The attainment of these new powers of exact vision further stimulated the animal's curiosity to examine and handle the objects around it and provided a more efficient control of the hands, so that acts of increasing degrees of skill were learned and much more delicate powers of tactile discrimination were acquired. Out of these experiments also there emerged a fuller appreciation of the nature of the objects seen and handled and of the natural forces that influenced the course of events.

With the acquisition of this new power of learning by experimentation, events in the world around the animal acquired a fuller meaning ; and this enriched all its experience—not merely that which appealed to the senses of sight and touch, but hearing also. Thus in the series of Primates there is a sudden expansion of the acoustic cortex as soon as stereoscopic vision is acquired, and the visual, tactile, motor and prefrontal cortex also feel the stimulus and begin rapidly to expand. This increase of the auditory territory is expressed not only in a marked increase of acoustic discrimination but also by an increase in the power of vocal expression. At a much later stage of evolution the fuller cultivation of these powers conferred upon their possessors the ability to devise an acoustic symbolism capable of a much wider range of usefulness than merely conveying from one individual to another cries expressive of different emotions. For when true articulate speech was acquired it became possible to convey ideas and the results of experience from individual to individual, and so to accumulate knowledge and transmit it from one generation to another. This achievement was probably distinctive of the attainment of human rank, for the casts obtained from the most primitive brain-cases, such as those of *Pithecanthropus* and *Eoanthropus*, reveal the significant expansion of the acoustic cortex. This new power exerted the most profound influence upon human behaviour, for it made it possible for most men to become subject to tradition and to acquire knowledge from their fellows without the necessity of thinking and devising of their own initiative. It is easier to behave in the manner defined by convention than to originate action appropriate to special circumstances.

Within the limits of the human family itself the progressive series of changes that we have witnessed in man's Primate ancestors still continue ; and as we compare such a series of endocranial casts as those of *Pithecanthropus, Eoanthropus, Homo rhodesiensis, Homo neanderthalensis,* and *Homo sapiens,* we can detect a progressive expansion of the parietal, prefrontal, and temporal territories, which are associated with the increasing powers of manual dexterity and discriminative power, of mental concentration and of acoustic discrimination.

The study of such factors of cerebral development will eventually enable us to link up the facts of comparative anatomy with psychology, and enable us the better to understand human behaviour.

Speech

At the present time the whole subject of the nature of the cerebral mechanisms concerned with speech and the interpretation of the significance of disordered speech is receiving a fresh illumination from the revolutionary work of Dr Henry Head. But as his memoir on the subject is now in the press, and will be in the hands of readers before this essay is printed, I need not stop to discuss the new doctrine here. I refer to the matter merely to call attention to the fact that Head's work enables us more fully to appreciate the meaning of the form and proportions of the cerebral hemispheres of extinct members of the human family. The problem of determining the exact situations of the damaged cortical areas in Dr Head's patients has been done in the department under my charge by the same investigators (Professors John I. Hunter, Raymond A. Dart, and Joseph Shellshear and Dr Tudor Jones) who were collaborating with me in the attempt to interpret the peculiarities of the endocranial casts of the Ape Man of Java (*Pithecanthropus*), the Piltdown Man (*Eoanthropus*), the Rhodesian Man and Neanderthal Man. The conclusion was forced upon us that the localised expansion of the acoustic territory, which is revealed in the most primitive members of the human family, must imply that the biological significance of hearing was suddenly enhanced at the time of the emergence of the human family. In fact, it seems a legitimate inference from the facts to assume that the acquisition of the power of communicating ideas and the fruits of experience from one individual to another by means of articulate speech may have been one of the factors, if not the fundamental factor, in converting an ape into a human being. All creatures endowed with a sense of hearing can communicate with their fellows by means of emotional cries : but man alone has the aptitude for acquiring a social heritage, of learning from his fellows, not simply by imitating their behaviour or following their lead, but by discovering by word of mouth their own interpretations of their experience, and transmitting it from one generation to another. Man, in fact, is the only living creature capable of building up a body of knowledge and tradition.

But there is an important truth buried in the cynical remark that "speech was given to man to disguise his thoughts." It is with this association of speech that I am primarily concerned in the second part of this essay.

The Thraldom of Catch-Phrases

One of the effects of the special trend of Primate development which gradually brought about the emergence of distinctively human qualities was the attainment of enormously enhanced powers of learning to perform an ever-widening range of highly complicated skilled movements. The essential result of the process of learning is the acquisition of automatic training to meet most of the ordinary needs of daily life. Having acquired such skill and facility, the performer's attention can be concentrated upon effecting subtle modifications of behaviour and quick adaptation to rapidly changing circumstances. So also in the domain of thought there is an inherent tendency in man to evade the exhausting process of mental concentration by devising formulæ to serve as automatic responses and as substitutes for serious investigation.

In two fields of scientific enquiry the sterilising influence of this common human practice has been very deeply impressed upon me this term—one in comparative neurology and the other in cultural anthropology. In the former subject I have been giving a course of lectures to students and trying to interpret the functional meaning of the evolution of the brain, rather than the mere dry bones of morphological doctrine. The difficulty immediately arose of recommending some book expounding the subject of my lectures and providing the relevant information. There are excellent books dealing with animal behaviour, with cerebral morphology, and with clinical morphology. For example, thanks largely to the investigations of Professor Parker of Harvard, we have a series of exact observations upon the behaviour of the dogfish. Morphological research has provided us with a vast apparatus of anatomical details concerning the dogfish's brain. But when one endeavours to explain to students the mechanism whereby a hungry dogfish, after scenting an attractive bit of crab-meat, becomes thrown into a state of violent emotion and begins to circle around in search for the source of the stimulus to its olfactory sense, the lacunæ in our knowledge become painfully apparent. But what I am especially concerned with here is the psychological problem of why these, the most vital problems of neurology, have been neglected, and how the issues involved have been evaded.

In the domains of comparative neurology and cultural anthropology at the present moment, while there is an intense zeal for the collection of facts there is a singular lack, on the part of most investigators, of any real attempt to discover their meaning. Most writers, dealing with the dogfish, for example, neglect to make any call upon the scientific imagination so as to picture what happens in the dogfish's brain when the olfactory nerves are stimulated. They are content to speak of certain parts of the brain as composed of " correlation tissue " and leave it at that, without explaining what it correlates and why certain events happen as the outcome of the correlation. The word " correlation" has, in fact, become an acquired automatism to evade the need for clear thinking and serious interpretation. This is merely one illustration of the increasing tendency to use what is little more than meaningless jargon and to lose sight of the chief aim of scientific study, to discover the real meaning of phenomena and truly interpret them.

But when one turns to the domain of cultural anthropology, the investigation of custom, and belief, which is coming to play an important part in the interpretation of all human behaviour, these vices of method, the abuse of catch-phrases and their employment as substitutes for serious argument, is much more rampant. In the sixties and seventies of last century the technical terms of biology, which were the weapons used in the great conflict started by the publication of Charles Darwin's *Origin of Species*, were somewhat hastily adopted by the ethnologists, and applied in ethnological controversy without any adequate attempt to learn the meaning the biologists attached to them. Ever since then the ethnologists have been using the term " evolution " for what is tantamount to the old claims for " spontaneous generation " ;

and within recent years " convergence " has become the fashionable phrase with which to dispose of all difficulties in interpreting identities or similarities of custom and belief. But far more insidious are the pseudo-psychological reasons given in attempted explanation of similarities of symbolism and incident in myths and folk-lore, in the phantasies of dreams and of the waking life, and in the beliefs of various peoples scattered throughout the world. The specious doctrine of " psychic unity," " the similarity of the working of the human mind," has no meaning unless it implies some reference to the instincts. But it is hardly necessary to explain to psychological readers that the arbitrary and artificial aspects of customs and beliefs to which this doctrine is applied are highly specialised features which have nothing whatever in common with human instincts. The claim involved in the catch-phrase " psychic unity " is as alien to the principles of psychology as it is unwarranted by the facts of history. Yet this sort of jargon has been used as a substitute for serious argument or real examination of the evidence for more than fifty years. And it is not only those ignorant of psychological methods that have been deceived by it. In his Presidential Address to the Section of Anthropology at the meeting of the British Association in 1911 the late Dr Rivers made a characteristically frank confession of his error in having accepted these fallacies, and made a public recantation of it. In the book on the *Pagan Tribes of Borneo*, by Dr Charles Hose and Professor William McDougall, attention is called to the remarkable survival in Borneo of the custom of inspecting the livers of domestic animals for omens, a practice which is certainly due to the diffusion of an element of ancient Babylonian culture to the East, as it is known also to have spread to the West as far as Italy. In their book Hose and McDougall suggest the true explanation just mentioned : yet in his book *Social Psychology* (second edition, p. 308, footnote 1), which gives so lucid an exposition of modern ideas concerning human instincts, Professor McDougall refers to the possibility of psychic unity as an explanation. I cite this, not to criticise, but merely to remind the reader that even the most eminent and advanced psychologists are apt to be deceived by such catch-phrases.

At a time when these false doctrines are beginning to lose their hold on ethnologists, Freud and his disciples have intruded into the domain of ethnology, and brought a contribution of catch-phrases that are fraught with more serious danger. Whatever view psychologists take of the doctrine of " typical symbols,"

I am quite at a loss to discover any consistency between the claim for such stereotyped (and wholly fictitious) automatisms of thought and the essential part of Freud's teaching, the dominating influence of the real instincts and of individual experience. Typical symbols come within neither category, and the claims put forward in support of their reality seem to me to be frivolous and irrelevant. But as an attempt to interpret customs and beliefs, as, for example, in Freud's *Totem and Taboo*, the appeal to this theory of symbolisation can be made even moderately plausible only by a gross misrepresentation of the ethnological facts, and the omission of all reference to the most significant circumstances that require explanation.

Yet the real explanation of how such customs and beliefs develop is the most vital problem for mankind. It is the issue with which every human being is daily presented when he has to interpret the conduct of his fellows and to understand how circumstances cause aberrations of behaviour. In neither domain of inquiry, biological or cultural, can we hope for any solution of the really vital problems until reliance on evasive terms and catch-phrases is entirely eliminated from the investigator's equipment.

The custom of using technical terms and phrases for the purpose of evading frank and direct examination of the facts has become so serious a menace to the acquisition of a sane understanding of the behaviour of men, whether we are dealing with the problems of psychology, ethnology or psychiatry, that it seemed to me the best use I could make of the opportunity of paying my humble tribute to a great physician with a rare understanding of the ways of men was to attempt to define the chief obstacle that interferes with progress at the present time.

ABNORMAL PSYCHOLOGY AND SOCIAL PSYCHOLOGY

BY

ERNEST JONES, M.D.

President of The International Psycho-Analytical Association;
Editor of the " International Journal of Psycho-Analysis ";
formerly Professor of Psychiatry, University of Toronto

ABNORMAL PSYCHOLOGY AND SOCIAL PSYCHOLOGY

BY

ERNEST JONES

In any reÒord of Morton Prince's contributions to psychological science the fact will always deserve mention that he was one of the first to perceive the intimate connection between social psychology and psychology of the abnormal, and to proclaim this by issuing a *Journal* devoted to these two studies. The purpose of the present paper is to inquire into the significance of the various points of contact between the two.

The title itself he has proposed for the latter of these branches of study does not seem to have been too happily chosen, to judge from the reluctance of other workers to adopt it. Apart from linguistic objections to it,* it would appear to lay unnecessary stress on the difference between the fields of the normal and the pathological. Without wishing to attach too much importance to the question of nomenclature, which, after all, is largely a matter of expediency and opinion, I should myself, for reasons that will presently be indicated, have preferred to use the term " clinical psychology." In England " medical psychology " is the term most widely used, but it is possible that professional prejudice may have much to do with this preference. In this connection an interesting suggestion made some years ago by Wilhelm Specht may be recalled. He proposed to restrict the term " psycho-pathology " to the study of abnormal mental phenomena carried out from a purely medical point of view, *i.e.*, the investigation of the causes, pathological significance, and modes of treatment of such states ; and to use the term " pathopsychology " for the investigation of the same data purely from the point of view of general psychology. Certainly this distinction is well worth noting, for much of the interest attaching to the intensive study of pathological mental states that has been carried out in the past

* Few workers have been willing to reconcile themselves to the admission that their psychology is abnormal, and still less to the risk of being themselves designated as abnormal psychologists.

quarter of a century is clearly due to the startling extent to which knowledge gleaned in this field has been illuminating for other fields as well.

The etymological association between the word " clinical " and beds has long ceased to operate. The feature of clinical medicine that distinguishes it from other forms of medical study is not that it is carried out at the bedside, for most often it is not, but that it represents a special mental attitude in the investigator. His attention is concentrated, that is to say, not so much on the elucidation of a particular disorder or the investigation of any given system of the body, as on the scrutiny of an individual human being considered *as a whole*. Now it seems to me that this is the very feature that most sharply distinguishes the medical psychologist from his more academic colleagues and also the one to which the fruitfulness of his results may fairly be attributed. One of the outstanding conclusions to which this methodological mode of approach has compelled assent is that the various forms of mental functioning are extraordinarily interrelated and mutually dependent, so that justifiable scepticism arises in regard to much experimental work which professes to isolate such processes as intellectual or memory ones from the rest. This is only one of the many respects in which the clinical method has come into some degree of conflict with the older methods, though the history of science gives every reason to believe that such conflicts can only represent a transitional stage in the development of psychology as a whole.

A reconciliation between the results achieved by different methods of investigation will only be possible when these methods are granted equal recognition and compared side by side. With this aim in view it would seem a reasonable extension of the term " clinical psychology " to apply it also in other fields than that of pathology. This would, it is suggested, be done when one intends to emphasise the special attitude of mind and mode of approach that we call " clinical " towards any psychological problem. In the present paper the term will be used partly in this sense and partly in its original, more restricted sense.

Before inquiring into the relation of this branch of psychology to the other branch called social psychology it will be necessary to enter to some extent into its characteristics. In seeking to define what are the most distinctive features of clinical psychology I shall probably find general agreement up to a certain point and then considerable disagreement after. This is inevitable with a writer representing the psychoanalytical school, for this school has developed the characteristics of the clinical method further than any other workers in clinical psychology.

The first characteristic, already mentioned above, is an aversion from, on the one hand, the generalities so common in the older psychological writings, and on the other the tendency to consider mental problems apart from the life of any actual individual. Put in an obverse way, this amounts to a preference for relating such problems to the life of the personality as a whole.   This in itself would stamp clinical psychology as a branch of individual psychology, and it certainly is that, though it is also much more besides.   It may appear odd that the branch of psychology which most devotes itself to the study of the individual should come to be also the branch which is establishing the closest contact with social psychology, but some of the reasons for this will appear presently.

The decision to make an intensive investigation of a (necessarily small) number of individuals proved to be a much more fateful one than it must have appeared at first.   The motive impelling the pioneers to make this decision was the necessity of doing something when confronted by the terribly urgent problem of suffering, and this motive enabled them to overcome just the obstacles that had hitherto been imposed in the way of any penetrating investigation of the mind.   The history of the investigation of the body was repeated in the sphere of the mind.   To examine the inside of the body had, for centuries, been forbidden as something taboo, not nice, not proper and not right.   But the extreme desirability of learning something about what, why or when men suffered from disease at last broke down this prohibition. Examination of the inside of the mind was still longer held up, and mainly by similar obstacles.   Even now discretion soon imposes a limit of permissibility on any psychologist who may seek to explore the mental processes of his subjects.   The curious result has been that psychologists have, till lately, been compelled to study anything rather than human beings.   They could investigate vision, hearing, speech, but only a careful selection of the things seen, heard or said—still less what the mind actually thought of these things ;   what animals do when they are angry or starved, but not what human beings do in similar circumstances.

With this tradition most clinical psychologists have definitely broken.   Faced with the grim tragedies of neurosis, they have had perforce to come to close quarters with the intimacies of emotional life, and, much to the horror of their contemporaries, including the more conservative members of their own profession, they have proceeded to examine dispassionately the facts in this way brought under their notice and even to publish the conclusions to which their investigations have led them. Their justification has been that the relief of suffering, on the one hand, and the march of knowledge, on the other, are more weighty considerations than excessive regard for wounded susceptibilities.

When now the study of the mind is approached in this way, with a propensity to consider every problem in reference to the whole personality and with the resolve not to shrink from exploration of the inner mental life, however intimate, wherever necessary, experience shows that it will result in certain characteristic views being taken of mental functioning. These, then, come to be rather distinctive attributes of the clinical method. Four of them may be selected for special emphasis ; they may each be memorised by a single word : genetic, dynamic, unconscious and instinctual, respectively. A few words will be said about them in this order. It will be noticed that academic psychology gives its assent in general terms to three of them, to all except the idea of the unconscious, but they are all taken much more seriously and applied much more rigorously in clinical psychology.

Everyone would, of course, agree with the statement that the mind develops, but a great deal more than this is meant when it is said that clinical psychology views the mind *genetically*. Here the continuity of the mind at different ages is regarded quite literally. It is held that the significance of any given current mental process is not completely known unless the full genesis of it is also known, unless its predecessors can be traced back in an unbroken chain to the beginnings of mental life in the infant. It has been found that many of the older elements of the genesis, and often the most important of these, are not completely transformed into or replaced by their successors, so that a certain amount of their original significance is still retained. The practical effect of this is that many of our impulses, interests, and ideas carry with them an extrinsic significance based on their genetic history, that they represent more than what they purport to. In extreme cases, of which unconscious symbolism is the most striking example, the subject is totally unaware of this surplus significance. The state of affairs just indicated is most pronounced in pathological conditions, the essence of which is that the patient is dominated by a still too living past, a past which, though forgotten, refuses to fade or to submit to transformation. The most advanced school of clinical psychology, following Freud, carries this genetic principle to its logical conclusion and maintains that all our later reactions in life are really elaborations of simpler ones acquired in the nursery. The power to modify the more fundamental types of reaction becomes rapidly less as the child grows, and some of us even think that no fundamental change in character can take place after the fourth year of life.

In its *dynamic* view of the mind, clinical psychology comes into decided opposition with the old associationist psychology. When one mental element occurs after another it is no longer possible to think we have explained this by saying that the second element, having been attached to the first through temporal contiguity, or inherent similarity, was aroused by the presence of the first. Dynamic factors such as those designated by the words motive, tendency, purpose, impulse, are sought for in every single instance, however minute, and no explanation is regarded as adequate unless a factor of this kind is demonstrated. This holds even with mental events, such as slips of the tongue and the like, that previously were supposed to " happen " without any ascertainable reason, and certainly without any motivation. Yet the older views die hard in some fields of work—for instance, in regard to dreams. Many psychologists are still satisfied if a dreamer says, " I was talking French in the dream, probably because my father, who appeared earlier in it, has just returned from France, so that the thought of him would make me think of the French language."

A thorough-going dynamic conception of mental events as essentially the expressions of the interplay of various forces* leads to many important consequences. One comes, in this way, to realise that a great number of mental processes come about as compromise-formations, various conflicting forces having contributed to the end result. The extent to which conflict between opposing tendencies takes place in the mind, and the importance of such conflicts, is a matter on which there is not universal agreement among clinical psychologists at present, but that intrapsychic conflict is of far greater significance than used to be thought is becoming very generally recognised. It is particularly hard to overlook its significance in neurotic disorder, for the manifestations of this are nothing else than the expression of such

---

* I am, of course, aware that " force " is one of those words not to be used in strict scientific speech, and only write it here as a convenient and easily comprehensible shorthand for more cumbrous periphrases.

C

conflicts. Freud himself has applied his "wish" theory of the mind in a great many different fields and, however much or little anyone may agree with the details of those applications, there can be little doubt, as Holt has well pointed out, that this line of work has given a considerable impetus towards the appreciation of the extensive part played by conative trends in regions of mental functioning, such as, for instance, dream formation, where their existence had been hardly suspected.

The subject of the *unconscious* mind is so vast—it is quite possible that in the future it may be ranked as the most important discovery of the past half century—that no discussion of it here would be in place. One word must suffice in reference to the empty objection that, since the word "mental" is equivalent to "conscious," no unconscious mental processes can be allowed to go on. *Ça n'empêche pas d'exister.* Its reality is attested by the work of many authorities, any one of which would suffice for the purpose ; one may mention the observations of Binet and Janet, and the experimental work on dissociation by Morton Prince, quite apart from the huge literature of psychoanalysis. Apparently the critics would have us write such phrases as : "the neural dispositions and synaptic changes, all of which are quite unknown, with which the corresponding mental processes, if they occurred in consciousness, would be expressed by the wish to murder a brother-in-law" ; whereas we are content with the less cumbrous phrase : "the unconscious wish to murder a brother-in-law." In the present state of our knowledge the whole question is a mere verbal quibble. When neurologists know enough to describe conscious processes in terms of cerebral physiology then they will have no difficulty in doing the same for unconscious processes, and everyone will be happy ; but the essential point is that the two kinds of mental processes are absolutely on the same footing in this matter. Nor can I repeat here the respects in which Freud's particular conception of the unconscious differs from that of other writers, fundamental as I hold them to be.

As befits a discipline of medical origin, the clinical attitude is close to the biological one, and most clinical psychologists feel that one of the chief goals of their work is to be able to state their mental data in biological terms, *i.e.*, in terms of the *instincts*. The interesting contributions that have appeared in the *Journal of Abnormal Psychology and Social Psychology* of late only go to show how complicated and obscure are the problems relating to the instincts, and it cannot be said that clinical psychology has yet been in a position to elucidate finally any of them.   But it has advanced two steps at least in this direction.   It has cleared the ground by showing that a number of supposedly inborn instincts with which other psychologists had operated are complex products, and so are capable of resolution into more primary elements.   This remark applies, for instance, to many in the list of instincts propounded by McDougall in his popular *Social Psychology*. In the second place, the analyses effected by clinical psychologists, particularly by Freud, of the conative aspects of the mind have revealed much of importance concerning the development, manifold fate, and products of the instinctual side of mental life, and it is reasonable to expect that further research along these lines will bring us nearer to the ultimate sources of mental impulse.

After this sketch, imperfect as it is, of the features characterising the clinical approach to psychology, let us turn to social psychology and try to ascertain something of the relationship between the two.   Social psychology itself has evidently been in great part developed because of the peculiar straits in which sociologists and all serious students of social problems find themselves.   It is impossible to proceed far in the study of social institutions without perceiving that the only work of a non-psychological kind that can be done in this field must remain on a purely descriptive or classificatory level.   The simple reason for this is that no problem can be raised concerning the origin, function or significance of any one of these institutions that does not immediately involve some psychological consideration.

The sociologists who have recognised this state of affairs have naturally turned to psychology for assistance and co-operation. They must in the past have been somewhat bewildered at the response, for until late years this has been decidedly a negative one.   The notorious lack of interest of most psychologists in such mundane topics as motive and meaning prevented a wide response of any kind, and the few who occupied themselves with the sociological data, such as notably Wundt, confined themselves either to the classificatory studies of the kind already familiar to sociologists or else to the vaguest generalities.

Three explanations have been proffered for this curiously unresponsive attitude on the part of psychologists.   The most charitable is that suggested by writers of the class of Le Bon, who suppose that the side of man from which light is needed to explain sociological phenomena, the side about which psychologists have been able to say so little, is perhaps one which is not present in the material studied by the psychologist, *i.e.*, in man considered as an individual. They have put forward the view that the mental tendencies concerned with social institutions are dormant in the individual and are stirred to activity only when he comes into close contact with a group of his fellows. They thus postulate a special class of instincts—the herd, gregarious or social instincts —which are manifest only in the relation of the individual with the group.

Of the many criticisms that can be made of the view just enunciated, one only may be mentioned here. The hypothesis would seem to attach far too great importance to the mere factor of number in human psychology. It would be very remarkable if instincts which are supposed to play no part in a man's relations to those nearest him—friend, enemy, wife and family—should suddenly emerge the moment he comes into contact with a larger number of people. At what point do they appear, and what is the magic number that has this effect ?

The second hypothesis, put forward by Wilfred Trotter, avoids this particular difficulty. He supposes that what psychologists have not borne sufficiently in mind is the biological history of man. He insists that man is throughout a gregarious animal, and agrees that we should postulate a special group of instincts, which he sums up under the name of " herd instinct," in accordance with this consideration. But he maintains that these instincts play an important part also in the simpler and individual relations of life, not only where group contact is present. According to him, man is at every moment, even in the privacy of his chamber, nothing but a gregarious animal, and much of his most individual behaviour is dictated by the indirect effects of his social instincts.

The third explanation of the general psychologist's lack of helpfulness in the social domain is that proffered by the psycho-analytical school of clinical psychology. It would agree with the two previously mentioned ones that something essential must have been overlooked by the general psychologist, and also with the second explanation that this something is, nevertheless, to be found in the study of the individual. But its indictment of the general psychologist is more far-reaching than either of the others, being to the effect that he has extensively ignored highly important aspects of his own field. As was already indicated above, we mean by this the intimate regions of the mind, those in which the final answers to most psychological problems are to be found.

To many it will seem an overweening pretension to maintain, as has been done in this paper, that the branch of psychology which is most concentrated on the study of man as an individual, and predominantly with the morbid states of the individual, should be regarded as the branch which has most to offer the student of socio-psychological problems. And yet these two grounds for objection are the very reasons why one ventures to put forward this pretension. For morbid states have special and overwhelming claims to importance as fields of psychological investigation. Individual suffering has momentous consequences for both the investigator and the subject which are paralleled by no other psychological situation. As regards the former, experience has shown that no other motive, not even scientific curiosity, is strong enough to overcome the various motives (largely of personal origin) which compel him to desist from intruding into the intimacies of another person's innermost life. And, similarly, no other motive than suffering has yet been found, except in the rarest cases, to induce a human being to submit to any really searching investigation of his own mind. The academic psychologist is thus, in regard to his study-material, at a permanent and unalterable disadvantage as compared with the clinical psychologist.

The second objection indicated above challenges the right to transfer to normal psychology conclusions arrived at through study of the abnormal. Such a critic, however, is being misled by the word " abnormal " and is evidently unaware of the real nature of neurotic suffering. As is now becoming more widely recognised, this is not due to disease in the ordinary sense of the word so much as to the adoption of a particular method of dealing with a social situation. The idea, which we owe mainly to Freud, that neurosis is one of man's ways of meeting various difficulties in his relation to his fellow man, i.e., to social difficulties, has revolutionised our conception of psychopathology in the past quarter of a century.

If neurosis represents a solution, however unsatisfactory, of various social difficulties, then it is impossible that an exceedingly intensive investigation of it, such as is necessary for therapeutic purposes, should be undertaken without throwing light also on the inner nature and meaning of the social institutions themselves in regard to which the difficulties have arisen. And there are ample indications in the literature of the past fifteen years that this expectation is being fulfilled, though even yet psycho-sociological studies proper are only in their infancy.

It will thus be seen that there are two fundamental points of contact between clinical and social psychology. In the first place, the study of social relationships and social institutions demands that special attention be directed to the questions of meaning, motive, significance, and the like ; in short, to the interpretation of the dynamic aspects of the mind. Now these are the aspects with which clinical psychology is perforce peculiarly concerned, certainly more so than any other branch of psychology. Further, clinical psychology is not in a position to be content with the superficial interpretations of motive that are customary. The correctness of its conclusions are constantly being checked by results, and to secure these it is necessary to deal with the real actual motives operative in a given case, not ·with the ostensible ones. In other words, it has to penetrate to the sources of motive in the unconscious, to the fundamental roots of all our impulses, emotions and conduct.

In the second place, as was hinted above, it so happens that the subject-matter itself is far more nearly identical in the two branches of psychology in question than might at first sight be supposed. The social institutions studied by the one discipline are the products of the same forces that create the neurotic manifestations with which the other is concerned ; they are simply alternative modes of expression. Let us consider for a moment a few of the chief topics that are the object of socio‑psychological investigation. One problem is the organisation of societies, the inner structure and external relationships of groups, clans and nations, with all the concomitant questions of government and authority. Another is the vast domain of sex relationships, the complicated questions surrounding the marriage and family bonds, the accompanying institutions of prostitution and concu-binage, and the endless variety of ritual, folk-lore and superstition that invest the themes of love and birth. A third is that of religion in all its forms and manifestations : theology, ritual, ethics and morality, and the conduct of life in general. One can safely say that every one of these problems has, at times, to be made the subject of a penetrating investigation during the eluci-dation of some neurotic manifestation. Many a neurotic symptom represents the individual's attempt to deal with the complicated relationship between son and father, a problem which, on the other side, connects with the great questions of government, leadership, authority, submission, and so on. That religion represents essentially a mode of appeasing the sense of guilt arising from various anti-social tendencies is becoming more and more widely recognised, and every clinical psychologist knows that conflict over these same anti-social tendencies may lead to neurotic or even psychotic disorder, so that his work is very largely taken up with the elucidation of them. That many clinical psychologists have also shown considerable intrepidity in investigating the manifold problems relating to the sexual life is familiar enough to the readers of Dr Prince's *Journal*.

It is impossible in a short contribution, such as the present one, to do more than call attention to some of the main points of contact between the two branches of psychology under consideration. The preceding remarks on the identity of content in the two cases may appear unduly categorical, but it would need a volume even to illustrate such an enormous theme. Fortunately, all that has been said here can be supported by reference to an already extensive literature on the subject, and I may conclude with the simple assertion that most of the keys to socio-psychological problems will be found in the realm of clinical psychology.

NOTES ON SUGGESTION, EMPATHY, AND BAD THINKING IN MEDICINE

BY

WILLIAM A. WHITE, M.D.

*Superintendent at St. Elizabeth's Hospital, Washington, D.C.;
Co-editor of "The Psychoanalytic Review" and the "Nervous
and Mental Disease Monograph Series"; President, American
Psychiatric Association; former President of the American
Psychopathological Association and The American Psychoanalytic
Association; Professor of Nervous and Mental Diseases, George-
town University, and George Washington University; and Lecturer
on Psychiatry, U.S. Army and U.S. Navy Medical Schools*

NOTES ON SUGGESTION, EMPATHY, AND BAD THINKING IN MEDICINE

BY

WILLIAM A. WHITE

I HAVE chosen the title of my paper because of the fact that Dr Prince has been one of those rare spirits in medicine who have departed in their work from the accepted and conventional standards of their day and dared to venture forth on their own account and to record what they saw. 'Tis true that many adventure on their own account, but few indeed are they whose records live or who find anything on the journey of value. It occurs to me, therefore, that it might be worth while to comment on the method pursued and the road travelled, to suggest the worthwhileness of examining the means at the disposal of the explorer in medical jungles. This, of course, is no new idea of mine. I merely thought that perhaps it might be worth while with respect to the specific matters mentioned in my title and appropriate because in the field wherein Dr Prince has lived in his thoughts these many years.

I shall not attempt to discuss exhaustively and thoroughly any of the topics mentioned in the title ; that would obviously be impossible in the limits of such a paper as this. It is merely my purpose to record briefly a few thoughts on these topics that seem to me to be of value. The fact that the thoughts are not original or that they may have been set forth many times in the past is, it seems to me, not significant. The significant thing is that, although perhaps recognised when attention is directed to them, they are rarely in mind and not infrequently quite out of mind at moments and on occasions when their presence would be of much value. They belong, no doubt, to the category of the obvious, but it is the obvious that so often eludes us, that may be right there in front of us and yet we do not see it, and even though we see it, we see it only too often with eyes that are almost blind.

The recognition of facts when they are brought to our attention

is not the important thing.   The average man would rate well in
such a performance test if the facts were well presented.   The important thing is to assimilate the facts so that they become part
and parcel of our bone and sinew, the very fibre of our being, available always when needed, going into action, as it were, with the
machine, because part of it.   It is only then, when they have become available for instant use, that we can be said truly to know
them.   And so it must ever be necessary to repeat and to emphasise,
to re-repeat and to re-emphasise the obvious, however distasteful
such proceedings may be to those of academic mind.   These are
my excuses, my reasons for what follows.

Suggestion

In the fields of psychopathology and psychotherapy probably
few terms have been so persistently and so outrageously abused.
If one looks back over the literature for, say, the last twenty years
it would hardly be far-fetched to say that he might conclude that
suggestion was " the be all and the end all " of psychological explanations.   The most diverse results were brought about by
suggestion ; the most diverse occurrences were explained by it.
Suggestion, as it thus paraded through the literature, producing all
these curious phenomena, seemed possessed of some inscrutable,
mysterious power which it wielded in quite an arbitrary way.   It
never seemed to occur to anyone to question the source of this
power nor to undertake to explain or to understand the way it
worked.   To pronounce the word seemed all that was necessary
to close the subject satisfactorily, to put the final stamp upon it
of approved explanation.

It is difficult to account for the slavish and almost mystical use
of the word *suggestion,* especially as it came from the most unexpected quarters.   Men used it who were students of human
behaviour and the human mind.   Probably the explanation is
after all the really profound ignorance of the nature and mechanisms of the mind, an explanation which is forced upon us in spite
of the fact that those who used suggestion to explain everything
made high pretence to profound learning.   Their use of the term
suggestion was to that end, for often they did not know much
of what was even then known of the mind.

Suggestion was used in those days, and still is, for that matter,
in the sense of the uncritical acceptance of ideas and their realisa-

tion in action ; and there was practically little improvement in the use of this term, despite the work of the French School and its followers, which gave some hint as to the nature of the hysterical and dissociated states in general.

The technique of producing the hypnotic state was elaborated, the phenomena of suggestion in relation thereto and also to the waking state were studied, as were also the phenomena of post-hypnotic suggestion, so that a pretty coherent body of facts was established, even sufficiently well hung together to make prediction possible with a considerable ratio of success under controlled conditions. Still, there was little effort to explain the " why " of the hypnotic state or the reason some ideas were accepted uncritically and others were not, and, in fact little appreciation that such problems even existed.

Of course, during this period, there were a few earnest workers in this field, but for the most part the state of the average medical mind that thought about the subject was about as described. Things remained, however, pretty much at a standstill until Ferenczi's paper in 1909 on " Introjection and Transference," which, for the first time, took up a study of the affective dynamic factors that lay back of the phenomena and an understanding of which was necessary for any deeper appreciation of the nature of those phenomena.

This paper of Ferenczi received all too scant attention, but it nevertheless did receive some notice, was translated into English, and has stimulated further studies since. This is not the place for a restatement of the results of these studies. I shall indicate the sources from which this information can be obtained in the appended bibliography. I will only make this comment in closing, namely, that the word *suggestion* can no longer be used in the loose and haphazard way of the past ; that even if we are not prepared to accept those explanations which have been offered by Ferenczi we must nevertheless acknowledge the fact that suggestion or suggestibility does not constitute an irreducible,* ultimate component of the *psyche*, that it is not, so to speak, an unanalysable element and that it can therefore be split up into further components. It might be said of psychopathology, in reference to this whole matter of the use of suggestion, what Lowie says of ethnology : " the obstacles to a clear understanding of reality lie in the bewitching simplicity of catchwords."†

* Freud, *Group Psychology and the Analysis of the Ego.*
† *Primitive Society.*

Empathy

Through all the long years that the so-called " insane " have remained outside our ken, it has been sufficient to dismiss their comments, ways of thinking, and conduct as simply " crazy," which implied that they were altogether alien to us and nothing more need be said. In recent years all this has changed, and it has changed apparently more or less contemporaneously in several fields, namely, the fields of genetic psychology, anthropology, and psychopathology. It has come finally into the field of conscious awareness, although often none too clearly, that we cannot hope to understand the child, the savage, or the psychotic by a process of projecting, so to speak, our own methods of thinking upon him and then trying to understand him in terms of ourselves. No one of these three classes thinks, feels, or acts as we do, and from the same motives, in any sense that permits such an identification. The child is not just a small adult ; the savage does not possess all our potentialities, only needing to be taught; and the psychotic is not just contrary, or mischievous, or vicious, or crazy. Again do catchwords intervene between us and reality, and because of them our opportunity to grasp the real is indefinitely delayed.

This method of interpreting others by ourselves is the natural one and has to be thought through before it can be improved upon. All these classes of individuals, children, savages, and " insane " have suffered enormously at the hands of adults, the civilised and the normal because of this way of thinking.

Here as elsewhere to recognise a problem is already to be well on the way to its solution. A problem stated is half solved, and this problem is now pretty well comprehended, and it is understood that because a child takes something that does not belong to it, or a savage demands pay from the Christian doctor for being treated for pneumonia, or a psychotic patient tears up his clothes, that an explanation that attributes such conduct to original sin, or ingratitude, or viciousness is of no value, that it will be necessary to go behind the returns and find out upon what such results are based in order to understand why they take place.

For a long time it has been pretty generally recognised that to an extent it was necessary to put yourself in the other fellow's place in order to really understand what was going on inside the other fellow. But this way of thinking has generally resulted in a sympathetic understanding, a form of sympathy which did much to rescue the child and the " insane " and the " criminal " from the cruelties that came of misunderstanding but which in the case of the anti-vivisectionist, whose form of query " How would you like to be cut open and experimented upon if you were a dog ? " was reduced to sentimentalism plus ignorance.

Now by empathy is meant " a process of introjection, since it serves to bring the object into an intimate relation with the subject."* It is perhaps best understood in the form of a literal translation of the German word *Einfühlung* ; namely, " feeling into." It implies a certain identification of the subject with the object. This identification does not necessarily imply sympathy nor does it partake of sentimentalism.

The point I wish to make is that our capacity to understand others is a function of the completeness with which we can feel ourselves into their ways of thinking and feeling, can introject ourselves into their situation, and that this capacity is based upon two factors which are dependent the first upon the second. The first is our capacity to intellectualise the total situation we are seeking to understand, and the second our capacity to recognise within ourselves those same components of feeling and tendency which are the dynamic factors in the situation we are studying. In order to understand the child, the savage, the insane and the criminal we must be able to identify the germs of similar motives in ourselves. The path to the better understanding of others, then, is the path of a developed intelligence plus an honest and clear-seeing vision of one's self.

Bad Thinking in Medicine

Bad thinking is not confined to medicine, but I suspect that errors of the same sort dominate wherever it is found. In medicine, of course, the most obvious error that dominates physician and patient alike and is largely at the basis of the success of charlatanism, is the error of wishful-thinking. The physician sees evidences of results which he wishes would come to pass : the patient wishes to get well and will take the treatment that someone says will cure him. This is all very simple, but it goes strangely unrecognised ; nevertheless even a casual inquiry will disclose how this type of error creeps into our thinking and to what an amazing extent it vitiates our results. So true is this that I cannot refrain from making the suggestion, although I know full well its practical

* See Jung, *Psychological Types.*

futility at this time, that the medical curriculum should include a course in " medical thinking."

The other error to which I would call attention is even less recognised than that of wishful-thinking. It is the error of logical thought. Just because a conclusion is contained in the premises and follows logically therefrom, is no reason why the conclusion is necessarily true. It is essential to separate process and content. The fact that the process is flawless does not mean that the content is true. The syllogism :

> All white flowers are lilies ;
> This flower is white,
> Therefore this flower is a lily,

is absolutely correct as to form. The conclusion follows logically from the premises, but if the flower that is in question happens to be a daisy, the conclusion is wrong, and it is wrong because the major premise is not true ; for all white flowers are not lilies.

Now it very often happens that bad thinking in medicine and the arguments and reasoning of the charlatan are quite logical. I remember reading a carefully-worked-out explanation of baldness that proved with logical rigorousness that it was due to a too tight sphincter ani. The contracted sphincter pinched the sympathetic nerve filaments. This pinching irritated the sympathetic filaments, this irritation was conveyed along the course of the sympathetic system up the cord to the head. The sympathetic system controls the capillary blood supply to the scalp. The irritation of the sympathetic caused a contraction of the capillaries of the scalp. The deficient blood supply resulted in baldness. Therefore, the cure for baldness is dilatation of the anal sphincter. I submit that this is faultless logic. The only trouble about it is that it is not true.

The arguments of the charlatan are made to those who do not know and who are seduced by the fine logic to think that when conclusion follows upon premise with such certainty there must be truth : and to those others whose critical faculty is obscured by wishful-thinking, by wanting to believe.

I shall close with an anecdote. A college graduate had finally come to settle down in the country and to lead the life of a farmer. A class-mate ran across him and in the course of the conversation that followed asked him how much value his college education had been to him. To this he replied that he used what he had learned in college very little, he planted his crops, improved his land and all the rest largely by guesswork, as did his neighbours, but in one respect he considered he had the advantage; when he did not know a thing he knew that he did not know it, and the ability to recognise when he did not know had been worth all the time and effort he had spent in acquiring a college education. Here again knowledge is the answer, and in this instance the beginning of knowledge was in the recognition of its absence. Such a man would not long remain in the magic stage of development of farming. He would soon project himself into the experimental stage and be on the highway to science.

BIBLIOGRAPHY

SUGGESTION

1. Ferenczi (S.), " Introjection und Übertragung," *Jahrbuch für psychoanalytische und psychopathologische Forschungen*, Vol. I, 1909, abstracted in *The Psychoanalytic Review*, Vol. III, No. 1, January, 1916; translated in *Contributions to Psycho-Analysis*, Chapter II, Introjection and Transference.
2. Freud (Sigm.), *Group Psychology and the Analysis of the Ego*, Chapter IV: Suggestion and Libido.
3. Jones (Ernest), *Papers on Psycho-Analysis* (3rd ed.), Chapter XIX: The Action of Suggestion in Psychotherapy and, Chapter XX, The Nature of Auto-Suggestion. Chapter XIX also appeared as an article in *The Journal of Abnormal Psychology*, Vol. V, and Chapter XX as an article in *the British Journal of Medical Psychology*, Vol. III, Pt. III, 1923.
4. McDougall (W.), " A Note on Suggestion," *The Journal of Neurology and Psychopathology*, Vol. I, No. 1, May, 1920.

EMPATHY

1. White (Wm. A.), Psychoanalytic Parallels, *The Psychoanalytic Review*, Vol. II, No. 2, April, 1915.
2. White (Wm. A.), Individuality and Introversion, *The Psychoanalytic Review*, Vol. IV, No. 1, January, 1916.
3. White (Wm. A.), Extending the Field of Conscious Control, *The Psychoanalytic Review*, Vol. VII, No. 2, April, 1920.
4. White (Wm. A.), *The Mental Hygiene of Childhood*, Boston, 1919.
5. Jung (C. G.), *Psychological Types*, London and New York, 1923.
6. Lévy-Bruhl, *Primitive Mentality*, London and New York, 1923.
7. Brill (A. A.), The Empathic Index, *Medical Record*, February, 1920.
8. Southard (E. E.), " The Empathic Index in the Diagnosis of Mental Disease," *Journal of Abnormal Psychology*, Vol. XIII, No. 4, October, 1918.

D

BAD THINKING IN MEDICINE

1. Bleuler (E.), *Das Autistisch-Undisziplinierte Denken in der Medizin und seine Überwindung*, Berlin, 1919.
2. Bourget, *Quelques erreurs et tromperies de la science médicale moderne*, 4th ed., Paris, 1915.
3. White (Wm. A.), " The Meaning of ' Faith Cures ' and Other Extra-Professional ' Cures ' in the Search for Mental Health," *American Journal of Public Health*, Vol. II, No. 3.

DOES THE WILL EXPRESS THE ENTIRE PERSONALITY?

BY

ED. CLAPARÈDE, M.D

Professor of Psychology at the University of Geneva

DOES THE WILL EXPRESS THE ENTIRE PERSONALITY?

BY

ED. CLAPARÈDE

THE brief discussion which is to follow is an attempt to show that far from expressing the aggregate of personality, as is currently received, the will always marks a division of the self. It is furthermore a matter much less of introducing a new conception of the will than of delimiting the term *Will* and restricting its use in such a way as to set the psychological notion of the will in accord with the facts of concrete and real life.

The chapter on the will is, in fact, remarkably anæmic in the modern psychological textbooks—not to mention the behaviourists who most frequently pass it by in silence. And yet in everyday life we have constantly to do with the phenomenon of the will. Is not this vital phenomenon in the very fore of the interest of educator, industrial leader, physician, etc. ? Developing the will, selecting for a given position an individual endowed with will, re-educating the will of asthenics—these are everyday preoccupations. But present-day psychology invests the concept of the will with a latitude so wide that it becomes practically useless. The practitioner has but very little to draw from the observation on the will which the psychological texts offer him.

Many writers define the will as "an act consciously directed by an idea." But is this really true of the will ? Assuredly not. The voluntary act is confused with the act which I call " intentional " and which is quite different from it. If I want to visit a friend, I should consider the most convenient or most expedient means of betaking myself to him (whether on foot, by electric car or by cab, etc.) and I adjust my behaviour to the result of this deliberation. But this is a simple intentional act and has nothing voluntary in it, in the sense given to this word in everyday life.

We are also told that volition occurs every time a *choice* is made or whenever there is *effort* or *delay* (that is to say, the preparation for an act which is to be realised only in the future). If it is true that these phenomena intervene in every voluntary act, they are not adequate for its characterisation. If I am offered the choice between a glass of milk and a glass of wine, I am not carrying out a voluntary act when I choose the milk, if I prefer it to the wine. Similarly, if I try to climb a tree in order to pick some fruit which I am fond of, it is again an intentional act with effort, but in no wise a voluntary act. Lastly, if, not being able to reach the fruit, I go looking for a ladder, I should accomplish an intentional delayed act, but no more would this act have anything voluntary in it; for no more than in the preceding illustrations will it revive within me this drama, little or big, which every voluntary act must represent.

I say a drama; that is to say, in reality every voluntary act is the expression of a conflict and struggle. If it indicates a conquest, it likewise betokens a submission. It denotes a sacrifice, a sacrifice which at times costs little, but a sacrifice just the same. Volition, one might say, is to refrain from doing what one has a tendency to do, and to do what one has a tendency to refrain from —or, as William James has so aptly said: it is to go in the line of greatest resistance. Every voluntary act then results from a conflict of tendencies, and the function of the will is precisely to resolve this conflict.

And it is here that we find the distinction—properly speaking— between the voluntary act and the intelligent act with which it is often confused. Both in the one case and the other, the individual finds himself in a problematic situation. But in the case of intelligence, the problem is one of *means* : it is a question of discovering the means to attain an end which the individual has set himself and which is not called into question. In the case of volition, on the other hand, the problem is one of *ends*. To what end must I direct my action? There is no question as to the procedure to take in each case in order to attain these various ends, but it is in regard to the problem which end to adopt that the dispute arises.

If there is any dispute as to the various ends, it is due to the conflict of tendencies. This conflict evidently marks a division of the personality. In the most serious cases this division is manifest : on the one hand, the whole group of tendencies which popular language (borrowed from ethics) designates as " low, coarse, inferior, egoistic"; on the other hand, the tendencies which are denominated " superior, moral, ideal."

Each of these groups of tendencies is affected by a certain co-efficient of selfhood, that is to say, the self partially identifies itself with them. For the most part, however, it is the ideal tendencies that the " true self " is identified with. Whenever these ideal tendencies are overcome by the inferior ones, the self sometimes gives the impression that it has been overpowered by a strange force (demon, etc.) or at least that it has been " carried away " by a force which it could not resist. It would be very interesting to study the variations of the feeling of self in the debates of the will going on internally.

Every act of the will, then, presents itself as the reaction of a part of the personality, of certain tendencies, that is to say, against another part of the personality. Considered from the functional point of view, it is the part of the will to stop this division of the self which impedes action, and to restore to mental activity the unity which is indispensable for the coherence of its adaptations. This is brought about by giving the upper hand to one of these groups of tendencies. If this mode of speaking is found too teleological, it may be said that the will is the name given to that process which leads to the re-enforcement of a group of tendencies and consequently to action.

In the general run of life, however, the will is referred to only when it is the superior tendencies (moral, ideal) which are re-enforced to the detriment of the coarse, egoistic tendencies. It is necessary, therefore, to indicate this characteristic in the definition of the will, at the risk of depriving it of the very thing which distinguishes it from the carrying out of a simple desire or the pursuit of the lower interests.

In certain cases the superior tendencies seem so ideal, so extra-mundane, that the subject can no longer get himself to regard them as belonging to his own ego. This is the reverse of the case which I have just indicated. Here, for instance, is an illustration which I am taking from an old book from the pen of the celebrated Protestant thinker of Lausanne, Alexandre Vinet (who, it may be said in passing, is a noteworthy forerunner of Pragmatism).*

In his *Essais de Philosophie Morale*, published in 1837, I find the following very interesting lines as testimony of an intimate psychological experience . . . " Man could very well feel that his will, far from being able to serve him as a guide, really, in its turn,

---

* *Cf.*, for example, this passage (p. 15) : " The simplest and most necessary truths have had a thousand obstacles to overcome . . . They had to live, and prove they are living, by action before being embraced by the intelligence."

needed to be itself regulated and rectified; that his will, in a word, was not good . . . In an absolute sense, it is not in our power to will ; our will is there only to carry out that of another. It is in the interest of this latter that we ought to will ; in other words, it is God who might be said to be willing in us . . . An irresistible impulse has led man to seek a will to which he could submit his own. He did not have to look for it very long. He has recognised it in God; or, if you prefer, he has named this will God. He has, immediately, conceived God as a regulating will . . . Man, then, has sought in religion the ideal, or the rule which he did not find in himself."

We see here that the author allows for two wills, one of which is to be subordinated to the other. What does it mean but that, in the act of true volition, there are two selves opposing each other, and one of which is to yield to the other ? The fact that only one of these selves is regarded by the subject who does the willing as his true self does not alter anything in the situation.

It is not necessary for me to examine here the nature or the origin of this ideal self with which the subject identifies himself or, contrariwise, from which he at times separates himself. I simply wish to underscore the extent to which this important fact is not recognised in the current conceptions of the will. Indeed, open any text in psychology at the chapter dealing with the will, and you will read there almost invariably that the will is a reaction which expresses the personality in its entirety. Let us give a few quotations at random. Fouillée, in his *Idées Forcées* (1893) writes : " It is my whole self which conditions my act . . . Every reason for acting in serious circumstances interests the entire personality, which as a whole determines the action." Parmelee observes in his *Science of Human Behaviour* (1913) : " The will or volition is usually regarded as an expression of the self." Warren, in his *Human Psychology* (1919) : " The prominent feature of voluntary control is that the action is determined by the man's *whole life*, not merely by present situation. Our volitional acts are the expression of *ourselves* ; we control them as personal beings." Bergson (*Données Immédiates de la Conscience*, 1889) maintains that : " We are free when our acts emanate from our entire personality." Even Paulhan, who has quite recognised the division of tendencies in the will, declares (*La Volonté*, 1903) that : " It is rather, for the action which engages more completely the aggregate of personality that we reserve the name of 'willing'." And Pierre Janet (*Brit. J. of Psychol.*, Med. Sect.,

1921) says also that the will " depends on the totality of the tendencies."

Experimenters like Ach, Michotte and Prüm have also observed that volition is a phenomenon attached to the feeling of subjective activity. But this does not invalidate the thesis of the division of personality, for, on the one hand, the subject, as we have seen, identifies his ego with the victorious tendencies—and on the other hand, most of the phenomena studied by these writers constitute intentional acts, rather than acts of the will in the full and active sense which I have given to this word.

It is hardly necessary for me to point out the consequence of this conception of the will for education and psychotherapy. If the awakening of the will is brought about by a split in the aggregate of tendencies, it would mean that the education of the will would above all render the will useless by avoiding that which would provoke this split, by avoiding in the process of education, the " abortive repressions," as Freud would say, and especially, by trying to sublimate rather than brutally counteract the inferior tendencies.

It seems to me that this examination of the will, as a function of the personality, is likely to throw some light on what Morton Prince has called " This troublesome problem of the nature of the will."* If we are still very far naturally from grasping its inner mechanism, let us at least begin to perceive its rôle in human conduct.

(Translated by A.A.R.)

* Morton Prince, *The Unconscious*, p. 458 (1914).

AN EXPERIENCE DURING DANGER AND THE WIDER FUNCTIONS OF EMOTION

BY

GEORGE M. STRATTON, M.A., Ph.D.
Professor of Psychology, University of California

AN EXPERIENCE DURING DANGER AND THE WIDER FUNCTIONS OF EMOTION

BY

GEORGE M. STRATTON

I

SINCE Cannon's work upon the physiology of certain emotions there has been widely recognised their invigorating effect upon the muscles useful in escape, attack, and defence. That certain emotions are sthenic, while others are asthenic, had long been known; but it remained for Cannon to reveal something of the bodily process by which the sthenic effect was produced.

In the accounts of emotion which we have from James, Shand, McDougall and others, stress likewise had been laid upon the motor connection of the emotions, their connection with the so-called instincts ; the emotions are by some of these writers regarded as ready to be awakened by certain instincts and to make use of certain other instincts in order to attain the end toward which the emotion may give a general impulse.

It is thus seen that the motor connections of emotion have, in recent times, been in the forefront of our attention. And yet, if one were to make a wider survey, taking account especially of the materials which lie at hand for students of the abnormal, we should (it seems to me) be in a position to see more justly the office which emotions hold in our mental and bodily life. After such a survey I believe we should return convinced that emotion has been too narrowly connected with muscular acts, and, indeed, that the relation of the emotions even to these muscular acts has not been quite satisfactorily stated.

It will be the purpose of the present paper to suggest what I venture to regard as a certain correction or enlargement of such accounts as connect the emotions chiefly, if not wholly, with motor activity, and more particularly with the mere energising of this motor activity.

Let me offer at once a certain type of evidence which may serve as our point of departure. A young man whom I have among my students, a highly intelligent person, served during the late war as an aviator in the United States Army. In the course of his extended service he suffered more than one severe accident, and his experiences during these times of especial peril were such that I shall draw upon them in some detail. From stenographic notes of his free narrative to me, and from my later questioning him, I give the following as the substance of his narrative.

" During my service as an aviator I had two accidents which were of psychological interest.

" The first of them was at Dallas, Texas, in June or July of 1918, while I was doing that part of my training which is known as ' stunts.' Before going up on this particular day I, as usual, examined carefully my controls, and found that they were working right. I then went up to a height of about 5,500 feet, having planned the order in which I should go through my stunts, so that I should make as good a showing as possible to my instructor on the field below. My first stunt was a loop, and this I went through all right and straightened out. Then I found that my elevator-control was stuck. I went up on the rise for a second loop, but instead of letting my ship whip-stall and thus running the risk of permanently damaging my controls, I kicked the rudder to the right and dropped into a tail-spin.

" It was at this time that a dual personality came into play. I had a rapid survey of my life, not as though I were looking at scenes of my past, but as though I were doing and living them again.

" Yet I was conscious at the same time of having to manage my ship. For as soon as I started down in the tail-spin I realised that I had a certain amount of time, and I went carefully over the different controls. I tried the rudder and found that it worked all right. I then moved ' the stick,' and its movements showed that the ailerons were working, but that the elevator was stuck. I thought that the elevator-wire might have become entangled in the leather slot where the elevator-wire goes through the covering to the outside. So I pushed the stick slowly and steadily forward to overcome such an obstruction. In shoving forward on my stick I felt the tension on my belt, which showed that the control was in some way entangled with the belt. So I reached around and found there the loose end of a wire used to support the triangle of the safety-belt, and which had been left too long and had become entangled in the wire which worked the elevator. I pulled this loose end out, and my elevator then worked perfectly, and I straightened out my ship. I was then at a height of about 1,500 feet, having fallen about 4,000 feet since the accident began.*

" During this fall I re-lived more events of my life than I can well enumerate. These were in an orderly series, very distinct, and I cannot recall that anything was out of its place.

" (1) One of the first things that I remember was my learning my A B C's. My grandfather was sitting in a tall easy-chair with castors attached to a frame upon which the chair rocked. I remembered him sitting as I am sitting now ; and I was on the floor. That was between the Christmas when I was over two-and-a-half years old and the February when I was three. That was the first picture I had.

" (2) Another was when I had to stay home when my mother had to leave me and teach school for a while. It was late in the fall, and I was looking out of the window and I saw her pass the window and go off to school.†

" (3) Next I was playing under a grape-arbor in the back yard at my grandmother's. In throwing things at the little chicks, I accidentally killed one of them. Then I buried it, feeling very sorry over what I had done.‡

" (4) Another one was during a very cold winter, when I went up to my grandmother's and had a long drive with a horse and buggy from the station, about seven miles, and there was a great family reunion.§

" (5) Another was of a very cold night in Kansas City when we were coming home from a play and got stalled on the street cars because the snow was so heavy.‖

" (6) Another was of fishing for small cray-fish in a little slough in a park in Kansas City.¶

" (7) Another was when I was on a journey, and my folks told me that we were coming to California. I thought we were going

---

* My aviator estimates the rate of his fall to have been about 150 feet a second, giving a total duration of about 27 seconds for the 4,000 feet.

† The original of this occurred when he was about three-and-a-half years old.

‡ When he was about three-and-a-half or four years old.

§ When he was about seven years old.

‖ When he was about nine years old.

¶ At the age of nine.

from Kansas City to somewhere else in Kansas. It was when we were out some distance. I remember the isolated group in the station-house when they told me where we were going.*

" (8) Another was when I was cutting some wood in the back yard in El Paso, Texas, after I had left California. It was a very clear moonlight night. It happened that at this time I was wondering what I was going to do some five or ten years later. It was just like I was there again. I cut the wood, and distinctly saw the moonlight, the axe, and the block again.†

" (9) Another was very distinct. It happened just a year before I went into the service. I went up here to Lake Tahoe with a party. We arrived about twelve o'clock, Sunday night, having come over a foot and a half of snow at the summit. There was hoar-frost all over the rocks, and ice on the edge of the lake. [Then follows in minute detail an account of swimming in the icy lake at midnight, as the result of a " dare."] I was doing it again ; I felt the cold air, and saw the hoar-frost."

On October 18th, of the same year in which he fell 4,000 feet, and before " straightening out " had the varied experience just described, this aviator had another experience of which we must content ourselves with a still briefer description. Upon this occasion, while in an area of artillery-fire, his engine stopped suddenly, and he, having to descend from an insufficient height of about 3,000 feet, and having, at the same time, to avoid the fire, set his ship into a flat glide for a particular spot ; but coming short of it, levelled his ship off above a field of broom corn where the ground was rain-soaked and bad, and landing here " cracked up " his ship. To quote his words :

" I knew I couldn't make anything like a good landing. Well, I remember the broom corn hitting the axle of the wheels, but from then on, until three or four seconds after we hit, it is a blank. I don't know just how the ship acted when we hit. I was not badly hurt. My back was badly wrenched. I got out to see what damage was done to the ship.

When I started down I was more or less amused, more or less laughing at myself for being foolish enough to get into a predicament of that kind ; of going over the field without sufficient altitude.

---

* At the age of nine.
† At the age of eleven.

" Meanwhile I saw a view from a notch in the Berkeley Hills up here on the other side of Wildcat Canyon, looking through toward Tamalpais and the Golden Gate. The notch is just on the other side of the canyon reached by crossing the hills after going up through Spruce Street. I stood right there at that notch and saw the view just as you see it at any sunset. As I remember it, the sun was setting north of the Golden Gate. It was not an exceptionally beautiful sunset. There were clouds up there, much as there are to-day, more or less distinct cloud-formations. I could see just a little reflection in the lake over there.

" This came to me while I was still gliding down toward the corn-field and I saw that I couldn't hold the ship off the ground."

I asked this aviator to compare the scenes recalled during these two accidents with others not recalled then but belonging to his childhood and youth, scenes which seemed to him as important as those which came back to him in his danger. He thought the danger-recollections to be about " twice as vivid " in recollection now as the others, vividness including for him, as he said, the colours of the scene. Asked whether his recollection during the danger came in alternation with attention to his machine, or whether the two went on at the same time, he answered that he believed them to be " separate but at the same time."

" There was no discontinuance of attention to the machine at all, because that was the first thing. The fact is, I do a great deal more flying on the ground than in the air. I figure out certain tight places that I may get into, and how to get out of them. Then when you get into a tight place, you automatically do the thing you figured out. Such was the case when I kicked the rudder and fell into the tail-spin. I had thought that out on the ground, and the rest was a matter merely of working it out at the time."

My aviator informs me that experiences such as he had are not exceedingly rare amongst airmen, that his companions in the service have repeatedly recounted to him similar experiences which they themselves have had. We also have at least one published account of such a dissociation during danger in the air.*

* Hoffman, " Ordeal by Fire," *Atlantic Monthly*, March, 1920.

E

II

Now the emotional condition in the experiences just described brought with it certain features which might be stated as follows :—

1. It is clear that there was no break-down of the motor integrations arrived at earlier both by actual practice in the air and by reflection while on the ground. There was no sudden incapacity to do the skilled acts which had been learned, but these were performed anew with sureness and mastery. The delicate motor adjustments, the motor co-ordinations which were needed to remove the obstruction to the control and to direct the ship before and after special difficulties were encountered were not disorganised, but they remained available and were actually employed.

2. Certain acts were selected from a large store of possible acts and were applied to the troublesome situation intelligently—although, so it seemed to the aviator himself, automatically—while the man took in the situation, analysed it, and put to the trial bodily and mentally certain of its possibilities of behaviour. From many acts practised beforehand, in fact and in imagination, there were chosen those which led to complete success in the first of the two accidents described, that in which, after a drop of 4,000 feet, the ship was straightened out ; and in the second, where there was landing on bad ground outside the field of the artillery-fire, there were chosen acts which at least led to escape from death by shells, although by accepting an alternative which involved, so the event proved, some damage to ship and man. Under the circumstances, and given the fact that in the second accident the man was flying too low, both crises were met, we must agree, with intelligently applied skill.

3. There evidently was a dissociation which approached, if it did not attain, that mental condition to which Dr Morton Prince has aptly given the name " co-consciousness." For it seems probable that the mental system which controlled the ship did not include that other mental system which was merely reminiscent. If, however, there was, during the period of dissociation, a wider consciousness wherein both of the dissociated systems were present, then the condition would not exactly accord with Dr Prince's definition of co-consciousness,* but was an approximation to it. But in either event, we have here in a normal individual an experience somewhere between those minor forms

* Morton Prince, *The Unconscious*, 1914, p. 249.

of dissociation which occur with everyone and in everyday life, and those major forms where, as in hysteria, there are relatively independent " personalities."

In the present case the dissociation is revealed in two relatively detached and smoothly functioning systems. There was (*a*) the system of ideas and impulses connected with the practical work in hand, namely, with those motor acts which directed the mechanism of the ship. And there was (*b*) the system in which there was a recollection of certain distant events of the aviator's life.

4. The emotional effect was not confined to the muscular field : it had its cognitive field as well. There was what we might call polarity in the emotional influence, a motor and an intellectual pole to its integrations. These two are clearly to be discerned in what has just preceded. But they are not equivalent to the two systems of the dissociation. One of these systems, namely, that of the reminiscences, it is true, was wholly or all but wholly cognitive. Images of earlier scenes arose with such astonishing detail and vividness that the aviator seemed to himself, not to be *remembering* but to be *re-living* them. The present situation, that of the peril in the air, seemed blotted out. There was nothing of that complication of past with present, which gives to our usual recollections their character of recollections because seen to be in temporal relation to what now is occurring. The past scenes were vivid and were without rivals. In sensory quality and intensity, in emotional tone, in impulses, the past experience returned as though it were a repetition—but not until later to be recognised as a repetition—of the very facts themselves.

But the cognitive effect was not confined to this particular one of the two dissociated systems, that of the reminiscences ; it reappeared also in the system concerned with muscular acts. For it is clear that the muscular acts employed during the two crises were not the outflow of motor habits so fixed as to be strictly mechanical, wholly without mental supervision and control. The aviator was meeting a novel situation wherein his movements were the outcome of an attentive exploration. He understood the needs of his case, and tried now this and now that form of action, in order to discover the precise character of the impediment in his airplane's controls. And he made, in the end, an accurate diagnosis of the trouble, and was able to effect a cure. In the other experience, when his engine stopped and there was danger of shells, he took account of the risks involved in the different courses open to his choice; and having made his decision, carried it out in full consciousness of what it involved.

The two-fold connection of the emotion is here clear : it stirred to movement, but it also stirred to thought ; it stirred to recollection of the past and to a consideration of the present, and of the prospects of success by one and by another course of action.

III

We might now inquire whether the features so clearly to be seen in the present case are present in emotion generally. Have we, indeed, in this extraordinary experience, something like a natural demonstration of the true course and function of all emotions, or at least of the sthenic phase of all of them? An answer to this question will require a glance at evidence lying scattered at many points, while we connect this evidence serially with the four features noticed in our aviator's case.

1. As to the maintenance of motor integrations.—Emotion, when it is not of extreme violence—for of exceedingly violent emotion I shall reserve the consideration until a later page— but moderate emotion, I would say, involves no general disruption of even complicated muscular acts. Certain movements, it is true, may become difficult or even impossible. A man's golf or billiards might be wrecked for the moment by an insult, or by news of a mishap to his business. But movements suited to the impulse then prevailing—movements of running or crouching, if fear be there ; or of vocal utterance, of vituperation, perhaps, together with the movements of bodily approach and of a deft blow with the fist, if there be anger ; or of caresses by hand or with tender words, if love ; or of whistling and singing and a sprightly step, if there be joy—such and many other complicated movements are not only possible during emotion, but come forth finished, as part of emotion's usual train.

2. As to there being more acts available for selection.—It is now well recognised that the movements performed during certain emotions are done with uncommon vigour. Closer examination, however, will make it clear that this is by no means emotion's only effect. It would seem true, rather, that there are more acts ready to be performed with vigour ; more acts are at the disposal of the impulses which may arise. Thus in the sthenic

phase of anger, fear, love, joy, sorrow, and mere excitement,* there is not only stronger action, but there is a greater variety of action, what we might describe as a greater flexibility of connections among the various motor units. I shall, of course, not be understood to hold that units of action, never before used in any connection, now come forth for use. But the existent units seem closer at hand or a fresh combination of them seems now more easily accomplished, so that integrations now occur which were hardly possible in calmer moments. Possibly the psycho-physical dispositions behind these movements are innervated in lowest degree. Or perhaps, without actual innervation, they are in some other way made more accessible, as though they were waiting nearer to the threshold of overt action.

This I may perhaps be allowed to illustrate from the behaviour of my dog. When I let him out from his confinement early in the morning, he may overwhelm me with the expression of his joy : he may jump up and upon me, scamper off, caper about and charge back upon me. Upon a recent occasion, when he seemed unusually glad, he picked up a stick and carried it along for a while uselessly, and then dropped it. Now he has not been taught to pick up or carry any object, nor is he accustomed to do it in any fixed relation to human beings ; so that the emotion seems here to have brought into life an act which, although practised by him in other connections, was yet unhabitual in this particular setting. The emotion led to some increase in the variety of things which were just then practically available for him.

And to continue with my dog ; in other circumstances which are emotional, but which give no great encouragement to running and wildly capering about, joy at my presence or attention may lead him to sit up and beg—this being a trick he has been taught in connection with offered food—but now performed where there is no slightest indication that I have the least of food to give him. And when we go into the hills—a region of uncommon stir for

---

* All these I should regard as either sthenic throughout or as having a sthenic phase. And, contrary to tradition, I am venturing to include excitement among these emotions, as something distinct, while yet it may also be present in them all. For excitement appears to me capable of existing as much by itself as any of the emotions, it being indeed an undifferentiated emotion, neither fear, nor anger, nor love, nor joy, nor sorrow, nor any other of the well-known and differentiated emotions. Excitement may precede or follow one of these, or it may rise and disappear without passing into any one of them. And yet there is doubtless some excitement in the sthenic phase of each of the differentiated emotions. An explanation and defence of this position I shall defer to another occasion.

him—his behaviour illustrates the principle which is now in my mind. Out in this wilder region are the signs for him of ground squirrels, field mice, raccoons, coyotes, not to speak of the various birds which there abound. There I have noticed that some not-loud sound made behind him, perhaps by my displacing a small stone, or by lightly clapping my hand, startles him as no such sound does when he is calm and at home. When he is pointing, let us say, at a squirrel hole, the start which my sound gives him does not actually draw him off from the act to which he has given himself. But it would seem that the threshold for a movement different from the one upon which he is already launched has been lowered, so that a slighter stimulus is now readier to initiate it.

Now this which is noticed in an animal's conduct is to be noticed also in men. Joy, love, anger, fear, and mere excitement, bring variety of action ; the entire motor mechanism seems to offer as into the person's hands a fuller store of such abilities as fit the instant's need. The lover may find language fluent that earlier was pent. Or other movements which might please his love are now performed, perhaps awkwardly, because with doubt or self-consciousness or with no practice ; but they lie readier for the attempt. So, too, a man in rage does not usually do the single act of offence which comes first and uppermost, but he gives evidence of having at hand a whole arsenal of acts to be thrown into the attack : he may advance with clenched fist as if to strike, he may gnash his teeth, may stamp upon the floor, and all the while be flooding his enemy with invective. It would thus appear that more variety of movement, as well as more energy of movement, is brought nearer to hand. The sthenic phase of the emotions thus makes available a greater scope of conduct. And out of this fuller offering the selection is made of acts to be performed.

3. Is there in emotion generally any characteristic tendency to dissociation ? There is evidence which hardly can be brushed aside. The analgesias of men wounded in battle would be in point, as would also be that analgesia which David Livingstone experienced when a lion seized him by the shoulder and crushed his bones. The shock, he says, produced a sort of dreaminess, without pain and without terror, an effect which he compares with that of chloroform.* So, in less degree, the lover's readiness to absorption in his great theme has as its counterpart a proverbial absent-mindedness, a narrowing of

* Horne, *David Livingstone*, 1913, p. 30.

the conscious field, and an exclusion of all that will not circle around his one idea. Dissociation, at least of a minor kind, must be involved in this. And so with the man in joy, in fear, in anger : he may later be amazed to find that, beside the occurrences which he noticed and the acts of his own which he consciously directed, there was much that he saw and upon which he acted almost as in somnambulism. Thus a friend who was recently in an automobile accident, when he himself was driving, told me that the adjustments in his wrecked machine, he found later, had been properly changed by him at the very instant of the accident, and yet with no recollection that these details had been included in the dominant system of his ideas. It would seem that in all those emotions which involve specific impulses—such as fear and anger especially—there are almost of necessity two foci, as in an ellipse. The self or the object of dread or anger is at the one focus ; and at the other is the end to be attained. In fear, these may clearly be diverse. With our aviator one of the personal foci of his emotion, his self, may have been the substantial meaning of his series of reminiscences, in which the aviator looked almost as though fondly and with regret at what perhaps was about to be lost, at himself as he had known this being from early childhood up to his recent years. On the other hand, the impulses to the action of the moment were able to bring forth the ideas and movements needed to realise the impulses and to organise them into an independent system. Here the two systems were straining apart, to the very breaking point.

Now a tension of some less degree would seem to be normal in all fear. And in anger also, if the angry man keep a hot attention upon the offender and the enormity of his offence, what is to be done to him must lie in the charge of some relatively detached system of ideas and their integrated impulses. The angry man, conscious primarily of his enemy and the wrong, finds himself saying and doing things as though automatically. These quasi-automatisms, it would seem, are the outcrop of a momentary dissociation.

4. As to the existence of an important polarity, a cognitive effect in addition to the muscular, there can be no doubt. The sthenic aspect of the emotions not only brings into activity certain impulses leading to movement, but also produces a profound change in cognition. In an earlier paper an account was given of the effect of emotion upon memory, showing that in normal persons there was often found, not only the well-known amnesia,

but also a strange and heightened liveliness of recollection extending behind the time when the crisis began.* This is in accord with the experience of our aviator, whose revival of parts of his life before his accident was with such vividness that he seemed not to be recalling but to be re-living them. He has given us but a fresh illustration of that retroactive hypermnesia, of which no more at present need be said.

Looking now beyond memory, one finds an emotional effect upon attention, perception, and imagination. Not only does emotion frequently have its rise in an activity of one of these powers, but it reacts upon them, bringing them to still more intense and prolonged activity. Fear, anger, love, and sorrow have their object ; and this object gains an important place in the cognitive system ; it is attended to, perceived, scrutinised ; and out of its slightest changes there comes to the mind a multitude of fresh interpretations, fresh anticipations.

But the cognitive stir works farther. In all simple emotions, except sorrow, perhaps, it leads to a certain fertility of ideas. Thoughts that otherwise would remain dormant, as mere dispositions, now awaken and are actual. Turgeniev, being asked why he had ceased to write, replied that he was now too old to be in love, and he had found that unless he were a little in love he could not write. Similar is the experience of those orators whose minds fairly coruscate when upon a great occasion they face a great audience, and get past their initial inhibitions. A man of eloquence whom I know once said that when he had entered fully into his speech, ideas came in such profusion that his task became then but to select from the wealth of thought which arose before him. In a very different connection, an experimental finding in our own laboratory seems to point in a like direction. Different groups of workers, equal in intelligence, were given, upon many days, carefully graded intellectual problems. It was found that those who were asked to assume an attitude of anger toward their problems, regarding each of them as an enemy that must be downed, had far greater success than did those who were asked to assume a merely alert and energetic attitude.† Further, one should bear in mind the effect of war-emotions upon the solution of intellectual, including scientific, problems connected with war ; and also should bear in mind the use which religion and politics

---

* " Retroactive Hypermnesia and Other Emotional Effects on Memory," by the present writer : *Psychological Review*, XXVI (1919), 474.

† From an investigation by Stella B. McCharles, a full account of which, I trust, will in due time be published.

have from time immemorial made of emotion to influence belief, to arouse and give potency to new or newly awakened ideas.*

From these and other facts which might be cited, I shall venture to offer a description of the cognitive effect of the emotions named. There is a cognitive disturbance, a commotion marked by something like a farther awakening of a mind already awake. In particular, and first, there is an increased rate of change within the cognitive field.† The intellectual processes move at a more rapid tempo than when there is no excitement. Second, there is a lowering of the threshold for the entrance of ideas. Thoughts come more easily ; they are aroused in greater variety ; there are more of them available. The intelligence is thus more fertile when under emotional stir. Third, there is an added strength of organisation, a more effective integration of certain of the ideas present. And fourth, there is with this heightening also some loosening of organisation, a disintegration amongst certain other constituents, so that these are omitted from the active system and are either suppressed or are left to form relatively independent and non-adaptive systems of their own. In this reorganisation, with its correlated association and dissociation, the cognitive activity runs a course not wholly different from that noticed by Cannon in the sudden reorganisation of the bodily response in the conditions which he studied. Some of these bodily responses are regrouped and intensified, others are uncoupled and weakened or repressed. The two contrasted effects observed in memory, in the article already cited—namely, a heightening and lowering of mnemonic power, when under emotion—seem, in the light of these further facts, more easily understood. In the retroactive hypermnesia and amnesia, which often go together in one and the same mind and in the one crisis, there is an exclusion of certain groups of impressions and the inclusion and vivifying of certain others. Such peaks and depressions are but the local manifestation of this selective and reorganising influence of the emotion, whereby it integrates some ideas and disintegrates and dissociates others. The remarkable changes in memory are thus but an instance of a wider cognitive consequence of emotion.

* That elation and depression in the mentally diseased bring disturbances of perception and of judgment, bring illusion, hallucination, delusion and cognitive disorientation, is so well known that I shall make no attempt to elaborate this aspect of emotion's effect upon cognition.
† This commotion may be of very brief duration, and be followed by a great mental calm, as in Livingstone's case already cited. But even this emotional calm is the outcome of a preceding turmoil, for which the description I offer in the text is perhaps more suited.

IV

The emotional seizure is thus an intricate and sudden re-organisation of all powers, both motor, impulsive, and cognitive, in order to meet a situation fateful for our interests. But such an account of emotion's office holds true only within certain limits of emotional intensity. Excitement may become excessive, and then the commotion or disarrangement of our usual mental combinations is not succeeded by a rearrangement which is more suitable and which helps us to meet the crisis with prospect of success. There here follows in the train of that disorganisation toward which all emotion tends no beneficent reorganisation. Thus we find that in intense fear there may be a paralysis, not simply of the muscular system, but of the impulses to movement, and probably also a freezing of the stream of ideas. The object of our horror here so fascinates us as to preclude all play of attention whereby the immediate object is properly related to its sur-roundings and to the imagined possibilities of action which fear ordinarily will arouse. It is probable that something resembling this occurs in moments also of intense anger. The outraged person may be incapable not only of motor action, but also of any free rise and play of images and ideas and judgments around the object of his anger. Nothing clearly suggests itself for him either to think or to do. His mind, at the height of its passion, is for the moment fixed, as though in stone. So also the excitement which some orators experience as a beneficent stimulation, may not at all have this character for the timid or unseasoned speaker. With him the excitement is merely disorganising, and the operations which in calm moments would move into free rearrangements are now kept in disorder or are blocked. This exceptional effect of excessive emotion is also to be illustrated by the absurdities which occur in high excitement. When Morgan's men were making their famous raid into the North during our Civil War, their conduct at certain moments was that of men beside them-selves. They would rush into some country-store and, in a whirl of greed, seize anything at hand. They would stuff their pockets with horn buttons, start off to southern climes with a string of skates, or with a chafing-dish on pommel, encumbrances only to be thrown to the roadside after some miles of gallop. They behaved it is said, like boys raiding an orchard.*

Other ridiculous things done in stress or panic would be here

* See the account in Nicolay and Hay's *Abraham Lincoln*, Vol. VIII, pp. 55f.

in point. During a recent conflagration in Berkeley a young man who risked his life to save the property of others, emerged from a flaming building with his pockets stuffed with bedroom slippers. And I myself noticed, in viewing the next morning the salvage that had been carried hurriedly to one of the fire-proof buildings of the University, that hard by a costly mahogany clock someone had rescued a pan of baked apples. The dissociative effect of emotion has in such cases remained as a too enduring effect. The explosive violence of the excitement has prevented the free functioning of the higher processes.

Now this exceptional effect is easy to observe, and, looked at too narrowly, has led to an entirely mistaken conception of emotion's function. Emotion has appeared as merely a break-down of organisation. It is as though one were to find the characteristics, let us say, of perception, not in its successes but in its failures, as when it arrives only at illusion or hallucination. The excesses of emotion then need not conceal from us the fact that normally there is, instead of a *break-down*, rather a temporary *break-up*, in preparation for a more effective reorganisation, with added resources now freely at our disposal.

Thus I should incline to answer in the affirmative the query whether the features of our aviator's experience are features of emotion generally. Emotions in their sthenic phase, it would seem to me, are not mere energisers but are also diversifiers, leading to a fresh or less usual organisation. Emotions are awakeners of dormant functions; and when awakened, these sleeping powers are given a special direction and objective. But emotions are also repressive; and, while some functions are awakened, others are rendered dormant or are forced into a dissociated action.

In all this it is clear, I believe, that the function of emotion is not confined to the motor region; it extends far beyond this, into the cognitive field. And in this cognitive field the emotions serve likewise both as energisers and as reorganisers. As energisers; for where a function properly connected with the emotional impulses is already active or becomes active, it becomes more vigorously active because of the emotion. But also as reorganisers; for, in the cognitive awakening which emotion brings, there is an increased intellectual fertility, with varied and novel ideas put at the disposal of the vague impulses. There is, however, no mere miscellany of ideas rising up, and in confusion.

There is, rather, a rise especially of such as promise some use in the present crisis. And among them there is a rapid selection and rejection, an organisation of some of them about the focus of present action, while others are dissociated and either vanish or become grouped about some other centre.

A wide service is thus rendered by emotion. For when so stirred, the individual finds himself at a new level of behaviour both in body and in mind, being enabled to meet his crisis with a more complete array and organisation of his powers, and these not of his muscles only, but of his entire psycho-physical constitution.

ON RECENT CONTRIBUTIONS TO THE STUDY
OF THE PERSONALITY

BY

C. MacFIE CAMPBELL, M.A., B.Sc., M.R.C.P. (Ed.), M.D.

Professor of Psychiatry, Harvard University; Director, Boston Psychopathic Hospital

ON RECENT CONTRIBUTIONS TO THE STUDY
OF THE PERSONALITY

BY

C. MacFIE CAMPBELL

" THE proper study of mankind is man," and of recent years, from many sources, this study has gained a new impetus and fresh inspiration. In the field of medicine, after almost complete absorption in the intricate mechanisms that regulate each constituent system, there is a return to the study of the organism as a whole, there is renewed interest in the personality of man.

In this renewed application to the study of personality there is a wider and more catholic point of view than in earlier studies ; not only is there continued interest in the detailed analysis of the subtle interplay of conscious and subconscious forces, in the study of which Morton Prince, P. Janet, and S. Freud have done such yeoman service, there is a wider interest in man in his diversity, in the individual man with his own special endowment, his own special needs, his own individual destiny.

The point of view which has been attained in this field has been influenced by the progress of medical thought in general. One has in medicine passed from the early stage of attention to symptoms, through periods dominated by structural lesions, pathogenic organisms, and biochemical anomalies to a standpoint, from which the original endowment of the individual, and the life-experiences which have influenced it, are seen to play a considerable rôle. The disturbing agent no longer receives all the attention, nor is the detailed process of invasion and defence the only subject of investigation ; much thought is now being given to the wide problem of those constitutional factors which determine that, of two women grinding at the mill, the one shall be taken and the other left.

That this is a field for practical research as well as speculation is shown by the establishment of a Constitution Clinic in an important hospital. Thus in all disorders the liability of the individual, as well as the rôle of the special environmental *noxa*, has begun to undergo scrutiny, and in no branch of medicine has this tendency been more prominent than in that dealing with mental disorders, where, after the period of special interest in morbid anatomy and the simple somatic processes, and the period of detailed analysis of special psychological mechanisms, the analysis of the contribution made by the congenital endowment of the individual has come to be the subject of intensive investigation.

That the study of the personality is important is clear ; it is not so simple to make this study in a systematic and profitable way. The personality is the individual in action, it is as complex as human nature with its traces of racial history and individual experiences ; the guiding lines of investigation are not at first obvious, and are apt to be determined to a disconcerting degree by the special interests of the investigator and by the material at his disposal. The worker who has been absorbed in the study of the endocrine glands, realises their influence not only on growth and metabolism, but also on the more complex functions of the organism ; he may come to the analysis of the personality, eager to see how far his simple formulæ may contribute to the clarification of the total picture.

> " Let me have men about me that are fat,
> Sleek-headed men, and such as sleep o' nights ;
> Yond Cassius has a lean and hungry look ;
> He thinks too much ;   such men are dangerous."

The enthusiastic endocrinologist will translate not only the bodily traits but the whole personality of Cassius into his endocrine formula, and with his glance focussed on the pituitary gland have little interest in the organisation of all the other forces which make up that sombre personality.   He may even simplify his formula into chemical terms, and then we find the absence of religious belief in Napoleon explained by the absence of the requisite chemical component, no hint of the formula for which is given.   For this worker not Wellington nor Blücher is the agent of destiny, but providence worked out its will by determining an early failure of the great man's pituitary gland.

This point of view is not without interest ;   it makes a partial contribution to a complex situation.   The danger is that the worker, absorbed in detailed researches, fail to keep in mind how much he has provisionally abstracted from the total problem and how partial is the situation with which he is dealing.   Still more dangerous are such formulations when they are based, not on accurate detailed research, but on facile hypothesis and unbridled speculation.

It is only in a small number of cases that these simple formulæ throw much light on the complexity of the total personality. In the great majority of cases we are left without any clear guide from such simple considerations as those referred to above. We face the bewildering variety of human nature, and grope hesitatingly in the direction of an analysis of its various components. For the study of the individual equipment several authors have worked out schemata which are of great use in making a systematic survey of the personality; one may refer not only to the broad outlines suggested by Morton Prince, but to the detailed inventories published by Hoch and Amsden, and by F. L. Wells. Such schemata owe their excellence to the authors' grasp of those functions which are of most importance in regard to adaptability. They pay particular attention to the overt reactions of the individual. They differ according to the individual taste of the author and they do not profess to be based upon general biological principles.

The first steps towards an analysis of the personality more along biological lines than the type of analysis above referred to have been taken, and at the present moment a programme of further investigation of bewildering extent is being developed. The results already adumbrated are not limited to the clinic but throw much light on the destiny of the normal individual. It is interesting to trace the change in emphasis on this line of investigation since Kahlbaum published his monograph on *Catatonia*. That work expressly aimed at delimiting a disease which was to be as definite as general paralysis and he denied any intimate relation between a special mental endowment and catatonia. It did not, however, escape his clinical observation that the personality of his catatonic patients was not an irrelevant consideration, and that individuals of a certain type seemed to be specially predisposed to this type of reaction, or to this " disease " as he considered it.

The end of the nineteenth century saw the Kraepelinian psychiatry in the ascendant, and under this dispensation interest in disease processes continued to be dominant, while the personality remained a matter of incidental concern. The beginning of the twentieth century has seen a change of orientation; interest in the disease process continues and leads to important discoveries, but the conception of the disease process no longer monopolises the field. German psychiatric literature of the past few years is full of discussion of the inadequacy of the conception of mental

F

ailments as diseases or nosological entities ; we find emphasised
the importance of formulating mental disorders in terms of types
of reaction, and the desirability of carefully attributing their
respective rôles to reaction-type, environmental stress, psychological mechanisms, disease process.   One finds no reference in these
recent communications to the fact that in America for almost
twenty years Adolf Meyer had preached this doctrine of emanci-
pation from a rigid and nosological scheme.   One reason for the
lack of adequate attention given to his view was the tremendous
development of interest in the new psychoanalytic doctrines.
These doctrines focussed attention on a much narrower field than
on that of the personality in general, and the wider problems were
somewhat lost sight of in the acrimonious discussion which ranged
round the ever-interesting subject of sex.   The wider issues have
been brought to the fore in the publications of Kretschmer.   In
his monograph *Der Sensitive Beziehungswahn* (1918) he takes
certain cases with ideas of reference and resolves the clinical picture
without any residuum into personality, experience and environment ; no necessity is felt for any recourse to a *deus ex machina*,
a disease, securely hidden behind the phenomena.   The main
thesis of Kretschmer's book had perhaps been more simply stated
by Hoch in a paper published in 1912 : " In paranoic states, too,
the contact with the environment is plain ; these persons are
sensitive, and markedly concerned about the rest of the world,
they expect something from it, and, with all their suspiciousness,
they are not without a certain open attitude in the sense of aggress-
iveness and a desire to seek contact.   Another equally important
difference between the paranoic state and the condition of dementia
præcox is to be found in the fact that sometimes the external situation is a much more potent factor in the causal constellation of the
former." In a later work (1921) Kretschmer deals with the
personality in a more comprehensive way.   In this book, *Körperbau und Charakter,** he takes up a review of the total constitution, including both physique and personality, and, starting from
the extremes met with in the clinic, he carries his analysis over
into the market-place and the salon.   From the physical standpoint
he divides the community into those who are sleek and of ample
circumference (pyknic), those who are slight of build (asthenic),
those of solid bone and muscle (athletic), while in a fourth hetero-
geneous group he places those who in their physical appearance

* English Translation, *sub tit.*, *Physique and Character*, London, Kegan Paul ;
New York, Harcourt, Brace, 1924.

show a great variety of deviations from the mean (dysplastic). When one takes two extremes of temperament represented in the clinic, one finds that the manic-depressive individual is as a rule a member of the pyknic group, while very rarely is the schizophrenic of pyknic type. This is an important biological correlation, and the introduction of the laws of genetics enables the author to deal ingeniously with the frequent mixtures of pyknic, asthenic and athletic elements. After laying this solid biological foundation for the differentiation of two most important clinical groups, Kretschmer proceeds to extend the application of his thesis. These two familiar groups of mental disorder include only the extreme representatives of two types of personality, of which less striking examples are to be seen not only in the borderland between mental health and disorder, but also well within the territory of the normal. Kretschmer, therefore, sets himself the task of a descriptive analysis of these two types, the cycloid and the schizoid, with their many mixtures and varieties.

In the description of the varieties of each type he presents us with a series of portraits of considerable literary merit, the enjoyment of which makes us overlook the fact that we are getting somewhat far away from the sound biological basis from which we started. Especially is this the case in relation to his description of various modifications of the cycloid type, where we seem to be as little on biological ground as in reviewing the characters of La Bruyère. As to the core of the cycloid personality in all its varieties, those dynamic and affective qualities which are of its very essence, the author insists on the sociable, friendly, amiable nature of the cycloid, which remains throughout life and can be traced in the exhilarated excitement as well as in the retarded depression ; the schizoid personality is more complicated than the cycloid, he has unknown depths beneath his enigmatical surface, he is a dual nature, with contradictory elements co-existing in variable proportions ; the biological determinant of his schizoid nature does not seem as in the cycloid to express itself continuously from the cradle to the grave, but to have a definite period of onset early (even prenatal) or late.

In discussing the various types of personality on a biological basis, Kretschmer naturally has recourse to genetic interpretations, which help to solve many difficulties. A personality which contains a subtle mixture of the two main types of reaction may be explained as due to the inheritance of different components from the two parents ; other difficulties may be smoothed over by reference to the fact that the overt personality, the phenotype, may only be the partial expression of the total congenital endowment, the genotype. Hence, too, variations in type of reaction during the course of the individual lifetime, nay, even during the course of a single interview, may be due to the varying fortunes of war between rival genotypal factors. Such considerations make the investigation of the heredity of the individual a complicated matter, infinitely more subtle and fascinating than the recording of the usual data with regard to the grosser anomalies of ancestors, siblings, collaterals and offspring ; but in a field of such extraordinary complexity compared with the investigation of *Drosophila* it is well to be on one's guard against the seductions of speculation.

If the psychiatrist intend to go over into the genetic field, he must realise the serious nature of the step and not merely dabble with the problem. He will have to accept the rigorous conditions of satisfactory genetic work, and will have to use terms in the same accurate way as the geneticist. He will have always to keep in mind the fact that he is working with phenotypal manifestations, and that it is no easy matter to be sure, without careful analysis of offspring and ancestors, that the same phenotypal manifestations are anchored in the same genotypes. The psychiatrist will have to use the term " constitution " less vaguely than is his wont, and will probably find it most useful to consider the constitution as the totality of the characteristics of the individual, so far as they are inherited or heritable, that is, anchored in the structure of the genotype.

This is essentially the formulation of Kahn, who claims that we are passing from the period of clinical psychiatry into that of biological psychiatry, in which due attention will be paid to the wider biological principles emphasised in genetics. Kahn endorses Bleuler's view that, while in general one must clearly define the clinical conceptions before constructing satisfactory genetic relationships, in psychiatry, on the contrary, it is the genetic study of the problem which will serve to define the limits of the clinical conception. While recognising the great merit of Kraepelin's clinical contribution, Kahn doubts whether, in view of the great variety of individual constitutions and modifying experiences (" Constellation "), one can hope sharply to delimit specific constitutions or group the functional psychoses into two disease units. According to him the usual psychiatric conceptions rest too much upon discussions of the phenotype.

The requirements outlined by Kahn, with the suggestion of a programme of severe genetic investigation, should promote clearer thinking on a difficult topic and do away with many careless references to the rôle played by heredity in regard to the personality.

It is pleasant, however, for the psychiatrist to let his thoughts roam occasionally ; *dulce est desipere in loco.* The restraint of severely directed thought becomes irksome, and even Bleuler has allowed his thought to play freely around the problem of the personality, its foundations, and the rôle it plays in the psychoses. Starting from much the same standpoint as Kretschmer, he does not think of opposed types of personality, but of personalities in which two definite mechanisms are present with different dynamic balance. In each individual these two mechanisms would be present ; in extreme cases the domination of one would allow the other little possibility of expression. These two mechanisms might be called the cyclothymic or the cycloid and the schizoid, but Bleuler prefers the term " syntonic " to the term " cycloid." "Syntonic" means well-balanced and harmonious. The affectivity of the syntonic blends with the atmosphere of the environment, and inside there is a harmony both of the feelings and of the strivings.

The discussion of the special qualities of the manic-depressive, or cyclothymic, or cycloid reaction, favoured the isolation of it from other aspects of the personality, and the next step has been the tendency to make this aspect of the total behaviour of the individual into an entity, the syntonic mechanism. We are, therefore, presented with a view of the personality as containing two different mechanisms, which are assumed to have a more or less independent existence. The degree to which these functions are thought of as actually existing mechanisms may be shown by the question, " Can the one component by itself become disordered in a psychotic way, while the other remains normal, or is one component stimulated to morbid reactions through the abnormal stimuli of the other?" Another question is: "Is the initial melancholia or mania of the schizophrenic condition a syntonic symptom elicited by a schizophrenia, or do such changes of mood form a part of the schizophrenic process?" Bleuler is careful to emphasise the fact that there are many other biological types among the psychopathic, besides those we call the syntonic and the schizoid ; there are many changes of mood which are not due to the syntonic mechanisms, but which arise, *e.g.,* on the basis of sex repression, but the great majority of the affective reactions tend to be referred to variations in the syntonic mechanism.

The other psychopathic types which are met with have not the profound biological significance of the schizoid or the syntonic, but are teratological or dysplastic anomalies. In the normal character of the average individual one can trace a mixture of schizoid and syntonic components with their origin in the ancestral endowment, and with varying domination of the overt personality of the individual at different periods of life. At one period the syntonic component may dominate the scene, at another the schizoid. Bleuler has rather interesting views on the biological or teleological significance of these mechanisms. We are apt to look upon the well-balanced syntonic as the normal individual, at peace with himself and in harmony with the environment ; while the individual dominated by the schizoid mechanism is usually considered abnormal or psychopathic. The schizoid individual, however, may have the greater social value. While the syntonic finds out nothing new and wishes no improvement, and is content with his environment, the schizoid maintains his independence and follows his own goal. Obstacles may lead to embitterment, but also to the finding out of new ways. His lack of respect for reality makes him wish to alter it or withdraw from it. His inner unrest may lead him to strenuous activity, which may be socially sterile, but on the other hand may be singularly fruitful. He is able to take a somewhat more detached attitude in regard to his own feelings than the syntonic ; he is the psychologist and the poet, the reformer and philosopher. It is by means of the schizoid mechanism that the individual rises above the present time and the actual environment, imposes his own values on it, contributes to it, sees the values behind it. In a way the syntonic mechanism represents the spirit of the past and of the race, the schizoid mechanism is the essence of individuality ; man is the innovator, woman is conservative ; man is more schizoid than woman. As to the relation of an actual mental upset to the personality or temperament of the individual, we are offered hypotheses couched in genetic terms. There may be a gen or gens for the total manifestation of the disorder, or there may be a gen for the disordered element *per se*, which needs to be added to the gen or gens determining the temperament, before overt or latent disease is constituted.

One may, in passing, mention that, not content with these genetic hypotheses, Bleuler pays homage to the power of the endocrine glands. Emotions set in action hormones, and these in their turn stimulate emotions, so that perpetual emotion would have been achieved were there not counter-hormones, chemical products which neutralise the original hormones. Bereavement produces grief, but the grief hormones produce such a defence reaction that a manic excitement may result. Bleuler talks not only of " grief hormones," but of " schizoid hormones."

With all the emphasis laid on the genetic and the hormonic aspects of the schizophrenic psychoses, Bleuler minimises the rôle of environmental influences or exogenous factors. Mental disorders after influenza may look like schizophrenic conditions, but they are not the true article. The schizophrenic pictures of wartime are not to be grouped with genuine schizophrenia with its genetic history. While Bleuler clings with great tenacity to the concept of a congenitally-determined deterioration, in relation to which environmental factors are comparatively irrelevant, he makes the most important admission that occasionally an environmental factor, such as being thwarted in love, may prevent permanently the escape from autism. In such a case we would be entitled to look upon the actual condition of the patient as completely resolved into personality and environmental influences, and the possibility that this formulation might be of much wider validity than is suggested by Bleuler would have to be kept in mind.

In a discussion such as the above, we are still kept near to the clinic, and feel that it is always possible to refer to documentary material to control the hypothesis brought forward. When we pass to the advanced formulations of Jung in his book on Psychological Types, we spend little time in the narrow confines of the clinic, but are soon engaged in grappling with broad problems of the evolution of human thought. The problem of the personality is dealt with from a different angle than that of the biological geneticist or the physiologist ; it is treated from the point of view of analytical psychology, but also from an historical and philosophical standpoint. Should we wish to control the formulations by reference to the original documents on which they are based, we are somewhat at a loss, for no one probably has a material systematically analysed from this standpoint which can compare with that of Jung, while the material on which he bases his conclusions is not so far accessible to any adequate extent. The formulations of Jung are conditioned, not only by his general philosophical outlook, but by his general psychological formulation, in which the collective unconsciousness plays so great a rôle. The collective unconsciousness is at the same time the womb of the future and the repository of the history of the race.   In the analysis of the various psychological types presented to us the occurrence of psychoses is a matter of incidental reference; we are dealing with a broader problem, with the most striking and typical of the ways in which the human mind can grapple with experience.   We are too much accustomed to think that there is only one correct way of dealing with experience, and that the angle, from which we personally come to experience, is the only one from which it can be approached.   We fail to realise the limitations of our experience imposed by our own personality.   The results and methods of others we are liable to see only as mistake and error, instead of merely as another way of dealing with experience.   We are not always true to our own nature, and sometimes try to deal with experience according to an unsuitable pattern offered by those of another temperament.   It is the special value of Jung's work that he has emphasised the complemental value of many psychologies, and his philosophical outlook is a useful corrective of a narrow and exclusive attitude.   It is not the psychology of the clinic or of the laboratory, it is a psychology of experience, the psychology of human nature with its infinite complexity and age-long history, grappling with the problems of existence.   It is a metapsychology rather than a psychology that fits into the framework of the usual scientific type, but the very fact that it is too complicated an instrument for the everyday needs of the clinic does not detract from its value.   It is no psychology for a personnel bureau, although there, too, it may be a leavening factor and even have its practical value, for human nature, after all, is not altogether shut out by the gates of the factory.

It is a far cry from Munich to Zürich, and to jump from the psychological types of Jung to the files of a personnel bureau requires a nimble intelligence.   It may not be possible for the one worker to make a synthesis of the views of Kraepelin and of Jung ; in order to get valuable stimulus from both he may have to oscillate from one to the other standpoint, and to realise that there is no resting point mid-way, from which the whole territory can be surveyed. On either peak there is sufficient foothold, but to the individual firmly balanced on the one it needs some courage to make the leap to the other, and it takes a period of adjustment before he grasps the situation with the new perspective.

The above brief sketch may give a slight indication of certain trends of thought during the past twenty years.   It is natural that the psychiatrist should have been specially prominent in the investigation of the personality, for his clinical material consists of the disorders of the personality, intrinsic or symptomatic. The clinician, however, has not been the only one who has shown keen interest in this field ; as the clinician may become emancipated from his disease concept, and consider the personality in its fullness, so the teacher may take an interest in the real child and forget the pedagogic unit, and the manufacturer may see in his workers more than the economic units of the text-books. In the school and the factory the systematic investigation of the personality begins to be recognised as a subject not merely of academic interest, but one which has a fundamental bearing on the social value of these institutions.

CHARACTER AND INHIBITION

BY

A. A. ROBACK, A.M., Ph.D.

National Research Council and Harvard University

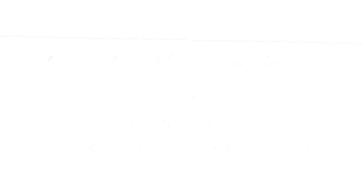

CHARACTER AND INHIBITION

BY

A. A. ROBACK

I

Introduction

" Von einem Menschen schlechthin sagen zu können : ' Er hat einen *Char-akter* ' heisst sehr viel von ihm nicht allein *gesagt*, sondern auch *gerühmt* : denn das ist eine Seltenheit, die Hochachtung gegen ihn und Bewunderung erregt."
Kant : *Anthropologie* **IV,** 3.

THERE is one department in psychology in which no progress seems to have been made for about two thousand years, in spite of the fact that it was perhaps the first topic to attract attention. It may be surmised that I am here referring to the interlocked subject of character and temperament which, though forming the core of any study of human nature, has continued to remain in the speculative stage, while other psychological material was being subjected to experimental scrutiny. Only recently have these siblings been examined anew under the more comprehensive head of personality, and in this fresh survey, the place assigned to *character* has been so circumscribed as to portend the eventual eviction of this concept from the study of psychology. It is for this reason, at least in part, that its claim to consideration should be championed.

Temperament has fared better, because of its falling distinctly into the psychological field, but it would be a difficult task to treat the one without introducing material properly belonging to the other, inasmuch as the concepts even to-day have not been sufficiently differentiated, as will be evident in the course of this paper.

The ancients have given evidence of almost uncanny insight in many of the scattered observations on both character and temperament to be found in the various books of wisdom. In a non-canonical tract of the Talmud called *Derekh-Eretz* (comportment) we find, for instance, a striking epigram in the form of a pun, the purport of which is that the scholar is chiefly recognised by his purse (b' khiso), by his wine-cup (b' khoso) and by his anger (b' khaso).*

These three words, in which only a change of one vowel has taken place, need perhaps a bit of interpretation, but it will not be difficult to see the connection between the pocket-book and the acquisitive instinct [and if I were a psychoanalyst, especially of Freud's school, I might find room for the sex instinct here too, for the word כּיס (kis) not only answers to our word *purse*, but also represents the scrotum ; and Freudians would surely regard this double meaning as significant on the basis of a psychoanalytic determinism]. The second criterion of character, according to the obscure Jewish sage of antiquity, refers to the whole situation of drinking, and includes doubtless not only the power of control and habits of temperance, but the manner of drinking, the quantity imbibed and, most important of all probably, the verbal consequences. The third mark, the anger response, again taps an instinctive source.

In this apparent pun there is revealed then the psychological approach to the study of character, and one which forms the groundwork of this essay. It matters little that the abstract word for character is wanting in the Talmudic *dictum*. The concept of character is implied in the circumlocution " A scholar may be recognised "—and the scholar in those days was first of all a gentleman.

Possibly there are many other like observations on character in the sacred books of the Hindus, in the philosophy of the Chinese sages, and the classical literature of the Greeks and Romans. Yet the psychology of character seems to have made no advance for centuries, and even after experimental psychology was making prodigious strides in at least some of its departments ; and, what is more noteworthy, after the subject of character had already become a central topic in ethics, religion and education.

But perhaps it is in the latter circumstance that the trouble is to be sought. Perhaps character, as some very recent writers maintain or at any rate imply, bears no direct contact with psychology, and is merely a concept to which are attached the possibilities of moral predication, so that it can easily be dispensed with in text-books on mind or behaviour.

Certainly this situation, at least in part, explains the neglect of

---

* Since writing the above, I have learnt that the original version of the saying so current among educated Jews, appears in a much earlier tract, viz., *Erubin* (fol. 65, col. 2).

this important subject, but it does not serve to excuse or justify it. While we must concede that character is not an introspective datum, nor even a subconscious fact, it nevertheless constitutes an integral part of personality ; and the study of personality has been rather in the ascendant than on the wane. From a psychological angle we can just as easily dispose of intelligence as of character. Even assuming that character possesses primarily an ethical denotation, must we not realise that this unity of behaviour or uniform response which in most cases permits of prediction and in any case serves to illuminate past responses, especially in the legal sphere, is psychological subject matter *per se* and furthermore is grounded in psychological causes? Whatever objections may be raised against the psychological treatment of character may also be brought against the discussion of intelligence in psychology.

Those who see in character nothing but a moral concept and a psychological fiction are oblivious to the fact that the unity and uniformity of certain behaviour forms, even in new situations (thus ruling out the mere operation of habit), cannot be considered in anything but a psychological light. Surely there is a definite integration, the result of innate dispositions and acquired tendencies, which corresponds to the concept under discussion.

I should not find it difficult even to subscribe to the notion that we are introspectively, or rather analytically, aware of our character, both before and after action. It is not because he is regarded as a gentleman that the man of character can readily place himself on the scale of social agents, just as the man of intellect does not require a series of intelligence tests in order to become aware of his mental capacity.

On the practical side of life the study of character will always have its advocates. The plea of Fernald which begins with the words " It is herein attempted to indicate that personality studies should recognise character as an integral field of inquiry " and ends with the conclusion that " character study then is entitled to recognition as a categorical entity ; since it is an integral field of inquiry having its own locus, mechanisms and event . . . "* is encouraging especially in view of the negative attitude taken by the more behaviouristically-inclined psychologists.

It is not to be overlooked, however, that the word *character*, as used by clinicians, social workers, administrators, and others who represent the practical sphere of life, have no clear-cut conception

---

* G. G. Fernald : Character *v.* Intelligence in Personality Studies, *Journal of Abnormal Psychology*, 1920. Vol. XV.

to work on, but understand by the term a conglomeration of numerous traits and qualities. Fernald, for instance, regards intelligence as the capacity or degree of personality, and character as the quality of personality, and on the strength of this division, he makes the rather suggestive remark that " character modifications continue to be reflected in behaviour after intelligence development ceases."*

The most general use of the word " character " in everyday life is invariably coloured with moral predicates. We may think of a man as having a poor memory, we may be aware that our friend cannot concentrate, that his perception is slow, without his incurring our displeasure, but no sooner do we discover some weakness about his character than we are led to take an altogether different attitude. Not only do we begin to rely less and less upon him, but we treat him as if he himself is to blame for the particular defect.

The popular mind has never distinguished more than two kinds of characters. It was either good or bad, strong or weak, noble or base, of a high or a low type ; and all these predicates are appraisals rather than statements of facts. To say that a man has no character is a euphemistic equivalent for the expression that he has a low type of character, and again, when Pope describes women as having no character at all, meaning that they are fickle and inconstant, the utterance again occurs in a slightly derogatory sense. All such references are calculated to evoke in the listener or reader a certain attitude or indicate that the speaker or writer has assumed such and such a position.

It seems to be this very circumstance, however, that proved detrimental to the growth of the study of character. Just because it was born or bred in an ethical milieu, the psychologist would be apt to disown it as spurious, while the moralist, on the other hand, after fully adopting it, would be prone to spoil it through sheer over-indulgence. Thus we see that between the neglect of a prejudiced parent and the exaggerated attentions of a zealous fosterparent, an arrested development has been the lot of our subject. And the more strongly moralists emphasised the cardinal importance of character for ethics, and incidentally in so doing encroached on the territory of other people, the more were experimental psychologists inclined to dispose of the whole matter with a word or two, sometimes barely mentioning such terms as

* G. G. Fernald : Character as an Integral Mentality Function, *Mental Hygiene*, 1916. Vol. II, p. 452.

character, temperament and even self and personality, although more recently the latter concept has come to swallow up the other three.

In this paper only the strictly psychological phase of character will be discussed. The ethical and pedagogical aspects that deal with character-building and for the most part contain hortatory appeals in behalf of the moral life do not enter here. Nor will the psychotechnical side of character be gone into at present. It is quite obvious that the theoretical examination of character must antedate both these inquiries, and more especially the latter.

II

Historical

The study of character, like many other things that have sprung into prominence recently, can be traced back at least to the enlightenment period of the eighteenth century, but it was left for the younger Mill to formulate the problem clearly and to pick out the difficulties which must beset the investigator.

In the Sixth Book of his *Logic*, Mill asks : " Are the laws of the formation of character susceptible of a satisfactory investigation by the method of experimentation ? " And he answers this in the negative. Still less weight does he lay on the method of observation in this connection, for, says he, " There is hardly any person living concerning some essential part of whose character there are not differences of opinion even among his intimate acquaintances."

Yet these various drawbacks do not prevent Mill from outlining the plan of his new science of character which he calls " Ethology." " The progress of this important but most imperfect science," says Mill towards the end of the chapter, " will depend on a double process : first, that of deducing theoretically the ethological consequences of particular circumstances of position and comparing them with recognised results of common experience, and secondly, the reverse operation : increased study of the various types of human nature that are to be found in the world ; conducted by persons not only capable of analysing and recording the circumstances in which these types prevail, but also sufficiently acquainted with psychological laws to be able to explain and account for the characteristics of the type, by the peculiarities of the circumstances,

G

the residuum alone, when there proves to be any, being set down to the account of congenital dispositions."*

This passage is cited not merely to give an historical background to the paper, but to show in what way the so-called science of characterology has sprung up, and how its motive force was primarily ethical.

Mill's advocacy of ethology has, besides influencing such men as Bain and Shand, occasioned a number of writers to make enthusiastic claims for the subject. It goes almost without saying that not a single one of the writers has advanced the projected science beyond the stage where Mill has left it, *viz.*, the embryonic stage. T. J. Bailey, to take one instance, under the promising title " *Ethology: Standpoint, Method, Tentative Results*," makes an attempt to link certain traits and qualities in a rather complicated manner, which is not simplified by the accompanying diagram, and finally has to admit that his sketch is " hopelessly incomplete and the most valuable technical features of the work have not even been mentioned."†

It is perhaps the growth of individual and variational psychology that has given the final turn to the study as we have it to-day. The positivistic tendency of the eighteenth and partly of the nineteenth century has been to slur over individual differences either as anomalies or as contingent and irrelevant matter. The *principles* of human nature constituted the desideratum of the positivists. It was the *genus homo* with which they were concerned, and not particular men.

But even in its most recent stage the subject has still its drawbacks. In the first place, as Mill has observed, it is a field where experimentation is footless. Even Ach's conclusions with regard to temperament are not derived strictly empirically, and it is only by courtesy that that part of his book *Denken und Temperament* can be called experimental.

In the second place, character and temperament have been so interlocked in their ordinary usage and more popular treatment in literature that confusion of the. two terms is almost invariably the result. It is easy to mistake the one for the other, as in either case a particular combination of traits is referred to, and sometimes, indeed, it is difficult to draw a demarcation line between the one and the other. In ordinary life we know what is meant by either

---

* J. S. Mill: *A System of Logic*, Book vi, ch. 5.
† T. J. Bailey: University Chronicles (*University of California Publications*), 1899. Vol. II, p. 31.

of the words, but when we come to pick out the principle of the difference, we are at a loss.

In the language of the street, character is often applied when speaking of more or less distinguished men, while temperament of one sort or another is something everybody is supposed to have without exception. Temperament is used in a more democratic sense and serves a social purpose, whereas character sets off the individual as a force by himself. Possibly the German view of associating temperament with the affective side of man and character with the volitional aspect will account for the ordinary usage of the two terms. We may remember how Kant made the will fundamental in ethics when he said " There is nothing in the world unconditionally good except a good will." Although the method of approaching our problem has changed considerably since antiquity, there is but little difference in our conception of what really character or temperament is. Many writers still go on pointing out that character etymologically means " an engraven mark," and that temperament is merely a technical term for a mixture or blend. This suggests, at least, that the general notion of character and temperament is the same as it was two thousand years ago. Even in the most recent works, the classification of temperaments is brought in accord with the time-honoured table of Galen, who had conceived his scheme on a metaphysiological basis.

But let us here confine ourselves to the examination of character. It is precisely because character originally meant a distinguishing mark that it has been regarded by some writers as synonymous with characteristic in the biological sense. Galton in his *Inquiries into Human Faculty* treats of character in this rather miscellaneous sense* in a brief and rather superficial essay which concludes with the injunction that schoolmasters, since they have a splendid opportunity of studying the character of schoolchildren, should not neglect making such observations. Otto Weininger's somewhat distorted account of character in his book *Sex and Character* may be cited as an exaggerated form of this tendency. According to this book, which both through its sensational claims and the morbid

---

* Klages in his *Prinzipien der Charakterologie* (third edition, p. 17) points out that there are at least three senses in which the word is used, the broadest of which practically coincides with the word " quality or property." He supposes that the circumstance is due to an animistic tendency hanging over from prehistoric days. It seems, however, just as likely that the concept " character " originally connoting a distinguishing mark was deepened in the course of time so as to designate the individual stamp of a person. The savage's notion of character differs very much from that of an educated person.

life and dramatic death of its youthful author has received a wide circulation, there are two principles in life, the male and the female, or, what is to him practically the same division, the Aryan and the Jewish. All characters partake of the two principles in varying proportions, there being very few individuals who are entirely masculine or entirely Aryan, or who, starting out as ordinary mortals, contaminated with the other principle have been able to conquer their femininity and rise to the pure stage of masculinity and Aryanism.

The dichotomous division which is the simplest form of classification, serves a useful purpose in science as a starting point. In this way it has a heuristic value.

In our particular instance, it is not difficult to see its origin. We are constantly seeing things in light and shade, we think in contrasts, and we recognise other people as different from ourselves, or what amounts to the same thing, we know ourselves through other people. And so we eventually come to learn of the two different types of people under various headings. You may call them the men of thought and the men of action, or spiritual and worldly, or you may talk of them as the intellectual type and the red-blood, but all these divisions are only another way of observing the fact that there are differences between men, that are recognised by the common people as well as by the special students along this line.

In the picturesque language of Jastrow : " The contrast persists : aristocrat and philistine, gentleman and vulgarian, Bromide and Sulphite, Athenian and Bœotian, are but different portrait titles for the same sitters, portrayed by different artists, with distinctive expressions and properties."*

In addition to the cognate categories which Jastrow has brought together, we may even accept the further divisions of H. G. Wells into poietic and kinetic, of James into tender-minded and tough-minded, of Jung into introverted and extraverted, or still further, the more technical classification of J. M. Baldwin into sensory and motor types, although here we are approaching the intelligence range rather than the field of character and temperament.

Yet in spite of this first clue that we got through experience and race intuition we are still at sea as to a satisfactory basis for a classification of characters. In the course of this essay we shall see how most classifications are either arbitrary or logical, at any rate, however, not psychological, and in the opinion of the writer

* J. Jastrow : *Qualities of Men*, p. 59.

the main obstacle seems to be that we have reached no agreement as to the essentials of character.

" It is a disposition of the will," says Wundt ; and this is the note struck by the German school in general, with Meumann as one of its foremost exponents. " It is the power to keep the selected motive dominant throughout life," is the view of Münsterberg (*Psychology General and Applied*). " Character is the system of directed conative tendencies," says McDougall (*Outline of Psychology*). " Character is life in action," according to Jastrow, which is a good metaphor but not a practical guide.

Shall we accept the statement that " Character is the power to keep the selected motive dominant " ? Münsterberg is careful enough to add that the motives might be egoistic as well as altruistic and that they might serve an ignoble as well as a noble end. But does such a view of character tell the whole story, and, above all, can it satisfy our inmost and firmest convictions ? We shall remember that, in an earlier part of the paper, the plea was to the effect that character is a subject that is taken from life and is handled in life. In cases of doubt, then, our life attitude must be the judge and decide, or else our whole problem will be artificially decked out with borrowed ornaments. Is it not, after all, the character of our daily social intercourse that we are studying and not an abstraction that has no place in the universe of our daily conduct ?

Character and principle must by all means go together, since we regard them as inseparable in our everyday judgments. The burglar and the mountebank have dominant motives ; yet we should not ascribe to them that quality called character. If we do call them disreputable characters or if we *do* say that a certain criminal is quite a character in the underworld, it is evident that we are using the word in a derived sense.

Caligula and Nero and, indeed, anybody who is obsessed by some *idée fixe* all through his life, can certainly keep his selected motive dominant if he is powerful enough, but we do not as a rule think of them as possessing character. A dog may be said to have as his dominant motive in life bone-gnawing in much the same way, and yet we should be chary of endowing the dog with that human property.

The contention in this presentation is that the predominance of a certain motive is inadequate. A substantial modification or amendment is suggested, *viz.*, that the impulses of the *will must be controlled and checked by certain inhibitions* that are evoked by the intellectual and moral make-up of a man. It thus arises from an interplay between the disposition of the will and that of the intellect.

The case of the great Italian statesman Cavour happens to occur to us and will furnish us a happy illustration of the view expressed here. Although Cavour was no more scrupulous a man than his vocation allowed, we do admire the firmness of his character not merely because he succeeded in keeping his selected motive uppermost, but because he was *actually guided by certain principles that he never flinched from*, though sometimes his resoluteness would bring him into sharp conflict with higher authority. The strength of such characters lies in the fact that, even though they may realise themselves to be on the brink of downfall, they would not save the situation for themselves by doing something they thought was not in accordance with their sense of dignity.

That is why the character of a *Tartuffe* is so repulsive, although he of all persons is bent upon carrying out his conceived plans. Were it not for the fact that he is capable of causing so much mischief, the attitude toward him would be that we take toward a jelly-fish. Nor does his whole outlook on life differ essentially from that of the lower animals. There is only this difference : the purpose of the former is explicit, articulate, while that of the latter is implicit, organic.

Far from the pursuit of one fixed motive, *character rather presupposes the possibility of change as our range of experience grows wider and richer*. A blind " will," heedless of a controlling intelligence, would be as devoid of character as Schopenhauer's universal principle.

When we begin to examine the implications of such a view, it is perhaps possible for objectors to detect a *petitio principii* in it, since it might be said that the occurrence of scruples or inhibitions to the agent already presupposes character. In answer to this, it may be pointed out that the " pure will " theory fares no better, since one can easily urge that a person's will-power will depend to some extent on his character, but, as is usually the case in such apparent circular proceedures, the influence develops on a mutual basis as soon as the first impetus is given, and the same holds true of the inhibitions that lead to the establishment of a character, and that in their turn are engendered by the reaction of the personality to the environment. There are certain facts in life that take shape gradually in spite of the " either-or " method in logic, else no one should ever have learnt to swim, else instruments should never have come into being and the construction of tunnels should have been a physical impossibility.

Friedmann* contends that we must have a scientific definition of " character " before we proceed any further, and he proposes the following one : " Character is a form-complex of reaction which keeps on recurring again and again and cannot be grasped as something general or inter-individual, but, nevertheless, appears as something typical among the most widely different constitutions."

Yet, curiously enough, toward the end of the article he tells us that we can *understand* those individuals only whose characters bear some quantitative relation to our own, but the question is : If character is merely a recurrent reaction, then why need we understand the reagent any more than we need understand the earthworm ? It seems that there is the confusion here of two points of view. Either character is not merely a type of reaction, but is something more than that, *viz.*, the outer aspect of personality, or else if it is a reaction complex, then it ought to be possible for us to study characters without having to live them as Friedmann requires. Friedmann is evidently immersed in the same dilemma which confronts the behaviourists to-day who eject introspection through the front door and take it in stealthily through the rear.

III

CLASSIFICATION OF CHARACTERS

The British School

We shall now go on to the classification of characters, about which there is much perplexity and disagreement. A classification that has enjoyed some vogue in the second part of the last century is that of Bain, who separated the characters according to the standard division of intellectual, emotional and voluntary constituents. In Bain, however, there is no strict attempt made to distinguish between character and temperament, and on the whole his position is too much that of the phrenologists in that he includes under character the most miscellaneous things, such as virtues, abilities, emotions, and general tendencies—all mixed promiscuously in one grand *potpourri*.

* R. Friedmann : Vorwort zur Charakterologie, *Archiv für die gesamte Psychol.*, 1913. Vol. XXVII, p. 198.

One service of Bain's *The Study of Character* has been, however, to emphasise the importance of finding a physiological basis for the various differences in character and temperament. The physical seat of spontaneous energy is, according to Bain, to be sought in the conformation of the muscular system.* Again some of that power is also due to cerebral currents flowing toward the muscles.† " If, there be any one point of physical conformation," says Bain in another place, " that regularly accompanies a copious natural activity, it is size of head taken altogether," and still further, " If we were to venture, after the manner of phrenology, to specify more precisely the locality of the centres of general energy, I should say the posterior part of the crown of the head, and the lateral part adjoining—that is, the region of the organs of Self Esteem, Love of Approbation, Cautiousness, Firmness and Conscientiousness—must be full and ample, if we would expect a conspicuous display of this feature of character."‡

This passage betrays the weakness of that whole school in trying to localise faculties rather than describing and explaining processes. That the influence of Bain is still felt in Great Britain can be seen from the atomistic account of character and temperament given in Shand's book which now in its second edition is an elaborate and painstaking expansion of an article published in *Mind* in 1896.

Shand, who may be regarded as a follower of Bain, also pursues an inductive method, though some of his results are not unlike the findings of the French school. He tries to build up types of character out of the various instincts, sentiments and emotions. A character for him is only the development of one affective element above the rest. Intelligence and will are totally neglected. He decidedly exaggerates the rôle of the sensibilities of man, and attempts to prove his thesis by showing how one over-developed tendency will have a marked effect on the whole moral and mental constitution of man by giving rise to new tendencies or at least giving them larger scope, and on the other hand by checking other more normal tendencies which interfere with the dominant one. " Every sentiment tends to form a type of character of its own,"§ is one of the numerous so-called laws that Shand formulates in his book.

By way of illustration the following paragraph may be quoted

* A. Bain : *The Study of Character, Including an Estimate of Phrenology*, p. 192.
† *Loc. cit.*, p. 193.
‡ *Loc. cit.*, p. 195.
§ A. F. Shand : *The Foundations of Character*, p. 123 (first edition).

from the same work: " Thus," says the author, " the miser's tyranny over those subjected to him seconds his parsimony, his industry, his vigilance, his prudence, his secrecy, his cunning, and unsociableness, which are the essential means of his avarice. He is secret because he is suspicious, he is suspicious because he pursues ends to which other men would be opposed, and because he has no counteracting trust or affection. He is cunning, because he both suspects and tries to outwit others. He makes a pretence of poverty that no claims may be made on him and that he may justify his economies. He is unsociable because he is secret and suspicious, being engaged in pursuing an object of which others do not approve and which alienates them from him.

" The qualities to which we have referred appear to belong to avarice in the sense that its thought, will, and conduct tend to acquire them because they are indispensable to the achievement of its ends."*

Now, the only fault about this treatment is that the fiction of our poets is erected into the ideal or standard type. Shand goes to literature for his illustrations, but, no matter how realistic the character of the miser in *L'Avare*, it is still the creation of Molière, and most miserly people are not nearly so morbid as Molière's character, so that all the other effects which extreme avarice brings on in its train might not be true of them at all. Now, shall we say then, that the true types of character are to be found only among neurotics?

Shall we, furthermore, deny the possession of any character to Kant, Spinoza and Fichte, simply because they did not have this or that sentiment abnormally developed? Unless we settle first of all the difference between the complex characters in literature and the real characters in life about which we are concerned, we should be involved in a hopeless mess. The study of abnormal characters portrayed by dramatists and novelists should be relegated, as Lévy has suggested, to psychopathology. We must begin with the normal characters first, though the abnormal types throw, of course, much light on the subject.

When we say that Raskolnikov in Dostoëvsky's *Crime and Punishment*, or Mishkin in the same author's *The Idiot* is a remarkable character, and that Carlyle had a remarkable character, we are certainly not using the term in the same sense. But in spite of scrupulous attempts at exact definition of the word, this confusion goes on unchecked. Definition, like the law, always admits

* A. F. Shand: *The Foundations of Character*, p. 124.

of some loophole. It is not rigid definition which is indispensable, but rather distinguishing the various usages of the term, so that we can be put on our guard against misunderstanding. In this respect Shand is by no means the only writer to be taken to task. Throughout the literature on the subject there are several contradictory trends. Particularly is this true about the word *will*, which some use as though it were only equivalent to energy, while others make out of it some entity, some faculty, which is innate and yet can be modified. Still others treat it as a source of good and evil. Such promiscuous use of the term has led to further confusion in the conception of character. We can only get our bearings by first consulting ordinary language, and here we find that energy and will are not synonymous, for we often have occasion to refer to a man who, though strong-willed, determined and resolute, is not possessed of a high degree of energy.

In dealing with the subject which is still in its initial stages, common usage should play a more prominent rôle than it has been doing in our psychological literature. Even Aristotle condescended to start his investigations with the popular notions of the subject matter under examination.

McDougall's Introduction to *Social Psychology*, which has exercised a remarkable influence in psychological circles since its appearance in 1908, may be regarded perhaps as the first systematic attempt to study the groundwork of character by examining its constituents and relationships. The merit of this work, which has much in common with Shand's, is the emphasis laid on content, and on the avoidance of formalism, so prevalent among the French characterologists. What McDougall has achieved in this direction is to lay stress " upon the systematic organisation of the conative dispositions in the moral and self-regarding sentiments . . . and to exhibit the continuity of the development of the highest types of human will and character from the primary instinctive dispositions that we have in common with the animals."

McDougall is not interested in the classification of *characters*, but in the *consolidation of character*, which he believes to be dependent on the " organisation of the sentiments in some harmonious system or hierarchy." Like Shand, he holds that the predominance of some one sentiment is crucial to the whole development of character. But, though character in the full sense of the word is not the result of a dominant motive or ruling passion alone, such as the love of home, the one master-sentiment " which can generate strong character in the fullest sense . . . is the self-regarding sentiment.''* But this needs further to be supplemented in that the " strong self-regarding sentiment must be combined with one for some ideal of conduct, and it must have risen above dependence on the regards of the mass of men ; and the motives supplied by this master-sentiment in the service of the ideal must attain an habitual predominance.''†

Since my own view bears a general resemblance to the foregoing, I might take occasion to indicate at this point that the chief difference lies in the method as also in the emphasis which in McDougall's treatment is laid on the moral side rather than on the intellectual.

Belonging to the British school, but without taking into consideration the much-needed information which other writers can supply, is Hugh Elliot's *Human Character*—a collection of essays rather than a unitary treatment. Since its chief merit is literary rather than scientific, I shall leave it out of account except to mention the fact that Elliot's discussion of what he calls "passions" and "emotions" is coloured by traditional British psychology with a strong tincture of Freudianism.

The French School

Turning to the French school, we find a more systematic treatment of the subject in Pérez, one of the earlier investigators. The basic principle with Pérez is movement or action. As a movement may be quick, slow or vehement, we obtain, through a series of combinations, six different classes of character. They are the active, the slow, the vehement or passionate, the actively intense, the slowly intense and, finally, the balanced characters.

Now, whatever of value there may be in such a simple classification, it is clear that we cannot adopt it, if for the reason alone that movement cannot be the pivotal point of personality and *a fortiori* of character. It was evidently the reaction that Pérez was emphasising as a mark of character. That it is easier to discern different kinds, or rather different rates, of movements in people than anything else in the way of reaction, is a fact which probably nobody will care to dispute, but the crux of the question lies in this : whether it is a safeguard whether movement is not after all merely an indication, and not the most essential indication, of one's inner make-up.

* Wm. McDougall : *Introduction to Social Psychology*, p. 267 (sixteenth edition).
† *Loc. cit.*, p. 261.

Are we not frequently baffled at seeming inconsistencies which we cannot clear up ? Do we not see people who are constantly in a bustle, rushing about from morning till night, and yet accomplishing very little ; while others who walk with a great deal of poise, speak with marked deliberation, and give the impression as if they were extremely slow and indolent, yet achieve wonders in comparatively brief periods ? In other words, appearances deceive ; and a quick external reaction may not be coincident with a quick internal reaction. We all know that quick apperception does not always go hand in hand with fluent expression. The rapid thinker is not always the glib talker, and to resort to the resultant as our last appeal is neither psychological nor philosophical. We might as well classify character according to noses and jaws, for we may assume on general principles that a certain type of nose and jaw goes with a certain kind of character.

In the study of character, more than anywhere else in psychology, our aim should be not merely to discover correlations, but to find out *the causes of the correlations*. If we see a man walking very quickly, it may be that he is naturally brisk, but there is also the possibility that, being slow and dilatory, he neglected something important which he is now trying to make up—hence his bustle. We can never be too sure as to which group a particular person fits into, for we do not know how much allowance to make for circumstances, and in that respect, therefore, we should never be able to compare any two individuals.

Paulhan in a more recent work, *Les Caractères*, approaches the subject from a different angle. He attempts to go to the root of the matter so as to discover the *modus operandi* of the apparatus which is responsible for differences in character—with the result that he lands in formalism.

Deriving his principle from the English Associationist School, Paulhan regards the organisation of character as the result of a systematic association process among the constituent elements of one's mind. These images, ideas, desires, and what not are welded together with reference to a certain end that characterises the individual. All that makes toward this end is reinforced, all that is antagonistic to the general purpose of the individual is inhibited. In this way we obtain a sort of metabolism which gives rise to various grades of character organisation in accordance with the strength with which certain tendencies are welded together and others driven apart. In the final analysis, character depends on just how well or how poorly the various elements can harmonise in the individual under the guidance of one main tendency. Thus Paulhan would have it that there are balanced characters and unbalanced characters, coherent and unified characters, and characters that are incoherent and not unified.

Fouillée in his *Tempérament et Caractère* devotes a good deal of space in criticism of Paulhan's doctrine ; and the objections may be summarised as follows : (1) Paulhan's classification is uninforming, though it is not difficult to accept it. (2) He puts the cart before the horse when he tries to derive difference in character from his law of systematic association. It is in virtue of the possession of a certain character that such a law would operate in an individual in one way and not in another, but to describe the reinforcement or inhibition of ideas, images and desires, by merely saying that such processes do take place, does not in the least explain why the law should operate differently in different minds.*

Fouillée himself, in an extremely suggestive book, develops a theory of character which seems to be based on his pet doctrine of *idées-forces*. The elements of character to him are ideas and will-power, with feeling as a mediator. Not unlike Bain, he has his three main divisions of intellectual, sensitive and voluntary characters, which again he divides into sub-classes : the intellectual types into the speculative and imaginative varieties, and again from the standpoint of their method of procedure into the intuitive and inductive minds ; the sensitive† class into (a) those who possess little intelligence and little will power, (b) those who are endowed with an energetic will but with little intelligence, and, finally, those who have little will-power but have a great deal of intelligence. The adjectives emotive, impulsive and reflective respectively may describe the three sensitive types. The same method of permutation and combination Fouillée follows in discussing the voluntary main divisions. Here we have : (a) those who have little sensibility and little intelligence, that is to say, the obstinate and perverted ; (b) those who have considerable sensibility and little intelligence, such as the headstrong and violent —a class from which criminals are recruited—and, finally, the " sensitives," who possess a great deal of intellectual power and have little sensibility. They are the cold and energetic calculators.

* A. Fouillée : *Tempérament et Caractère*, p. 122 *et seq.*
† " Sensitive " perhaps is not so good a rendering as " sentimental " or " emotional." " The *sensitifs*, from the physiological point of view," says Fouillée (*loc. cit.*, p. 136), " are those whose nervous system, and especially the cerebral part of it, is originally constituted in such a way as to ' play ' practically alone with an intensity which is often out of proportion to the external excitations."

All through the book Fouillée emphasises the part played by the intellect in shaping and determining a man's character as against the views of Schopenhauer and Ribot that intelligence is a negligible factor in its relation to character, and that the very concept of character presupposes an innate disposition that is fixed and immutable.   Illustration after illustration is adduced in confirmation of his thesis that intelligence has actually changed the behaviour of many notable men ; and there can be no doubt but that Fouillée's contention is sound, except that it suggests that originally there must have been some disposition in these men to want to change.   Intelligence acts only as a means, but the will takes the initiative.   It involves really the hoary issue whether or not determinism in the ultimate analysis implies fatalism.

The classification of Malapert is along the same line as that of Fouillée.   For him there are primarily four classes of characters : (a) the intellectual, (b) the affective, (c) the active and (d) the voluntary.   The supplementary classes are the apathetic whose sensibility is very small and the perfectly modulated type in whom there is no predominance of this or that character element.

In the four main divisions, there are the following sub-divisions. The sensitive may be fickle and vivacious, emotional or passionate. The intellectual may be analytic, reflective in a practical sense or speculative and engaged in constructive work.   As regards activity, there are the inactive, active and the reacting types.   Lastly, among the purely voluntary types, we find the men without will power, *i.e.*, those who carry on a routine life or the amorphous and unstably impulsive.   Again, we have the incomplete " voluntaries," comprising the weak-willed, the wavering and capricious, and, finally, the men with great will power who are complete masters of themselves.

Ribot in his treatment of character leaves out of consideration the factor of intelligence entirely.   The two functions that are fundamental for him are feeling and action.   In this way he derives his two large divisions of character : the sensitive and the active, according as feeling or energy predominates in the individual. The apathetic class, possessing a low degree of both elements, is added by way of supplement.   Out of the more comprehensive classes he builds a hierarchy of character types.   Among the sensitive may be enumerated (a) the humble, marked by excessive sensibility, shallow or mediocre intelligence, and no energy, (b) the contemplative, characterised by a keen sensibility, acute and penetrating intellect, and no activity, (c) the emotional type, combining the extreme impressionability of the contemplative with intellectual subtlety and activity. Two sub-classes belong to the active characters comprising the mediocre minds and the powerful intellects, technically called the mediocre active type and the extremely active. The apathetic class is composed of the purely apathetic with little sensibility, little activity and little intelligence ; and the calculative type is endowed with little sensibility and activity but with a practical intellect. More combinations yield us the sensitive-active kind, the apathetic-active, the apathetic-sensitive, and the temperate.*

It will be seen that, after relegating the intellect in the first place, Ribot smuggles it in to make room for new groups and varieties that could not have been introduced on the basis of feeling and action alone.

Ribot's scheme is no more psychological nor less logical than those of his predecessors, but the notion of a hierarchy that he suggests seems to be a valuable innovation which may be used in the future after we reach some more satisfactory classification.

In a book called *Psychologie du Caractère*, by Lévy, we find another basis for classification. He recognises that all attempts at classification of character must necessarily remain artificial, but, since that is the case, he says, we ought to fit our scheme into the three great manifestations of mental life, *viz.*, intelligence, feeling and will. The resulting classification would then hinge on the amount of blend there is in the individual. To Lévy it does not matter so much whether it is intelligence or feeling that is predominant so long as we recognise the fact that some one faculty is more marked than the rest.

Thus he obtains three classes : (1) the exclusive or unilateral types, characterised by the predominance of one of the three so-called faculties or functions ; (2) the mixed type where two of these faculties are highly developed at the expense of the third, and where there is possibly a conflict between the two elements, the one having the upper hand at one time, the other at another time, with intermittence of vigour and apathy at intervals ; (3) the perfectly balanced characters which may be the result of great

---

* It would seem that Jastrow is influenced by Ribot in his classification of temperaments, when he divides them into (a) the *sensitive*-ACTIVE, corresponding to the *sanguine* type of the original terminology ; (b) the SENSITIVE-*active*, representing the *melancholic* temperament ; (c) the SENSITIVE-ACTIVE, answering to the *choleric* temperament ; and (d) the *sensitive-active*, familiarly spoken of as the phlegmatic kind. (*Character and Temperament*, pp. 255–256).

deficiency of all the three elements or else may indicate a beauti-
fully harmonious organisation.

Lévy would add under another rubric the morbid characters,
for, he says, there are diseases of character, such as hypochondria,
melancholia, hysteria, etc. But these, he concludes, come under
the head of psychiatry rather than ethology.

Finally we may mention, among the French character studies,
the doctoral thesis of Ribéry, who follows pretty closely in the
footsteps of his teacher Ribot, carrying out the idea of a hierarchy
of characters more consistently perhaps than the latter. At the
top of the table may be set down the amorphous, *i.e.*, those without
any definite characteristics. Then come the sensitive, divided
into two groups : (a) the affective, (b) the apathetic. The passionate may be either stable or unstable, and the apathetic may be of
the feeble or the intense sort. A combination of the active and
the sensitive yields us a new class—the sensitive-active with its
sub-classes; the affective-passionate, the emotional-passionate and,
lastly, the perfectly balanced or modulated character.

Ribéry admits that these are only empty forms which the
innumerable individualities may fill out in a general way only.
The number of conceivable combinations and permutations is
legion, but what Ribéry endeavours to do is to provide us with a
formula that we can use to our heart's content. His general classification follows the botanical or zoological scheme with its classes
and sub-classes, orders and sub-orders, its species and varieties.
The method is deductive, the combinations being derived, according to the author, from general psychological principles.

The German School

Passing on to the German characterologists, we notice that they
have not been so prolific in this field as the French psychologists ;
and the little that has been done by them has not been taken
account of in the French works. The Germans laid more stress on
temperament, perhaps because it affords a more definite scope for
physiological explanation. Hence we find Julius Bahnsen in an
elaborate work on Hegelian principles (though his guiding *motif*
came from Schopenhauer) attempting to deduce the various types
of character from the temperaments—a procedure at which Meumann shakes his head in disapproval.

Wundt has not much to say on the subject of character, except in its relation to other qualities, such as temperament.* More promising, however, is the account of Meumann in his *Intelligenz und Wille*, where he expounds a physiological theory of character. Meumann, like Wundt, defines character as a disposition of the will, and thinks character quite independent of the feelings.†

After discarding the attempt to derive character from any form of affective life, he says, " We should come much nearer the truth if we traced back the intensity or energy of the will to an elementary strength of the will dispositions themselves. It must then be a physical basis that lends its force to the will act. In the last instance it is to be sought in the nervous energy of men. He who is endowed with great energy for motor innervation and movement and in addition possesses an intensive and easily evocable association between the sensory parallel processes of his goal ideas and between the external movements has in these qualities the foundation for energetic physical activity. And the man whose central nervous system, especially whose cortex is the seat of numerous sensory cells with a large stock of physical energy, whose functional sensory dispositions are possessed of great energy, will have thus the foundation for mental energy."‡ The corollary to be drawn from this suggests that men with weak nervous constitutions have little will energy ; and the flagrant negative instance of Kant is explained away by Meumann in assuming that Kant's physical weakness stopped at the brain, and that the philosopher's central nervous system, but especially the brain and those parts of it in which the parallel processes leading to mental activity took place, were endowed with an enormous amount of energy.

In the above we have, according to Meumann, the first of the fundamental properties of the will, which gives rise to pure volitional types of character.

A second property is the time relation. The " will " activity may be transient or lasting. He who can manage to expend a relatively equal amount of energy and develop for all tasks a lasting intensity possesses an enduring will. Here, too, Meumann, profiting by the results of Mosso, Kraepelin and Stern, traces this property back to the way in which the stock of nervous energy operates in different people, and their aptness to be easily fatigued or not, and to the various stages of the work at which fatigue is likely to set in §

A third property is to be found in the degrees of development

---

* W. Wundt : *Physiol. Psychol.* Vol. III, p. 637 (fifth edition).
† E. Meumann : *Intelligenz und Wille*, Part II, Chapt. III.
‡ *Loc. cit.*, p. 237.   § *Loc. cit.*, p. 243 *et seq.*

H

that the will attains in various individuals. The will that is guided by one principle or a system of principles to which all other things are subordinated will form the consistent character. Sporadic outbursts of activity will form the inconsistent character.

The disposition to act instinctively and impulsively on immediate ends and its opposite tendency, *viz.*, acting with reference to more ultimate purposes, yield us a fourth property of the will. Aligned with that is the attentive type of the will, the root of which is a concentrated attention and the perseveration of goal ideas (static, as opposed to dynamic, activity).*

Another type of pure will form is derived from the manner in which people will approve or disapprove of a certain course of action. Some will be led to behave in a certain way through the co-operation of their feelings directly, while others will not act until they have considered and turned over in their mind all the reasons by which their course might be ratified. In this way we obtain the wavering type and the one who quickly makes up his mind.

Finally, among the pure will forms, may be mentioned the habitual or mechanical or routine characters, that is to say, the individuals who have a tendency to get into certain grooves of conduct. So far we have dealt with *pure* will forms.

The second large division of will forms is the affective order, and it is here that Meumann finds eight fundamental properties in the feelings. (1) With reference to quality, they may be either pleasant or unpleasant. (2) As to intensity, they may be of various degrees. (3) In respect to time, they can persist in consciousness for a longer or shorter period. (4) The feelings may be excited with greater or less ease. (5) Their effect may be transitory or more lasting and reverberate in consciousness. (6) They may be classed as to the manner in which they develop, some feelings having a more objective basis than others. Again, the content of the idea may influence us, or the particular form in which we experience it may excite the feeling. (7) Connection with other contents of consciousness or the degree of fusion forms another category. (8) Their relations to us may be different. We can objectify our feelings ; for instance, when we say a " cheerful day," or a " pleasant neighbourhood," we read our own feelings into those objects, or else we can subjectify the feelings by ascribing them to our own inner condition.

* *Loc. cit.*, p. 238, 239.

Through such an analysis, Meumann is able to construct an elaborate scheme of the temperaments according to the combination of the different attributes of feeling a man possesses.

The third large class of will forms is called "intelligence forms of the will," by which Meumann means forms of the will that have their origin in the effect of certain fundamental intelligence forms of the will ; for, says Meumann, properly speaking, intelligence forms of the will are only forms of intelligence that are translated into action, just as the affective forms also are to serve the purpose of the will or activity.

In this third class there are three categories : (a) that which is responsible for differences in mental productivity, reproductivity and unproductive thinking in man, (b) comprising differences in intellectual independence and dependence, (c) embracing differences between analytic and synthetic thinking and between intuitive and discursive thinking.

It will easily be seen what an immense stock of character types can be had out of the manipulation of so many forms in different combinations.

Meumann has perhaps overstepped the limit in the drawing up of numerous classes and forms, but he, more than anyone else in Germany, has given us a solid foothold for our problem and has pointed out the direction in which we are to attain our object.

Lucka's view* is somewhat interesting, not only because he takes the point of view of the worldly man on the subject, but because he has recently been recognised as one of the most prominent fiction writers in Germany. Character to him is not so much what differentiates one man from another as the attitude a man takes toward the external world. He sponsors the philosophical aspect of the subject. It must be on the ground of worldly experience that he divides men into four, or perhaps two, wider classes and two narrower sub-classes. We begin with the naïve who make no distinction between reality and value, who are always on the spot to act because they, as a rule, do not realise the import of their acts. They make the soldiers, the speculators and the adventurers. Then there is, secondly, the mediate class, the reflective people, who not only have experiences, but ponder over them. They often waver and hesitate, because they see so many relations of which

---

* E.Lucka : Das Problem einer Charakterologie, *Archiv für die gesamte Psychologie*, 1908. Vol. XI.

the naïve man has no idea.* The man of the moment is our third type. For him there are only incoherent experiences. He lacks the continuity of the subject. He is perfectly passive without being able to create anything new out of his impressions. He is reproductive but not productive. His life is made up of impress-ions alone. (4) The productive type, represented by men like Goethe, whose very memory is a recasting of experiences, constitutes just the opposite. His life is directed outward, beginning with his own personality, whereas the reproductive type brings the outward world into his own. Spontaneity marks the productive individual who never merely learns, but is continually experiencing.

Lucka, though he is abreast of the literature on the subject more than any other German writer, disregards the *psychology* of character entirely, and trusts to his insight into things alone. His view of character belongs to the class of observational accounts, approaching in content, though not in form, to the scattered brilliant *aperçus* contained in La Bruyère, La Rochefoucauld, Jean Paul and Schopenhauer. The newer school to which Lucka's views seem most aligned is the *Struktur movement*, and in some measure there is an overlapping between Lucka's types and those of Spranger, who will be considered in the next part. To Lucka "character" is "the disposition of an individual psychical organisation to receive impressions from the world about (in the widest sense) in a definite way, and to react to them in a definite manner." Character is to be translated as a "characteristic attitude toward the world," in Lucka's vocabulary.

Though Klages' *Prinzipien der Characterologie* might properly be brought into relation with the other German treatments of character, it would take too much space even to give the merest outline of Klages' classification which is marked by a complex architectonic. The capacities of men, he believes, form the stuff or texture of character, while the strivings or conations constitute its quality. Furthermore, the structure of character is determined by the organisation of the material.

When we begin to look into Klages' tables, we are confronted by a rather perplexing list of differences which are pigeon-holed into various categories, such as differences of quantity (full and empty) ; differences of distinctness (warm and cold) ; differences of mobility (heavy and light) ; differences of quality (deep and shallow). Klages is very careful to find a place for every quality

* We immediately perceive in these Jung's introverts.

and trait, but his mode of procedure smacks of Hegelian dialectic, and the presentation lacks clarity, so that, with all his discerning observations and eagerness to save us from general fallacies, he is apt to be confusing. The confidence with which he makes certain statements, such as that, though we say " *Es* reizt mich," we never use the same quasi-passive construction in the case of willing, would be shaken if he took cognisance of other languages.* Similarly his tabulation and schemes do not carry conviction. Under deficient self-preservation, he lists in the ethical category— injustice, unreliability, " characterlessness," and unscrupulousness. It would seem that the very people who possess these negative traits were born with an exaggerated instinct of self-preservation.

A Dutch Account

The laborious comparative study of Heymans and Wiersma in which the character traits of thousands of persons were treated statistically on the basis of both biographical and questionnaire material resulted in, or rather began with, the selection of three fundamental criteria for the rating of character, *viz.*, activity, emotionality and the preponderance of either the primary or the secondary function, and the statistical tabulation of numerous traits or responses relative to the above criteria. The criteria of activity and emotionality need no explanation, but the curious designation of " primary functioning " refers to such qualities as " easily comforted," " changeable sympathies," " ever interested in new impressions and friends," " easily reconciled," " apt to change occupation or course of study," "often takes up with great plans which are never realised," etc. The preponderance of the " secondary function," on the other hand, called for such data as tenacity, " clinging to old memories," " hard to reconcile," conservatism, " influenced by future prospects rather than by immediate gain," etc.

On the basis of the three divisions according to the fundamental

---

* It is well to examine a concept from the point of view of its popular usage or etymology, but Klages places too much emphasis on linguistic forms. As a matter of fact, the untutored person scarcely uses the verb *to will*; and *willing* is most frequently employed by the man in the street in the sense of *desiring*. In Yiddish, the quasi-passive construction with the verb " to will " is often used, but in the sense of desiring. " Es vilt zich mir " is the equivalent of " I should like," with the implication of the desire being due to organic sources.

criteria, Heymans and Wiersma have set up eight types of characters after this fashion.

1. *Amorphous*—the non-emotional non-active with predominant primary function.*
2. *Apathetic*—the non-emotional non-active with predominant secondary function.
3. *Nervous*—the emotional non-active with predominant primary function.
4. *Sentimental*—the emotional non-active with predominant secondary function.
5. *Sanguine*—the non-emotional active with predominant primary function.
6. *Phlegmatic*—the non-emotional active with predominant secondary function.
7. *Choleric*—the emotional active with predominant primary function.
8. *Passionate*—the emotional active with predominant secondary function.

The chief value of this extensive investigation lies in the detailed delineation of a given type by affixing numerous qualities to the individual in varying degrees. The application of the results of the questionnaire to the miser is in itself a very interesting study which appears to approach the truth more nearly than a similar study by de Fursac.

What the Dutch authors have done is to supply us with a ready chart, which brings to light correlations among the hundreds of traits catalogued and at the same time affords a grouping scheme according to the basic criteria and correlations. The eight separate classes which they obtained fit in well with the results of the French school, except that a much more empirical method has been employed by the former.

In other respects, however, we miss a theoretical basis both for the concept of character and its categories. We must proceed on an arbitrary plan in the first place, and in the last analysis the correlations are of statistical value more than of practical application in individual cases. The spendthrift, for instance, is domineering in 31% of cases, mercenary in 20% of cases, unselfish in 48% of cases, but how about *this particular* spendthrift under examination?

* G. Heymans and E. Wiersma : Beiträge zur speziellen Psychologie auf Grund einer Massenuntersuchung. *Ztft. für Psychologie*, 1906–1909. Vols. XLII–XLVI, XLIX, and LI. ›

IV

RECENT TRENDS

The Psychoanalytic Approach

Since 1908, when Freud published his paper, *Character und Analerotik*, a number of his disciples have attempted to show that certain traits of character are connected with the sex impulse and the excretory functions. Freud started out by relating three traits to anal-eroticism, but within a few years of the publication of his original article the list had been increased to a score or more. The whole problem of motivation which Freud has raised may, of course, be considered as a vast contribution to the study of character,* treating it from a hitherto unknown angle, but it is evident that I must confine myself to the more specific references which seem to centre about this peculiarity, so much made of by psychoanalysts.

It would not be profitable to review the literature on the subject of anal-eroticism, especially as Jones has covered most of the ground in his paper, *Anal-Erotic Character Traits.*† We should, however, dwell at greater length on the views of two of Freud's former disciples and now leaders of separate schools, *viz.*, Jung and Adler, both of whom have been dealing especially with character types.

Jung's well-known classification of psychological types into introverted and extraverted individuals has received considerable recognition not only in educated lay circles, particularly journalistic and literary quarters, but even among psychologists. But that is as far as the latter will go with him. The breaking up of the original dichotomy into eight sub-divisions does not lend itself to ready acceptance, and, furthermore, the compensatory principle which he introduces to explain the vast majority of cases that elude the ordinary classification is plausible in theory but scarcely applicable; for, granted that there is a primarily conscious introverted type with a complementary unconscious trend of extraversion, and conversely a conscious extraverted type with an unconscious trend

---

* The extent to which psychoanalysts are prone to employ a definite term in a colourless way can be inferred from the mere title of van der Hoop's account of the psychology of Freud and Jung; for, though the book is called *Character and the Unconscious*, there is hardly a direct reference to the first term of the title in the whole presentation.

† Jones: *Papers on Psycho-Analysis* (second edition), Chap. XI.

of introversion, our utmost ingenuity will be taxed in discovering the criteria in the first place, and secondly in reaching an agreement as to which fit whom. Illustrating with instances from literature and history, on which the Neo-Platonist of psychoanalysis draws so energetically, is not a wholly satisfactory method ; for, as in the case of the illustrations to be found in the various books on character analysis, they are *post ex facto* constructions, and out of innumerable possibilities one is apt to select just those which best suit the particular theory advanced.

Since Jung's latest utterances on this subject appear in the present volume, there is no need of presenting here a detailed exposition of his views. The reciprocal interplay between the conscious and unconscious elements in one's personality is, to my mind, the most interesting feature of the doctrine. In other respects, especially in the use it makes of thinking and feeling as bases of the sub-divisions, it resembles the classifications of the French school.

Adler's contribution to the study of character, as developed in his chief works, *The Neurotic Constitution, Organ Inferiority and its Psychical Compensation* and *Individual Psychology*, is woven around the now famous inferiority complex and its compensatory mechanism. The gist of Adler's doctrine is really contained in this compact statement, " All manifestations of neuroses and psycho-neuroses are to be traced back to organ inferiority, to the degree and the nature of the central compensation that has not yet become successful and to the appearance of compensation disturbances."*

Knowing, as we do, the tendency of all of Freud's disciples, both present and former, to assign to every person a fair share of such manifestations at least in some mild form, we may readily see why, according to Adler, all the various aberrations in man's conduct, from the serious offences down to the mere peculiarities in everyday behaviour, would be linked with an hereditary, often latent, inferiority of a certain organ and its nervous superstructure. Character, then, must be understood in such terms ; but though Adler's detailed interpretations and diagnoses are highly ingenious, they fail to connect the specific conclusions and inferences with the doctrine in general. In Adler's texture we may find threads from Nietzsche (Will to Power—Superiority Goal) and Weininger (Male Attitude in Female Neurotics) in addition to the material which contains the warp and woof of psychoanalysis at large.

* A. Adler : *The Practice and Theory of Individual Psychology*, p. 316.

White* in this country (U.S.A.) has approached the problem through the psychoanalytic avenue more directly, though in a highly eclectic way, claiming that character is merely the resultant of an interplay of unconscious factors in which conflict plays the most important part ; the resolution of this conflict then becomes the desideratum of man. And to that end White places at our disposal all the mechanisms of Freud's, Jung's and Adler's schools, interwoven with a number of other factors. Van der Hoop's exposition of the theories of Freud and Jung, under the somewhat misleading title *Character and the Unconscious,* is based on the same presuppositions as those which White has set out with.

Kempf, both in his *Autonomic Functions of the Personality* and *Psychopathology,* particularly in the latter work, harps *ad libitum* on the psychoanalytic theme, but his own contribution, *viz.,* the linking of the autonomic functions with the affective side of man and his temperamental make-up, brings him into position with the seekers of character determinants in physiological and especially chemical processes ; and though not primarily concerned with the glands, he suggests a definite location for some of the Freudian and Adlerian mechanisms (even if he comes far from making actual specific connections). Thus he affords a sort of synthesis between the mental approach of the psychoanalysts and the physical approach of the endocrinologists.

A host of Freudian writers may be mentioned as authors of observations on this topic. Many of these observations display an insight into what is ordinarily called human nature. Some of the writers give evidence of penetration in special fields, such as Adler and Stekel in their descriptions of various sorts of neurotics and Pfister in his accounts of children's peculiarities, but on the whole, the psychoanalytic attack consists of sallies. It does not represent a carefully worked out plan based on solid foundations, and for this reason it may be said that, while the intuitive scintillations are appreciated particularly from an artistic viewpoint, the scientific groundwork upon which they purport to stand cannot provide a foothold for the logically-minded investigator who must have his concepts clearly separated before they can be related to one another.

One serious criticism which applies especially to the Freudian phase of psychoanalysis is the exaggerated importance attached to experience in the formation of character. While admitting that no individual is entirely immune to the effect of emotional stimuli,

---

* W. A. White : *Mechanisms of Character Formation.*

I should take occasion to point out that *since different people are affected differently by apparently similar stimuli, it would be reasonable to maintain that character in reality precedes and determines the nature of the effect, instead of being the resultant of the multitude of experiences to which man is subjected.*

If character is formed in such an utterly mechanical way, there is no reason why we should not attribute this quality to a radio apparatus or to a steam engine.

On the surface, Adler's type of doctrine would claim to escape this criticism, since his defection from the orthodox camp of Freud was due primarily to his hankering after a doctrine that would champion the cause of freedom against the extreme determinism of his master ; but on strict analysis it will be seen that, though the organ inferiority itself is held to have an hereditary basis, the compensatory reaction is a process developing out of the inferiority complex in relation with the environment.

Suggestions from Psychiatry

If the difference between the abnormal and the normal is only one of degree rather than of kind, we may well hope to obtain valuable data from the field of psychiatry to elucidate the more obscure regions of psychology, and it is only recently that the seemingly regressive method has been adopted. Again, I shall not attempt to catalogue all the references showing what psychiatrists have to offer to the student of character but will content myself with the more direct treatments.

Offhand it might seem that psychoanalysis and psychiatry could go hand in hand in their approach at least, even if their findings should turn out to be divergent, but in reality the presuppositions and standpoints are different from the very start. The psychoanalytic camp is inclined to stress the cause of the disturbance as a determinant of the disorder ; the orthodox psychiatrist, though in the past seeking the entire cause of the evil in a special incident or series of incidents, has at last come to recognise that the same stimuli would react differently on different individuals. Now, if there are different types of diatheses in organic as well as in mental diseases of a functional nature, it stands to reason that each diathesis is correlated with a certain personality type.

Boven* proceeds from the facts of character to diagnose psychoses

* W. Boven : Caractère individuel et aliénation mentale, *Jour. de Psychol.*, 1921. Vol. XVIII.

on the supposition that the diversity of psychoses corresponds with the diversity of characters; allowing, of course, for combinations of traits and temporal factors, one might, according to the French writer, say that the particular type of character an individual possesses will be responsible for the psychoses he develops.

As Jastrow* expresses it, " A temperament becomes a more or less marked liability to a specific type of abnormal complex."

The same general principle operating, however, in the reverse direction leads Rosanoff† to deduce a theory of personality in conformity with the classification of psychopathic types, which, according to him, consists of (a) the anti-social; (b) the cyclothymic, behaving like a swinging pendulum; (c) the shut-in or autistic, and (d) the epileptic personalities. In the normal individuals the various personality types are more or less mixed, and it must be remembered that not only is the normal individual safeguarded because of the low index of the peculiarity or the fortunate combination producing a more desirable blend, but also on account of the inhibitory factors and greater stability of the nervous system.

The psychiatric treatment of character and temperament is not a sporadic attempt. It has a number of representatives and seems to be spreading. In a carefully worked out monograph which has passed through three editions in two years, and which is to appear shortly in an English translation, Ernst Kretschmer finds a distinct relationship between what he calls character and physique. Taking a large number of clinical cases for material, and charting the chief physical characteristics of the patients, he establishes the following four types : (a) asthenic, (b) athletic, (c) pyknik, or plump, (d) hypoplastic, or regularly undersized for the most part, though, as in infantilism, certain parts are apt to be especially small. The temperaments are divided into *schizo thymic*, from which the schizophrenic patients are recruited, and *cyclothymic*, which forms the basis of the circular psychoses. Each of the two classes is sub-divided into several popular types, such as the " gushing jolly people," " the quiet humorists," etc.

The author apparently does not think that he is invading psychological territory with psychiatric methods; for, says he, " It must be pointed out clearly from the very start that the designations schizothymic and cyclothymic have nothing to do with the question of sanity, but are terms for large general biotypes . . ."

* J. Jastrow : *Character and Temperament*, p. 320.
† A. J. Rosanoff : A Theory of Personality Based Mainly on Psychiatric Experience, *Psychol. Bulletin*, 1920. Vol. XVII.

" The words, then, do not indicate that the majority of all schizothymic persons must be psychically dissociated and that the majority of all cyclothymic people are subject to periodic fluctuations."*

Kretschmer's application of his classification to both ordinary individuals and men of genius, though teeming with suggestive characterisations, suffers from the defect of all books on character analysis, viz., the characterisations are made *post ex facto*, and the most solid theoretical observations will be of no avail so long as there are no fundamental principles to guide us in making individual judgments.

Before we leave Kretschmer's account, it would be well to reproduce here his definitions of the concepts *constitution, character* and *temperament*. By constitution he understands the collection of all individual qualities which depend on heredity. Character is to him the mass of affective and volitional reactive possibilities of an individual as they have come about in the course of his life development, and include therefore not only hereditary dispositions but also physical and psychical influences derived from the environment and experience.

Naturally, after broadening the concept of character to include practically all mental traits, Kretschmer is obliged to reduce the term " temperament " to a heuristic concept (" *noch kein geschlossener Begriff* "). In common with other writers he bases temperamental differences on chemical reactions in the body, and claims the cerebro-glandular apparatus to be the organs of the temperaments.

As to the two main temperamental divisions, Kretschmer's cyclothymic temperament, from his description, would correspond to Jung's extraverted type, while the schizothymic person may easily be recognised as the introvert.

Of perhaps equal importance with the preceding book is the discussion of character in relation to nervousness by the Hungarian psychiatrist Jenö Kollarits,† which I know only from a meagre review.

But we should bear in mind that, after all, personality types are not exactly the same as character types, though there is a tendency to identify the two orders of facts in most accounts. It is really here that we have an opportunity for revealing a significant difference between the two. It is this : While much may be inferred

* E. Kretschmer : *Körperbau und Charakter* (third edition), p. 154.
† J. Kollarits : *Charakter und Nervosität*.

from a patient's psychosis as to his original temperament traits, there is little information to be gained as to his character, except through a method of extensive reconstruction. It is precisely for this reason that the insane are considered irresponsible. In a word, the affective pattern of the normal individual has merely been thrown into bolder relief when he becomes insane, but his character complex has been so twisted that it loses its very essence. *There is no character to the insane.*

The Endocrinological Attack

For the last quarter of a century the interesting results obtained in experiments with the ductless glands have turned the thoughts of many a worker in the borderland territory between physiology and psychology to conjectural expectations as to gross mental changes in consequence of processes going on in certain glands. The astonishing transformation brought about as a result of operations on the sex glands and the thyroid as well as the less spectacular findings of Crile, Carlson, Cannon and others, in regard to the emotions as affecting and being affected by the humoral processes in the body have been responsible for many a bold statement which scarcely bears examination.

The thesis of the endocrine enthusiasts, the most articulate of whom is Berman, claims that an individual's personality is regulated by the glands. According to this writer, " Character, indeed, is an alloy of the different standard intravisceral pressures of the organism, a fusion created by the resistance or counter-pressure of the obstacles in the environment. Character, in short, is the gland intravisceral barometer of a personality.*

Aside from the extreme haziness of such a definition, the essential mark of character is missing in it. Manifestly we cannot envisage character as a pressure. This were ludicrous. What the author, I suppose, means is that character depends on these various pressures, etc., but he has not told us what character is.

The most conservative of us are probably ready to concede that our personality would undergo slight changes in consequence of alterations in the functioning of the ductless glands. A treatment of the subject of character and temperament, such as Jastrow's, without the mention of endocrine secretion, must be regarded as deficient in that respect ; but to base character entirely on meta-

* L. Berman : *The Glands Regulating the Personality*, p. 107.

bolism and secretions is, in spite of Bertrand Russell's speculations in regard to the possibility of transforming emotional dispositions through physiological manipulation,* a mere romance of modern science.

The Behaviouristic Detour

If the problem of character presents so much difficulty to the traditional psychologist, the behaviourist, naturally, could not be expected to even attempt a solution, and, like the fox in the fable, denies the value of the object. At least this is the attitude of Watson, who may be taken as the spokesman of the behaviourists, and who is usually clear and consistent in his views.

In a footnote he tells us that " Character is generally used when viewing the individual from the standpoint of his reactions to the more conventionalised and standardised situations (conventions, morals, etc.)."†

Apparently he makes short shrift of this term on the ground that it is an ethical and not a psychological concept. *Prima facie*, we might be inclined to apply in support of the behaviouristic contention the remark of James in his famous chapter on *Habit*, to the effect that there is, physiologically, no difference between a good habit and a bad one. But, as has been said earlier, a character is more than a habit. It is a system of tendencies which permits a considerable amount of predictability. And certainly one system of tendencies is far different from another system, while in many cases the tendencies do not hang together so as to deserve a unifying mark.

But it is possible to expose the *ratio ignava* of Watson's school in a more direct manner. The behaviouristic fallacy of giving an environmental turn to everything conceivable is apparent here as elsewhere. Whoever would say that a person like Herminia Barton in *The Woman Who Did* was without character simply because she chose a path which in the eyes of her community and indeed the world at large was considered irregular ? On turning from fiction to grim reality, would not the very judges who sentenced the Irish patriot Roger Casement to the gallows testify to the noble traitor's

---

* Bertrand Russell : *Icarus*, pp. 53–54. Russell's tone in this booklet is hardly a serious one. It is rather in the vein of a *feuilleton* when he writes : " Assuming an oligarchic organisation of society, the State could give to the children of holders of power the disposition required for obedience. Against the injections of the State physicians the most eloquent Socialist oratory would be powerless."

† J. B. Watson : *Psychology from the Standpoint of a Behaviourist*, p. 392.

well-knit character? Is it necessary to call attention once more to the elementary distinction made time and again between reputation and character?

Character is a relation which holds not between a man and his community, but between his reason and his own acts. It is because character emanates from one's own self that it transcends the community and *presents an objective problem.* To be sure, in the last analysis posterity is the judge, but its criterion is not what Watson implies it to be, *viz.,* the conformity to conventionalised situations, but the living up to one's own convictions in spite of social pressure.

A mere acquaintance with the lives of universal heroes will convince us that the man of character was usually he who combated the prevailing notions of his time by word and deed. Were the community in which he lived to be asked about his character, the consensus would be decidedly condemnatory. When, in response to Napoleon's captious remarks about his music, Cherubini replied, " Your Majesty knows as much about music as I know about battles," thus bringing upon himself the disfavour of the redoubtable Emperor, with the consequent humiliation and disgrace, it matters little really whether or not Napoleon had an ear for music or whether Cherubini's music was not of a high order. Still less does it matter what Napoleon's court or his worshipful subjects would think of such *lèse-majesté.* The remark of Cherubini will have to be considered for all times, even if his operas and masses should pass into oblivion, as an indication of the man's character.

We need not linger on this negative platform, which confuses a psychological issue with the ethical judgments surrounding it, and were it not for the fact that so many psychologists find it expedient to dispose of a troublesome subject cavalierly rather than to take account of it, we should have passed over the behaviouristic denial in silence.

From the Angle of Struktur and Gestalt Psychology

Though we are repeatedly reminded by writers that the *Gestalt* school is not to be confused or even too closely connected with the *Struktur* movement, in that the former practically ignores personality problems,* I see no reason why the two apparently concentric groups

* G. W. Allport, in " The Study of the Undivided Personality," (*Journal of Abnormal Psychology and Social Psychology*, 1927, Vol. XIX), suggestively criticises the analytic approach of personality studies, in favour of the *Gestalt* method.

cannot be treated together on the basis that the difference is more in the selection and concentration of the subject-matter rather than one of method or fundamental presuppositions. While realising therefore that the objection made in this section against the general movement can hardly hold with regard to the sub-school, or perhaps companion school, which shuts its eyes almost to everything in psychology except the problem of perception, we may gather from intimations, such as the allusion by Koffka* to some lectures on personality by Wertheimer, one of the leaders of the *Gestalt* school, that not all its representatives share the circumscribed views of Koehler.

The principal feature of the *Struktur* school, whether it approaches the study of perception, after the fashion of the *Gestalt* group, or dwells on the problem of personality, the *pièce de résistance* of the movement consists in the emphasis it lays on the complex as a totality. The parts or elements receive their proper attention and evaluation only in the light of the whole. For our present purpose, I think, we need not consider the important difference between the *Gestalt* theory and the allied *Struktur* doctrines, which, according to Koffka, consists in the separation of mind and body in the latter, while his own school regards personality as a natural phenomenon, not a mental or spiritual fact.

It is most significant that even the *Gestalt* psychology, which is a strictly experimental movement, must make room for an artistic and intuitive current in the treatment of personality. And this streak is especially noticeable in the writings of the *Struktur* psychologists. The psychographic methods of William Stern are pushed into the background to allow for a life *cliché* as taught by Dilthey and Spranger, whose philosophy concerns itself with the pulse of life, not with congealed elements.

In contrast with the various analytic personality investigators, Spranger in his *Lebensformen* and William Stern in his *menschliche Persönlichkeit* set out to look for a form of structure which would polarise a personality, setting it off as a distinct entity. And it is noteworthy that, at the risk of injecting metaphysics or even mysticism into psychology, they and others of the school tend to recognise the uniqueness attaching to personality in its value aspect. As Erich Stern, one of the younger representatives of this wider school, states it, " In what a man sees value, especially in what he sees the highest value of his life, that value, in fact,

---

* K. Koffka : Psychical and Physical Structures, *Psyche*, 1924. Vol. V (n.s.), p. 84.

which makes life important to him, that is what we must know, if we are to be capable of understanding his personality."*

Spranger sets up six types of personalities on the basis of their value tendencies : The economical, the theoretical, the artistic, the social, the political and the religious. To place an individual somewhere in this scheme is to understand him. Inability to do so implies that the person is beyond our comprehension.

In criticism of this view, I should submit that Spranger is judging in terms of interests rather than on the basis of values. Value implies linear measurement. But the artistic form of personality is certainly on a par with the theoretical or the religious type. The forms are not commensurate and one form is just as valuable as any other in the scheme. And what affords to value its distinctive mark is the possibility of appraisal and contrast which it carries with it. In this case then the term value which is to serve as the touchstone, if not the dowsing rod, of personality, may be regarded as a misnomer. The question then reduces itself to this : Can we discover uniqueness by collating a number of interests and colligating them under some predominant bent of mind ?

If psychology cannot help us to gain a foothold in these elusive regions, it is rather hazardous to turn to philosophy for an entrance since, through such an avenue, our very entrance would be an illusion, and we should not even know that we were unsuccessful, whereupon we might devise other means of gaining access.

V

Inhibition as the Basis of Character

Having devoted considerable space to the historical development of our subject, I shall set forth my own views as briefly as possible.

In the first place, though the discussion necessarily included the concepts of temperament and personality, yet since it is not always possible to isolate the subject of character from a general treatment of personality, which in some presentations is identified with it, it is necessary to remind the reader that character is regarded here as one aspect of personality, the others being intelligence, temperament, physique and other mental and physical qualities.

* E. Stern : New Ways of Investigating the Problem of Personality, *Psyche*, 1923. Vol. III (n.s.), p. 364.

I

If character is a psychological entity we must endeavour to examine it by means of psychological methods and place it on a psychological basis.

But there is another condition that must not be lost sight of, and *that is the cumulative meaning of the word throughout the ages*, a meaning which psychology cannot supplant without actually talking about a different thing. The concept may, of course, be grasped in a different setting in order to be invested with authority, but its nucleus must remain intact.

The reason why the tripartite division of mind is inadequate to furnish us a classification of characters is primarily the overlapping of the divisions with respect to the two allied subjects—character and temperament—as well as the resulting confusion. I think it is well to keep the temperaments in reserve for the affective side of man. To talk of an affective character is not instructive, and to institute further divisions by hybridisation such as " cognitive-affective " or " active-sensitive " reveals the weakness of the position, and serves but to escape the necessity of pointing out definite categories on which we can put our fingers when we come to apply the findings in real life. In the last analysis, instead of psychological types, we see before us verbal categories ; and the core of character in its original denotation is missing to boot.

Nor can we be satisfied with the resort to speed and intensity as the foundations of character. Perhaps these criteria would be suitable for the classification of temperaments, and it is remarkable that, over two thousand years ago, these principles were mentioned in the Talmud to differentiate the four mental types of man, as may be seen in the following passage from *Pirke Abot* :—

" There are four types of mental disposition : (a) He who is easily irritated and easily reconciled, thus offsetting his liability by the asset ; (b) the one whom it is difficult to anger and difficult to appease, thus counterbalancing his gain by his loss ; (c) he whom it is difficult to provoke and easy to pacify—the saint, and (d) the one who is easily provoked but reconciled only with difficulty—the villain.

We thus have the speed of the reaction in the time it takes for the anger to develop and the intensity in the time it takes for this emotion to subside under proper conditions.

ארבע מדות בדעות: נוח לכעוס ונוח לרצות, יצא הפסדו בשכרו; קשה לכעוס וקשה לרצות, יצא שכרו בהפסדו; קשה לכעוס ונוח לרצות. חסיד; נוח לכעוס וקשה לרצות רשע. (Abot 5 : 14)

Speed, energy, intensity, perseverance—these are all significant traits, especially in the matter of engaging employees, but in our relationship with friends and in the appraisal of historical personages they do not loom so large.   Character counts for much more ; and it is the distinguishing mark of this character that we are in quest of.

Often we are deceived by the use of such terms in that they have practical application only when coupled with an objective.   The indolent scholar may turn out to be an energetic professional baseball player or a hustling politician.   The slow eater and awkward manual worker may nevertheless be a quick thinker and writer. *The persons who display most of the article we call character are the ones to offer the most contradiction in their make-up. The contradiction, however, lies not in them, but in those who do the judging and who are not provided with a key to the objectives.*

But to what psychological entities, then, can we hitch character ? The answer is : *The Instincts.* We shall soon see that through such a procedure we can meet the requirement of the man in the street, and at the same time move safely on psychological territory without taking recourse to hazy categories combined in sets of two or three. An instinct, after all, notwithstanding the attempts made in certain quarters to evict it from the psychological purview, is a definite mechanism which operates visibly enough to convince us of its existence.*

Roughly speaking, one of the major differences between men and infra-human beings is that the latter do not inhibit their instinctive impulses except after a painful training ; and that is the chief reason why character cannot be ascribed to animals.   If speed, intensity, perseverance and other such traits were to be the basis of character division, we should expect animals, since they present marked individual differences in regard to such traits, to partake of the classes of characters drawn up for man.

The view proposed here also makes use of the tripartite division of mind, not, however, in a way to break it up into strips, eventually to be pasted together in various combinations, but in a synthetic manner, so that each character may be said to consist of cognitive (intellectual), affective, and conative elements.

My definition of character accordingly is as follows : *An enduring*

* A reading of McDougall's two papers, one entitled The Use and Abuse of Instinct, in the *Journal of Abnormal Psychology*, 1922, Vol. XVI, the other Can Sociology and Social Psychology Dispense with Instinct ? in the *American Journal of Sociology*, 1914, vol. XXIX, will be sufficient to prove the anti-instinct movement without foundation.

psycho-physical disposition to inhibit instinctive impulses in accordance with a regulative principle. Each of these conditions must be fulfilled before character can be attributed to the individual. The possession of instinctive urges is of prime importance. The inhibition of the urge stamps the agent with character, though of varying degrees. Not until we have the regulative principle as a clue can we determine to what extent the man or woman we are judging possesses character.

Since every instinct is grounded in both conation and affection and since inhibition is wholly a matter of conation, and finally since the determining factor of this inhibition is or has been reflection of some kind, we perceive that the older categories still have a place in our scheme when properly arranged so as to form a synthesis, the affective part furnishing the condition, the conative supplying the raw content and the cognitive factor colouring it with significance, giving it status and suggesting a possibility of measurement.

To the objection that our knowledge about the instincts is limited and that controversy is rife as to their number, one might easily reply that it is not necessary to have detailed information about every instinct before we can work with any of them, any more than we have to give up talking about the elements in chemistry until we shall have discovered their exact number for all times.

It is quite sufficient to base our study of character on the more palpable instincts, such as self-preservation, sex, acquisitiveness, self-aggression or the will to power. We must remember also that not all instincts are of equal intensity. Many, if not most of them, can be placed on a scale according to their universal intensity. Thus it is quite certain that the instinct of self-preservation is more potent than the mating impulse or the food drive. The inhibition of the latter is therefore not so expressive of character as the inhibition of the former, other things being equal.

As regards the logical principle regulating the inhibition, it must be pointed out that inasmuch as different people will be guided by various principles or sanctions, there will be different degrees of character. Little boots it to say that we all rationalise our actions. *It is the type of rationalisation which counts.* In our everyday life we can recognise this especially in our dealings with men (and perhaps women, too). Some excuses we accept as reasonable, others we reject as chronic alibis. The Freudian over-emphasis of rationalisation then is apt to mislead and in fact has misled many educated people. In calling attention to the tendency of the average man and, we may add, the average woman to rationalise their actions, Freud has universalised a truth which was noted in the past by acute observers in their own spheres ; but if, on that account, the barrier must be broken down between Socrates' reason for refusing the opportunity to escape an unnatural death and that of a soldier's wife attaching herself to a paramour while her husband is at war, if one reason is no more of a *libido** manifestation than the other, then it is better perhaps that the universalised truth should have remained restricted to the unscientific area of individual sages than to appear in such a distorted form.

Instead of classifying the characters according to affective or intellectual predominance or traits, such as quickness, firmness, energy, etc., we should on our scheme range them *as to kind* in accordance with what instinctive tendencies are or are not inhibited by the individual. As a rule, the *man of character in the full sense of the word exercises a distributed inhibitory power in keeping with a general principle which subsumes under its authority more specialised maxims*. But we do find irregularities manifesting a weak spot in some specific direction, as in the case of Byron, noble in many ways, but lax in sex relations, or as exemplified by Beethoven, whose character (not his temperamental make-up) seems to have been unimpeachable but for his unreliability in the matter of adhering to contracts, especially in his dealings with publishers. The epigram about the famous actress Adrienne Lecouvreur, who was regarded as Voltaire's mistress, that she " had all the virtues but virtue," strikingly illustrates the point that the contour of character may be broken at some particular spot.

There is no reason why we should not look for a general character factor and specific sub-factors, such as Spearman contends to be the case in the sphere of intelligence. Perhaps the strength of a single instinct is greater in one individual than in another, but for the most part I should ascribe the cause to the relation between the impulse in question to the guiding principle.

We all like comforts and what is vulgarly called " good times," and we all know that the acquisition of money is the only road for attaining that object; but then, if our ruling principle is not to " do" the other man, or, in the more dignified language of Kant, to treat every person as an end and not a means, we shall not indulge in telling lies, a practice which is condoned in business, or what is perhaps even worse, engage in flattery in order to gain

* Jung's term is more appropriate here than Freud's.

advantages with influential people, so as eventually to satisfy our material cravings.

It may be urged that the inhibition of one instinct is only the furtherance of another, *e.g.*, in shunning society for the sake of accomplishing a cultural piece of work, we are swayed by the will to power in downing our gregariousness. That such a reciprocal interplay between the instinctive impulses goes on is perhaps beyond question, but it hardly touches our problem. For what gives the stamp of character to an individual is not the mere fact that some instincts have been subordinated to others, but the nature of the guiding principle, whether, for instance, the man's purpose in life is to add to the sum total of knowledge, to benefit humanity in some way, or merely to increase his fame, to become, in the slang of the street, an intellectual " go-getter." The difference between a Spinoza and a Voltaire with respect to inhibiting certain social pleasures for the sake of achievement—and even the latter was obliged to repress at times his gregariousness, or else his output would not have been so vast—is an instance of like inhibitions inspired by different reasons.

Nor are we to infer that character is attached to the operation of the so-called higher, altruistic or other-regarding instincts as against the baser, egoistic or self-regarding congenital urges. Whether such a division of instincts is at all useful is unimportant here. What I should like to emphasise is that characters are evaluated *from the point of view of such principles as truth and justice rather than on the strength of altruistic tendencies.* The masses who mistake disposition, mood, or what not for character are often inclined to make false judgments in this connection, especially as their judgments are based on the attitude the person takes towards them. A " good " railroad conductor is frequently one who takes but a fraction of the fare from passengers, which he keeps for himself, thus cheating the company out of the full fare. A " good fellow " in politics is one who cherishes no principles in life and whose corruption is shielded from view because of the many individual favours he is willing to grant those who assert themselves. On the other hand, many a criminal thinks of the " hard boiled " judge who sentences him for a long jail period as a hard character.

The truth is, however, that character is not dependent on human emotions. Many persons of touching sympathy are devoid of character, and, conversely, most of the great characters known have been ruthless in dealing with evil. The man of high character (and there is just as much reason for talking about high character as about a high intelligence quotient) is exemplified by the Roman father who sentenced his fiendish son to death, thus inhibiting the paternal instinct in deference to the principle of justice. Firmness is the quality which typifies character at its best ; and firmness goes peculiarly well with inhibition, for the greater the inhibition the greater the firmness.

In this light we can readily conceive the insight contained in Goethe's famous couplet

Es bildet ein Talent sich in der Stille;
Sich ein Charakter in dem Strom der Welt.

The man who leads the life of a hermit has fewer opportunities to inhibit his instinctive urges. His inhibitions cannot compare either in scope or in number with those of the man of affairs in the bivouac of life. It is on this account that only statesmen are potentially able to realise the highest there is in character, though, unfortunately, they nearly all slip before they reach the summit. And that is what marks the greatness of Lincoln, and perhaps also of Wilson—the uncompromising political idealism in the face of a *force majeure.*

One objection to my conception of character, I fancy, would be the apparent negative definition to begin with. It may be said that the mere inhibition of an instinctive tendency does not lead to action, as is classically exemplified by Hamlet. If this should constitute a serious objection, it would of course be possible to give a positive twist to the original definition proposed here, but we must be mindful of the fact that the material to yield an estimate of character consists of both acts and restraints. Now, in many cases—for instance, in the matter of refraining from being dishonest—the inhibition is sufficient to warrant the making of a notch on behalf of the agent. But even the case where the man is called upon to act in the face of death is covered by our definition, since naturally the inhibition there centres around the instinct of self-preservation, and unless he does act in a manner to renounce his life if necessary, there is no evidence of such inhibition.

We also know that the inhibition of one tendency will lead to the expression of the opposite tendency, so that absolute inaction as a result of inhibition is restricted almost exclusively to neurotics and characters in fiction. Even the waverer *par excellence*, the much ridiculed Prince of Denmark, was throughout his inhibitive " pandering to thought " waiting for a better opportunity to undo the villain that slew his father. In justice to the scorned Hamlet, it should be mentioned, too, that he was not absolutely certain of the crime.

The Index of Character

Turning now to the application of the inhibitory view of character, we shall be able to test its validity through the instances cited. Since the character of an individual is to be *described* in terms of the instinct which offers most trouble to the inhibitory mechanism and further *evaluated* according to the ruling principles through which the inhibition of the other instincts has been effected, we have two distinct tasks before us. Below, there is the criterion of inhibition ; above, there is the analysis or interpretation of the inhibition. The one without the other is practically valueless.

Each particular inhibition of an instinct *derives its significance only from the logical motive* which governs the restraint. The highwayman, especially of the type depicted in the romantic novel, certainly inhibits his instinct of self-preservation, as does the circus dare-devil in his hazardous stunts. They are not, however, governed by a *principle* but are rather led to their eventual destruction by a *less important instinct*, whether it be acquisitiveness, display, or the will to power. Hence, though the most potent instinct has been suppressed by the bandit, the estimate of his character is on the minus side because of the violation of absolute principles. Similarly, the North American Indians, though possessing the making of character in their self-control and physical discipline, cannot, because of their deficiency in principle, be credited with character of a high type.

Again, he who inhibits the prime instinctive tendency as a result of military or social pressure must be accorded some measure of recognition, but character in the proper sense he has not necessarily on this account. Higher in the scale is the religious martyr who dies for his belief, yet expecting to reap some benefit in another world. But the only perfect evidence of character in connection with the self-preservation instinct is that to be found in the thinker who gives up his life for a principle which he would not renounce merely in order to satisfy authority.

Let us seek confirmation in another direction. The sex instinct is no doubt a powerful congenital tendency. Yet the inhibition of this instinct does not evoke so much admiration, nor does the expression of this instinct, even in illicit modes, call forth so much condemnation *per se, i.e.,* without reference to violations of absolute principles like justice and truth, as in the case of other instincts. Only a Philistine would consider Oscar Wilde, in spite of his unfortunate practices, low in character and less of a gentleman than an officially respectable grafter or fraudulent broker. The reason is not far to seek. *The sex instinct is not governed by absolute principles.* The exercise of the sex function in a legal and legitimate manner has no bearing on the estimate of character. Nor is the celibate who represses his sex life completely credited thereby with a superior character, though, of course, the capacity to subdue such a potent force, assuming that there is no psychophysical defect in that regard, is indubitably a mark of character in the rough. When, however, a Roman Catholic priest, vowed to celibacy, indulges in sex relations even with a woman whom he has secretly married, his character is rightly called into question, but not on account of his worldly indulgence, as every clear-sighted person will admit.

It is possible to carry a similar analytic course into other instinctive impulses. The inhibition of the reactions which attend the emotion of fear comes under the category of character only if effected on logical grounds. But if the tendency to flee has been thwarted by a pugnacious impulse or the self-administration of a drug, the inhibition loses its force.

Fanatics and Don Quixotes, in spite of their frequently self-denying inhibitions, lack the higher type of character because their guiding principle is often stubbornness. We shall see later that the *highest types of characters can be realised only in the highest types of intelligence,* and if, as Webb has tried to prove in his dissertation, there is a character element in intelligence—what corresponds to persistency of motives*—the converse of the proposition should not be lost sight of, *viz.,* that there is an intelligence factor in character.

The observation made by so many thinkers about the characterlessness of women also brings out this conclusion. The typical woman in some respects manifests even stronger inhibitions than the average or even superior man, but her inhibitions are imposed upon her not by the dictates of reason but by public opinion, convention, fashion, and instinctive urges.

The rating of character will always remain a pesky problem, and it is idle to deceive ourselves that any quantitative procedure

* E. Webb : Character and Intelligence, *British Journal of Psychol. Monograph Supp.,* 1915. Vol. I, part III, p. 58.

could ever be devised to approximate the method of testing intelligence. Rugg has in a series of articles* shown the magnitude of the task and the drawbacks attached to it even when carried on under conditions which the rigours of a great war have laid at the disposal of the investigators. In one place he observes, " The unordered—yes, the chaotic—character of the judgments appears, irrespective of what traits are considered or of what kinds of scales are compared."

Let us note, however, that what may be termed the " discrete " character investigations are fraught with disadvantages that do not apply in the more restricted treatment of character. The " discrete " view assembles a number of traits arbitrarily, or in accordance with practical demands, and proceeds to the rating of individuals as regards that particular trait. But these single traits are often very complex. Leadership includes so many qualities ; and besides, the concept of leadership is by no means standardised. The Y.M.C.A. notion of leadership, the revivalist's idea of a leader and the intellectual's requirements of a leader are vastly different things, so that each judge will rate this article according to his own temperamental inclinations.

The interesting scale of tests which Downey has devised for constructing a will-profile, though a valuable contribution to the subject, suffers from the further limitation that the only general criterion to serve as guide is that of motor co-ordination in the form of writing under various conditions, which can hardly cover or correspond to all the important types of situations by which a man would be judged in actual life. Of course, we may hold that as in small things, so in great things ; but we must first be certain that there is an actual correspondence and not merely work on that presupposition. If a high correlation is proved by the results, there will be the further question to settle as to whether the most important traits have been included in this profile.†

Of a less satisfactory nature is the method of self-questioning, unless checked up by others, and even then we have no reliable ways of establishing the validity of the ratings. *What we think we should do on a given occasion and what we actually do on such an*

---

* H. Rugg : Is the Rating of Human Character Practicable ? *Journal of Educ. Psychol.*, 1921 and 1922. Vols. XIII and XIV.

† Incidentally, the factor of inhibition figures considerably in her tests, and the most important traits are judged on the ability of the examinees to overcome their original impulses, as shown especially in the motor inhibition test. (J. E. Downey : *The Will-Temperament and its Testing*, pp. 132–134).

occasion often do not coincide. Light on such hypothetical situations can be had with greater reliability in dreams. In the questionnaire method there are the following obstacles to guard against : (a) the disconnection between a given question and a particular trait which the question purports to prove, (b) the personal bias, (c) the imaginative bent which is unequal in the various examinees.

By omitting the purely affective and temperamental phase of personality from our conception of character, and taking the instinctive tendencies as our field of operation, we not only are in a position to deal with something definite and traditionally continuous, but in addition can treat character as a unitary pattern, in which each of the points considered has its position, and not as a pincushion where the different traits are stuck helter-skelter.

To be sure, our scheme would not be so useful in rating the ordinary man and woman as in judging the outstanding individual who, in the first place, would possess a more typical character in our sense, and, secondly, whose actions would be better known than those of the ordinary mortal. The students of history and biography would be the gainers on such a basis rather than the executive and the administrator, but now that the admission of the limitation has been made, let us not underrate the importance of a restricted but definite guide.

In charting an individual character we might mark off our scale of motivating principles as ordinates, and the instinctive tendencies, *sufficiently differentiated as to make allowance for the objectives of the tendencies*, as *abscissæ*. The scale of guiding principles would include the well-known sanctions, such as the physical, legal, social, religious, æsthetic, ethical, logical ; and the highest type of character would be found in that individual whose inhibitions are brought about by motives of the ethico-logical class only. It is questionable whether the legal sanction is sufficient to prove character. Certainly the physical is not ; and it is herein that we discover another feature of character, and one which clearly differentiates it from a characteristic. While a characteristic is *immutable,* character suggests *variability in accordance with a rule or principle.* The wetness of the water or its tendency to run downhill will forever remain its property in consequence of natural law, but a man of character, not only is subject to a lapse, but his conduct will differ according to principle, so that, to the outsider, his behaviour may seem at times contradictory.

There is one other observation to be made in this connection. The higher the sanction which regulates the individual's conduct the more integrated, better-knit, and more pronounced is the character, though, as already stated, there is no reason why we should expect a perfectly unbroken or regular pattern, even in the highest type of life. Conflicts unfortunately cannot be avoided, and their bearing on the appraisal of character should be clear to everyone, but, unlike Holt, who thinks their very occurrence is culpable,* or what would amount to the same thing in our discourse, prejudicial in the appraisal of character, I should hold that the *mental conflict is rather indicative of character*, so long as the stronger instinctive tendency has eventually been overcome in obedience to the higher sanction or maxim of conduct.

But lest it will appear that this essay is written in the interest of ethics and is a moral exhortation in disguise, I shall take the opportunity to emphasise the fact that we are not concerned with ethical acts in the evaluation of character. The mention of ethical sanctions is no more than a reference to *logical principles in relation to behaviour*. The mother who is constantly watching over the welfare of her child will probably be regarded as an ethical being in that respect. But she will not gain an iota from such behaviour so far as her character evaluation is concerned. Similarly, the benefactor who in a burst of sympathy for a crippled beggar creates a fund for him so as to maintain the unfortunate in comfort will be hailed as a moral hero, and will by his deed call forth the approbation of at any rate by far the majority of people ; but his philanthropy has not set him one whit higher as regards his character. If anything, it has lowered him, for, instead of inhibiting a congenital impulse (though sympathy is not necessarily an instinct) he yielded to it without consulting the principle of justice or fairness, which would dictate a more equitable distribution of his beneficence. In his case, the individual whim has not been overruled by a principle which claims universality. But then, suppose he discovered a starving refugee and gave him no aid, let it not be inferred that on our view such behaviour would be indicative of character ; for the instinct of acquisitiveness is here allowed to *express* itself in the form of miserliness, and this is a more potent inborn tendency than that of sympathy. Besides, there is no logical principle citable to call forth such conduct, which is in direct contravention of the dictates of justice.

* E. B. Holt : *The Freudian Wish.*

Thought and Character

There is probably enough implied in our presentation to show that character is not so much linked up with morality as with reason or intelligence, on the one hand, and instinct on the other. Webb,* in his interesting study on the relation between intelligence and character, has come to the conclusion that there is a volitional ingredient in intelligence, what he calls an ω factor. Now, we are apt to overlook the truth of the converse proposition, *viz.*, that there is an intelligence factor in character, or, to put it more explicitly, other things being equal, *the highest type of character will be manifested only in those individuals of the highest type of intelligence, or rather intellect;* for it is doubtful whether the mental alertness conception of intelligence has anything to do with character. But it is not to be gathered that, therefore, a mighty intellect would necessarily give evidence of a high type of character, though from biographical material it would be possible to construct the view that profoundness of mind correlates highly with a well-knit character, and the psychographic results of Heymans and Wiersma tend to show that the predominance of what they call the " secondary function " (comprising such qualities as seriousness, persistence, depth, etc.) is an indication of a solid character.

The reason why character in its highest forms is to a certain extent dependent on intelligence should be almost obvious. Judgment is indispensable in the shaping of a character. The mind which conforms to the rule of the tribe, it is true, partakes of character, but in a lower degree than that mind which sees thousands of years ahead and acts in such a way as to set a guiding ideal before humanity. The prophets belong in that category, in so far as they were the apostles of truth and justice. In other respects they might have fallen short of the highest standards.

In every great system of ethics, intelligence took its place as a virtue. Socrates made knowledge the basis of all virtue. Plato recognised it as a cardinal virtue. Aristotle included judgment in his ethical system ; and if we turn to the Chinese code, we shall again meet with wisdom as a fundamental.

Nevertheless, the positive relationship between character and intellect is by no means to be taken for granted, and it would be a serious omission to ignore the position of Schopenhauer on the

* Cited earlier.

subject, who at times is inclined to agree with Goethe's stricture,

Er nennt's Vernunft, und braucht's allein,
Nur tierischer als jedes Tier zu sein.

Schopenhauer's various discussions of the affinity of intellect and character, though teeming with pregnant remarks, are not untainted by his dominant desire to prove the primacy of the will over the intellect. The passages which are to be cited will presumably reveal at least the somewhat wavering attitude in this respect of the otherwise pertinacious philosopher.

In his essay *On Human Nature* the great pessimist writes : "No one can live among men without feeling drawn again and again to the tempting supposition that moral baseness and intellectual incapacity are closely connected as though they both sprang from one source. . . That it seems to be so is merely due to the fact that both are so often found together and the circumstance is to be explained by the very frequent occurrence of each of them, so that it may easily happen for both to be compelled to live under one roof. At the same time it is not to be denied that they play into each other's hands to their mutual benefit ; and it is this that produces the very unedifying spectacle which only too many men exhibit, and that makes the world to go as it goes. A man who is unintelligent is very likely to show his perfidy, villainy and malice; whereas a clever man understands better how to conceal these qualities."

Yet in his *Ethical Reflections* the same sage allows himself almost to contradict the above by claiming that " genius and sanctity are akin." " However simple-minded," we read, " a saint may be, he will nevertheless have a dash of genius in him ; and however many errors of temperament, or of actual character, a genius may possess, he will still exhibit a certain nobility of disposition by which he shows his kinship with the saint."

The most explicit statement on the connection between the two chief personality factors is contained in the essay entitled *Character*, wherein Schopenhauer furnishes us the key to the situation and in reality cedes his point, when he discriminates between " two kinds of intellect: between understanding as the apprehension of relation in accordance with the Principle of Sufficient Reason, and cognition, a faculty akin to genius, which acts more directly, is independent of this law, and passes beyond the Principle of Individuation. The latter is the faculty which apprehends Ideas, and it is the faculty which has to do with morality." The next moment his oscillation again becomes apparent, for he fears that " even this explanation leaves much to be desired. *Fine minds are seldom fine souls* was the correct observation of Jean Paul, although they are never contrary."

What can account for Schopenhauer's indecision in the matter ? To my mind it is the conflict between his insight and his metaphysical dogma of the omnipotence of the will. It is Schopenhauer, the subtle metaphysician, combating Schopenhauer, the keen psychologist. The two kinds of intelligence mentioned at the beginning of this section tell the whole story, and, recalling what has been said there, we are in a position to secure confirmation of Schopenhauer's point of view as expressed in his essay on character.

The implication is that, while intelligence and character show no correlation, intellect and character are far more closely connected in that the higher types of intellect involve a character factor and *vice versa.*

The attempted sharp dichotomy between the will and the intellect in Schopenhauer's earlier and crowning work need not detain us, except for the quotation of one passage, where the author points out that " it is not the really great minds that make historical characters, because they are [not ?] capable of bridling and ruling the mass of men and carrying out the affairs of the world ; but for this persons of much less capacity of mind are qualified when they have great firmness, decision, and persistence of will, such as is quite inconsistent with very high intelligence. Accordingly, where this very high intelligence exists, we actually have a case in which the intellect directly restricts the will."*

The issue which Schopenhauer has raised here is too ponderous for examination at present. But it is needful to guard against the insidious identification of certain concepts, like character and will ; and it is in illustration of such possible confusion that the argument used by Schopenhauer has been adduced. In reply to Schopenhauer's observation it must be urged that the man of will-power and energy is not necessarily the man of character in the sense described in the present treatment, and, furthermore, it is just because *the man of affairs possesses more will than character that he can get into the position of ruling the masses ;* and, *conversely, it is for the reason that the man of character who may at the same time be*

---

* A. Schopenhauer : *The World as Will and Idea,* Second Book, Chapter XIX, Sect. 5.

an intellectual giant is not prone to waste his time and lower his principles on the follies and vices of man that he chooses not to rule the destiny of the masses directly, but indirectly, yet with greater permanence. Let us not be misled by the notion that the ability to forge ahead or, as Münsterberg put it, that the power to keep the selected motive dominant is the essence of character.

Psychological Source of the Regulative Principles

I am aware, of course, that the problem of character is not pre-empted by making it hinge on the instincts on the one hand and rational principles on the other. One might ask whether the possibility of a certain instinct being much stronger in one person than in another might not call for a greater amount of inhibition and, therefore, warrant a higher rating, if such an instinct has been successfully modified.

Another question bears on the genesis of the inhibitory force. What explains the different capacities to inhibit instinctive tendencies in different individuals? If a congenital affair, then are we not claiming *ex hypothesi* that character is an instinctive tendency dominating other instinctive tendencies? And if, again, we are born with this disposition, then is not Schopenhauer justified in denying the possibility of modification in a person's character, contending, as he does, that we are but the tools of Fate? And if such is the case, are we not bound to reduce the proportions of the dignity and greatness attached to character?

It would take us too far afield for our present purpose to examine each of these questions at length. Yet a word is necessary to show the psychological origins of character, and particularly that element of it which has been referred to as regulative principles.

In the first place, as regards the varying strength of the instincts in different individuals, there is reason to believe that even the miser can under certain conditions curb his stinginess. Most prisoners, no matter how refractory and intractable they are in ordinary life, are, as is known, held in check by the jail wardens. We have also the testimony of some of the noblest characters in history, such as Moses Mendelssohn, to the strength of their passions, which, however, they were able to rule with perfect ease. Furthermore, the biographies of great men have in a number of cases revealed the subjects to have been given to profligacy in youth, though in later life devoting themselves to the loftiest purposes. (St. Augustine, Tolstoi).*

Any instinct, then, no matter how intense, *can* be overcome ; and it is in this regard that character is so disparate from intelligence, for no amount of effort would turn a moron into a superior intelligence, but the most defective character can be changed at least for a short time, provided its possessor makes up his mind to take a firm stand, that is to say, provided sufficient inhibitory force is exerted. But then, what about those whose inhibitions are feeble compared with those of others ?

That some persons are capable of controlling themselves better than others goes without saying, but it is not so generally known that even children at a tender age may be differentiated according to the seriousness with which they take instructions. The influence of the environment, tradition and customs cannot be invoked to account for the perceptible germs of character displayed by three-year-old children. *We may reasonably assume that some persons are born with greater nervous plasticity than others, and plasticity in this sense does not mean merely resiliency of the tissues or elasticity, but organisation in such a way as to allow the nerve currents to take different paths without serious disturbance.* Naturally the psycho-analytic schools would eagerly point to the many neuroses and psychoses as evidence of the impossibility of such an organisation ; and I do not feel it incumbent to dispute their doctrines. All that is set forth in this connection is the fact that with our apparently fixed instinctive mechanisms,† we inherit also an element of modifiability, not in the form of a lever or a muscle, like, say, the tensor tympani on the tympanic membrane, but in the actual concatenation of the instinctive steps. Mechanically, the greater inhibitability would call for greater slowness in the instinct to run its course.‡ *Brakes and gears could be put on at more points and with greater effectiveness in the more inhibitive individual than in the less inhibitive.*

So far, then, we have seen there is no necessity to posit an inhibi-

---

* *Cf.* also H. Begbie's *Twice-Born Men.*

† The word " mechanism," as employed here, merely represents the physical basis of the disposition and is not meant to indicate that instincts are merely mechanical forces devoid of purposiveness and adaptability. A mechanism is the enduring arrangement which engenders a particular disposition and is invested with the potentiality of modifying the given disposition in accordance with various circumstances. It is clearly not a machine.

‡ The " all-or-none " principle which Rivers has taken over from physiology (Symposium on " Instinct and the Unconscious," *British Journal of Psychology*, 1919, Vol. X), applying it to the course of an instinct, is of little service even if it were proven to hold true of instincts in general.

K

tory mechanism as such. The variability of the instinct is to be looked for in the instinct itself. But, besides the facility of inhibition, there must be a something to bring about the inhibition. Now, this agency may be another instinctive urge operating in an opposite direction. Anger may be turned aside through fear. The threatening finger of the law is sufficient to inhibit the acquisitive impulses of many people within certain limits. Such inhibitions, arising out of purely instinctive sources, cannot be considered as revealing the earmarks of character. It is doubtful whether even the social inhibitions can be claimed as a criterion, but since in most cases it is scarcely possible to discover the real motives of conduct, we can afford to be charitable and give the benefit of the doubt to all whose actions do not betray evidence of merely seeking social approbation. Similarly, the religious and æsthetic sentiments exercise their inhibitory power over the primitive instincts, but it is only the ethico-logical principles which count in full measure toward according to character its proper value.

Certainly these principles are not implanted upon us by some mysterious force. They may be regarded as sentiments, that is to say, affective complexes, deriving their nourishment out of the individual's social milieu, but I think it is worth while emphasising the universality and absoluteness of these principles, which are more logical than psychological, inasmuch as they attach to cognition rather than to affection or instinct.

Lest, however, the impression be gained that these principles represent a sort of *deus ex machina* device which has no psychological basis, I should remind the reader that even striving in the cause of truth and the religious exercise of justice are not beyond the possibility of inheritance. But, as McDougall has observed, " The innate structure of the human mind comprises much more than the instincts alone . . . There are many facts which compel us to go further in the recognition of innate mental structure, such facts as the special facilities shown by individuals in music, in mathematics, in language and other æsthetic, moral and intellectual endowments."* These principles differ from instinctive drives particularly in this respect, that, while an instinctive expression is no more than a *particularisation* of an act involving one's own self, the guiding principles which are under discussion represent *universalisations*, involving naturally also the individual who is acting, but directed toward humanity in general, of which this or that

* Wm. McDougall : " Instinct and the Unconscious," *British Journal of Psychology*, 1919. Vol. X, p. 37.

person appears as a case. Anger, too, is directed against somebody else, but no universalisation takes place in expressing this emotion. It must be remembered that justice has been distinguished from sympathy in another section, and the difference holds here, too, and consists in the fact that *sympathy, though, as Adam Smith taught, it may be the root of all our moral sentiments, is primarily a particularised act, immediately generated by an impulse suffused with feeling, while a just act is more impersonal, less immediately generated and mediated through reflection, momentary as it may be.*

It will have been noticed by this time that the use of the words " principles " and " sanctions " is not clearly demarcated, the former being employed sometimes to cover only the purely ethical determinants, such as truth and justice, and at other times with reference to the standards of action. The reason for this apparent looseness in language is that all recognised standards of action are merely popularised versions of the ethical standards diluted with the appeal to fear and the incentive of reward so as to gain a hold on the average man and woman. Even though the social sanction often encourages flattery and hypocrisy, it without question originally took rise in the community desire to safeguard the interests of its members, which could not be realised without invoking the primary ethical principles as a *sine qua non*. In spirit, then, all approved standards of action are the same, though they sadly differ in application. The purely ethical appeal may, therefore, be looked upon as containing the various other sanctions in their ideal form, while these other standards may be considered as a graded stratification of the ethical principles governing action.

But even these ethical principles have two sides to them. It is one thing to recognise that fairness should be the mark of all dealings, but quite another to observe this rule in practice ; and character value depends on the observance, not the mere observation of the maxim, because it is in the practice that the crucial test lies. That all normal people, that is to say, *all*, excluding the aments and the demented, possess a sense of justice, can be readily seen from the fact that they seize on every opportunity to set forth their claims when they believe themselves to have been unfairly dealt with. The next to receive such consideration is their kin, then their affiliated groups, etc., but what must appear so puzzling to a logical mind is the disinclination of the vast majority of human beings to apply the same measures to themselves and to others.

Now there are two paths open to us in explanation of the two divergent approaches. One alternative is to assume that the recognition of right and wrong is not sufficiently potent to actuate most people in the cause of others. But then, if the notion is dynamic in one's self-interest, something else must be sought to account for its inertia, otherwise. It is within reason, I think, as our other alternative, to postulate a *consistency* urge as the basis of all conduct typifying the person of character. Like other connate tendencies, this urge requires sufficient time for maturation. Young children seldom give indications of this tendency, yet it is possible to detect significant differences in reactions to others on the part of even five-year-old youngsters, and that in spite of their being brought up in the same environment.

To attribute the differences to education is to put the cart before the horse ; for the fact that some children will benefit by the strict injunctions and others will not ought to convince us that there is something in the child which accepts the consequences, rather than that it is the nature of the injunctions, which brings results. In some, the argument : How would you like me to take that toy away from you, as you did from that little boy ? produces a ready and desirable response, while others, though they seem to understand the injustice of their act, make no effort to mend their conduct, and still others find some either wholly fictitious or else totally irrelevant excuse to justify their budding rapacity. Women too, are, as many great novelists and essayists have remarked, incapable of acting with consistency, and, unless moved by pity, are prone to commit many unfair acts on various pretexts, chief among which is that, being the weaker sex, or the weaker of two of their own sex, or having " gone through " more than their rival or expecting to enjoy life less than someone else, they ought not to lose at least this opportunity of making up for the hardship either already endured or in store for them.

We hear it said and repeated almost *ad nauseam* that women are prompted by their feelings rather than by their reason. But such a hollow statement possesses no scientific value. Many women reason well enough at the very time they are supposed to be guided by their feelings. Their reasoning, however, lacks consideration for others. It is the element of consistency alone which is lacking —a gap which is sometimes filled by the substitute of pity. If the above time-honoured and apparently universal belief about the mainsprings of women's conduct is to be invested with any psychological meaning, we should necessarily hold to one or the other of these alternatives ; either that women, on the whole, are born with stronger instinctive tendencies, or else the consistency urge is weaker in them than in man. The former alternative does not seem plausible, more especially as the maxim of parsimony would lead us to explain the phenomenon through some weakness in the one factor rather than in the many. It is, therefore, not in the relative strength of the instinct that we shall find the reason for the lack of objectivity in female conduct, but in the relative weakness of the fundamental principle of conduct which has its root psychologically in some mechanism making for consistency. In fine, then, consistency in action, which is one of the chief determinants of character, can be traced to original connate tendencies; and if this smacks too much of Descartes' innate ideas doctrine, I might point out that there are vast differences between the two classes of concepts. Men differ as to the relative strength of instinctive tendencies—granted; but they also differ as to their nervous constitution in respect of inhibitability, application to others of what they consider to be fair for themselves, and above all in the strict adherence to an abstract principle, like liberty, for instance, in the face of great danger to the acting individual. It is in connection with the recognition of the issues to be championed that intellect is of service, so that it becomes indispensable in the make-up of the most typical specimens of character.

Conclusion

Although this paper has grown far lengthier than originally intended, I cannot represent it as anything but an attempt to indicate the direction in which the study of character is to be undertaken if we wish to retain its original core and at the same time set it down on the solid ground of psychology. It is easy to dispose of character entirely, as the behaviourists are inclined to do, and it is almost as easy to treat it from an exhortative point of view, as religious teachers and moralists are wont to do. But, in making character the function of (a) instinctive tendencies, (b) certain properties of the nervous organisation which facilitate inhibition, and (c) principles which claim as their psychological basis a mechanism yet to be investigated, I realise that there will be no end of protests on the ground that antiquated doctrines are being appealed to.

I am aware, too, that the description of the rating method on the scheme here outlined has been left in its initial stages. It is to be hoped that someone, with a leaning toward quantitative treatment and a knack for the manipulation of charts, will work out on a far more elaborate scale the evaluation of some well-known historical characters in accordance with the definition of character as the psychophysical disposition to inhibit instinctive tendencies in keeping with fundamental principles of action. The stratification of the various characters in an hierarchical system, so as to make allowance for the different levels of principles (legal, social, religious, æsthetic, ethico-logical) would further have to be undertaken at the behest of the conservative critic. Once, however, the method is clear, we should find little difficulty in removing obstacles.

Lest some readers still misunderstand my position in the belief that I regard instincts as something to be repressed, as containing the germ of sin and wickedness, I must remind them of what has already been stated before, namely, that we have nothing to do with the ascetic doctrine. The machinery of character involves the inhibition of original or inborn tendencies, just as musical composition necessitates the mastery of a certain technique ; but the inhibition in itself, just as the technique as such, possesses very little value. It is the direction which the inhibition or the technique takes that is all important. Both man and beast work along the lines of least resistance,* but it is for *man to change high resistance into low resistance* by adhering to a rational guiding principle —a purpose. The courageous man's very difficult course is to him a course of least resistance, once he has firmly espoused his cause. If time-binding may be considered, according to Korzybski, the chief characteristic of man, we must not neglect the characteristic of resistance-reducing. In fact, it might be claimed that man is a time-binder only by virtue of his capacity to reduce resistance. Consider how much inhibition was necessary in order to assume permanently an erect posture on the part of our primitive ancestors. Now, the original tendency to walk on all fours is neither base nor immoral, but the subsequent change through a process of inhibition, until the new habit became fixed, may well be considered a mark of character.

As for the rest, the position taken in this paper is based on a view of instincts like the one described by McDougall, but calling for a more detailed differentiation and specification in relation to the stimuli evoking them. The perceptual determination of the instinct I should emphasise even to a greater extent than does McDougall.

---

* *Cf.* A. A. Roback : Interference of Will Impulses (*Psycholog. Review Monograph Supplements*, Vol. XXV).

And if the numerous " anti-instinctivists " in the United States were to direct their energies toward the goal of discovering what tendencies develop in early childhood, without the aid of education, instead of spending all their efforts in explaining away theoretically and by means of *non sequitur* arguments manifestly instinctive behaviour, we should now be in a more enlightened state regarding one of the most important subjects in a whole group of sciences.

Ordinarily we do not credit young children with the slightest germs of character, but no one who has watched them at play can deny that they exhibit signs not only of the knowledge of right and wrong, but even of the observance of certain rules. The prophets of Israel, and probably those to whom they preached, seem to have evinced a greater interest in that subject than we in the twentieth century, for many are the passages in which an event is prophesied to take place before a symbolic child grows up to know the difference between right and wrong.

Character and behaviour pertaining to the moral sphere can and should be studied genetically and comparatively as in the case of other capacities and behaviour. The sociological researches of men like Westermarck, Lévy-Bruhl, Boas, McDougall and Hose in this regard are valuable indeed, but they cannot take the place of ontogenetic investigations, for the chief reason perhaps that the primitive impulses of the savage tribes are coloured by tradition and custom.

It is only by pursuing an analytic method that we can avoid the nihilistic tendency so current to-day and drawing illegitimate support from modern logistic development—of employing a term in a sense for which it was never intended, and thereby breaking entirely away from the past. The most clear-headed thinker of antiquity, if not of all times, admonishes us in his *Nicomachean Ethics* to consider first the popular notion of a concept before we attempt to define it; and his suggestion should serve as a methodological beacon-light for all times.

By preserving the unitary and essentially unique mark of character instead of breaking it up into a number of unrelated qualities we enjoy the advantage of attaching it to some body of scientific facts and subsuming it under rules and principles, without which even the technical arts are under a serious handicap. The unitary basis of our conception does not prevent us from seeking after elements, factors and determinants, but saves us rather from the fruitless effort of beginning our search blindly or, as in the exuberant mood of some psychologists, contenting ourselves with the feeling that we are looking for what we are looking for—an attitude which may be recommended only for Alice in Wonderland.

There is probably not a single one of the various approaches to the study of character which is without at least a grain of value for the clarification of so complex a subject. The recent experimental methods are particularly hopeful signs. Each point of view may be regarded not only as a contribution *per se*, but should serve as a touchstone for the others. In this way the particles of gold in each finding may be sifted out, but it is necessary to be provided with a field of operation in the form of a general method before the particles can be assembled and properly arranged so as to cohere into a tangible substance.

ON MEMORIES WHICH ARE TOO REAL

BY

PIERRE JANET, M.D., Litt.D.

*Member of the French Institute ; Professor of Psychology
at the Collége de France*

MEMORIES WHICH ARE TOO REAL

BY

PIERRE JANET

THE feelings of reality and unreality which often attach to certain psychological phenomena are of great importance ; for they indicate the more or less considerable degree of activity which accompanies these phenomena. A feeling of unreality is often observed in connection with the perception of objects among patients who might be called psychasthenic doubters. In several places I have had occasion to point out that this feeling does not depend on a disorder in sensation but on the waning of the tendency to act in response to these perceptions. The same evidence has occurred to me in even a simpler form while studying the unreal memories of these very patients at the J. J. Rousseau Institute at Geneva,* and the same problem might be examined in a somewhat inverse manner in trying to understand the exaggerations of the feeling of reality which in every case accompanies the memories. A rather striking observation suggests to us these reflections on the degree of reality which we attribute more or less correctly to our representations.

I

A young man, thirty years old, Léon, whose parents were very psychoneurotic, and who (himself a twin) had been subject since his twenty-second year to fits of depression, preceded by a more or less lengthy period of excitement and euphoria, which seemed to be better designated by the English word *elation* than by the French word *excitation*. These spells appeared wholly in connection with exhaustions caused by excesses in work or emotion. The patient had already had a very serious and interesting crisis of this type at the age of twenty-two ; but we shall study here only the last spell, which began at the age of thirty-five.

During the war Léon had been entrusted with a commission in a foreign country ; although he had already been worn out by a

* " Les souvenirs irréels," *Archives de Psychologie*, 1924, Vol. xix.

serious attack of the grip and overcome by the death of his brother, he had given himself up to his work with incredible zeal. His health had been excellent, and he felt full of energy, courage, and self-confidence ; and in his patriotic ardour he thought " that he could never work hard enough for his country " ; but at the same time he was taking an interest in everything—walked in the country, frequented museums, admired landscapes and works of art, was studying foreign literature as well as historical and political questions, etc. At the same time he took for a mistress a woman " whose beauty had produced on him a tremendous effect," and his love for his mistress was just as much exaggerated as his passion for work ; although he vaguely felt that all this was excessive and abnormal, " he was enjoying to the full this superhuman life," and he was in a state of continual joy.

After six months he was beginning to feel as if he were giving way, and he realised that for a number of reasons it would be wise to part with this woman. As he was recalled to France, " he had the courage to break away, or rather to flee," but " this last effort shattered him " and he rapidly fell into a state of depression very different from his previous elation. If I am not mistaken, this breaking away and departure would not be considered as a " huge effort on the part of his moral will," but as the first effect of the growing depression which had already inspired him with feelings of dread of action.

In this new state his health and appearance become transformed, and there appear such things as lack of desire (*inappétence*), digestive and circulatory disorders, insomnia, buzzing in the ear, etc. Let us only recall this rigidity of the face, this fixed countenance so frequently seen in depression, which suggests some interesting correspondences with diseases determined by lesion in the corpus striatum. Our patient begins to feel his face annoyed by continual irritations, and this annoyance impels him continually to look into the mirror. He also feels a stiffness in all his movements.

The feelings are entirely transformed : Léon takes no pleasure in anything, joy is no longer his ; he has no artistic enjoyment ; " nothing is good or pleasant, and he never feels at ease " ; he no longer has any interest : " I could not listen to a play at the theatre or look at a flower ; the one interests me no more than the other. I desire nothing ; I need nothing." Previous to that, he had a keen desire to see his mother again ; he found her without feeling anything, and could not enjoy her company. In spite of his efforts, he did not succeed in becoming interested in a young girl who had been his fiancée.   He was otherwise indifferent to all women—which surprised him : " I who had been so curious about things and people."   Persons and objects had not become so unreal as we have seen in the case of other observations of the same kind ; but they had lost all charm and all interest.

The feelings which persist belong to a category of feelings of fear of action which I discussed at the Congress of Psychiatry in Atlantic City.*   He shows fear and disgust in regard to every action, which gives rise to fear of the future and distressing thoughts : " Ah !   If I could only regard the future calmly, but the life before me frightens me."   He explains this feeling by saying that he no longer feels good for anything, that he is no longer capable of doing simple addition, that he is bewildered by the fear of errors, that he is clumsy and ridiculous even in saying " How do you do ? " to anyone, " he is only afraid of making blunders, or paying out too much money, or losing his umbrella."   It is this collection of sentiments, constituted by secondary actions, flight of action, inhibition of action and economy of action, which forms essentially the state of grief into which he is constantly plunged.

These feelings, although exaggerated, are accurate enough : his activity is really very much reduced ;   Léon is evidently incapable of continuing his ordinary work ;   he no longer has any system or initiative ;   he remains undecided in regard to the most trivial question ;   and he experiences a constant need of assistance from others ;   " I no longer have any method," he repeats with a groan, " I can't tell the place of things, I no longer have any real life ;   I should like to remain with you all the time.   I am bullied for everything, and I can no longer do anything about it.   The slightest bit of a letter to write is too much for me and I used to be very keen about it at one time."   Let us note further, that he can hardly retain in his mind events of the present.   He does not recall anything that is of consequence ;   and above all, he no longer has any visual representation of objects which he has just seen.

Parallel with these same negative characteristics there are also some features which consist in superadded behaviour.   He has numerous tics, a mania for tearing the skin of his fingers or brushing his clothes.   He repeats *sotto voce* some verses.   He relates incessantly some memories of his childhood or youth, and he cannot get rid of them.   But above all, he presents a remarkable symptom which lends a special characteristic to this fit of depression.   He is

* " The Fear of Action," *Journal of Abnormal Psychology*, June–September, 1921, Vol. XVI, p. 190.

continually tormented by an obsession which presents itself in the form of a visual image with an almost hallucinatory intensity.

At every instant he stops absorbed by an obsessive contemplation. He sees rising before him the apartment in which he had been living during his stay abroad—the apartment where he had been so active and so happy with his beautiful woman : " Ah ! This sacred apartment . . . I am in the hall. I see an open door, and through there the main room where I would keep myself —I feel that the woman is there. I could tell where she is to be found . . ." Sometimes he would see one room, at other times another ; sometimes from one point of view, at other times from another. The woman would appear variously dressed, or in various positions or hidden in the bed . . . the images change without being extremely varied. They always represent the principal aspects of the apartment, and the woman in various attitudes ; and the scenes which keep coming up always centre about the previous happy period.

The memories to which these images are attached are not forgotten memories which reappear. He can call them forth perfectly at will, but he never does so unless I ask him ; for spontaneously he would not do so. The reappearance of these memories is painful: "That is a happy period and I can only experience suffering while thinking of it." When the image is called forth voluntarily in this manner, it has some special characteristics to which I shall return ; but more often the image appears without his having searched for it, suddenly, for no reason, just like a picture which you find is before you and which you must endure. The memories then are all of an extraordinary and ridiculous precision : " I see myself again in this room, and such persons and all the details of the evening pass before my eyes again." These images are always excessively impressionistic. From the very moment that they begin to appear they are accompanied by a sort of surge and temptation : he desires to enter the apartment, to see the woman, to speak to her. He feels his mouth muttering some phrases he used to say formerly on entering the hall: " I am going to fix up my things in the wardrobe, to put my coat here . . . ." But these initial acts would stop immediately as soon as he would give himself up to these memories of the past, just as he would apply to these memories of the past his present fear of action. He never continues the scene ; he doesn't hear the woman speak to him ; he doesn't hear the sequel of the interview ; by an effort he turns back ; " again this good woman who has come back ! " and he tries to think of something else ; but several moments afterwards the spectacle reappears under another aspect.

This inhibition of action probably prevents the vision from becoming altogether hallucinatory.   Never do these images mix with the actual perceptions ;   they confine themselves to momentarily obliterating them.   These images are never taken completely for present realities.   The patient feels that he is no longer capable of resuming this life, that he no longer has the strength for it, nor has he the power to repulse it.   He could not begin it over again, even if he wished to accept it.   The image also is always recognised as a memory.   But it is a very special memory which, though a memory of the past, has attached to it a peculiar mark of the present. " To be sure I almost always know that it is only a memory of the past, but it is a past which is so close to me   .   .   .   Of course, I know that these things have taken place more than a year ago, but when the image appears, it seems to me that it was yesterday, that only a month before I have been in this apartment, and that I spoke to the woman."   In a word, these memories are extremely rich.

II

These too real memories contrast in a curious manner with the unreal memories which I have described as occurring among many other patients.   In the minds of the latter there are only empty reports, with no imagery or attitudes surrounding them, calling forth no feeling of joy or of sadness ; and arousing no interest or desire for action, in the way of either drawing them out or cutting them short.   Sometimes these unreal reports are not even accompanied by belief, and the patient cannot affirm that these visions have had a real existence in the past.

An important feature of these unreal memories is the fact that they always refer back to a very distant past.   A patient, who had come out of a sanatorium only a week before, said that he had come out of it 25 years ago, and similarly referred the birth of his last child, two months old, back to 25 years ago.   In my opinion, the unreal character of these memories depends precisely on this absence of reverberation or echo ; on the suppression of all the processes which ordinarily surround and complete our perceptions and reports.   In all our behaviour there is a primary act which is the reaction to external stimulation.   To these exteroceptive reflexes, as M. Sherrington would say, there are attached some interoceptive reactions determined by the primary act itself. Reactions which prolong the act reinforce it, establish it and transform it into belief or else inhibit it, avoid it or transform it into its opposite, etc. These are the secondary acts which give to the report its particular flavour, and its degree of reality. The largest portion of these secondary acts disappears with exhausted and asthenic patients through a sort of shrinking of the report which reduces it to its core.

If that is the case, we ought to allow for the too real memories an explanation which is the converse of the previous one. These memories are accompanied by many affirmations, many images, and very powerful feelings. That is just what we have seen in the observation of Léon, who is certain to the most minute exactitude of his obsessive memories, who images them vividly and experiences in connection with them very keen interests and sentiments. These memories then should represent a great psychological force capable of surrounding them with a very large number of these secondary acts. But right here arises a difficulty which puzzles us: Léon presents these memories during a period of great asthenic depression. His whole present behaviour, as we have seen, is enormously reduced. How then could the memories alone preserve such a force amidst the exhaustion of all the other functions?

Let us note in the first place that the wealth and power of these memories are very relative, in reality. Léon has never gone far enough with the acts called forth by these memories. He has only taken very few steps in regard to them, confining himself to some gestures of protestation. If this memory appeared so rich, it is apparently as a result of the comparison with the poverty-stricken acts of his present life. It is, moreover, on account of this poverty of his present behaviour that these visions did not develop into hallucinations and delirium.

Notwithstanding, i.e. in spite of this observation, the strength of his visions is much greater than that of the other memories, and we should be astonished at this disproportion. The solution ought probably to be drawn from the strength of the state during which these memories have been organised. All these obsessive memories have been registered during a period which was not normal, nor was it a period of depression, but rather one of elation. It is probable that there had been at this stage a state of hypersthenia in contrast with a state of asthenia of the depressive period, and that a great quantity of force had been employed in all these actions. The formation of a memory is analogous to the formation of a tendency, although we are dealing with an altogether special tendency. This form of tendency does not only consist in organising series of movements in response to a certain stimulation, but its function is also to invest this tendency with a certain quantity of reserve force which will permit it to become activated later on when the occasion should arise. This hypothesis of force deposited in the tendencies at the time of their formation allows for an explanation of the reservation of force and the recourse to the reserves, which play such a large part in the excitations, as William James has so well presented it in his little book *Energies of Men.** Our observation confirms this hypothesis, and shows us that the memory tendencies organised during the period of hypersthenia are powerfully endowed with reserve energy. It is on account of this original force that they form a contrast with the acts organised in the present period of asthenia. It is probable that facts of the same sort might be observed in connection with all the memories and tendencies organised during life epochs when the psychological force is superabundant. The habits acquired in infancy when the force is great are preserved and often survive almost alone in periods of depression. Léon himself remarks that his obsessive memories could sometimes reproduce episodes of his infancy and youth. This force of memories acquired during hypersthenia might be considered as a counterpart of the curious phenomenon which I have described elsewhere under the name of psychological scars,† where we see tendencies formed during psychological illness or depression preserving a certain weakness throughout life.

Finally, as a concluding reflection, this force of the tendencies acquired during the periods of hypersthenia does not manifest itself in the asthenic period and does not show any contrast to the other tendencies except in one respect, viz., that these strong tendencies function alone without their becoming related to or combined with the other tendencies in the behaviour adapted to the present moment. I have noted toward the beginning of the paper that one might ask Léon to call forth of his own accord the memories of the woman in answer to our questions by adapting these memories to the present moment. He could do so, although it would be disagreeable to him, but it is curious to note that under these conditions the memories have lost their peculiar character. They are reduced, faded, and the subject readily refers them to the

* *Cf. Les médications psychologiques*, 1920, III, pp. 219, 220.
† *Cf. loc. cit.*, Vol. 2, p. 289.

past. He finds himself then in the same state as our other asthenic patients who have weak recollections because they call them forth voluntarily. The memories of the woman only assume their abnormal strength with Léon when they appear beyond the actual volition of the patient, without any connection with the present, that is to say, when they function in a dissociated manner.

Many conditions then are necessary for the realisation of this curious syndrome of super-real memories : (1) it is necessary that they should be acquired in a state of psychological hypersthenia. (2) that they should be called forth in a period of asthenia. (3) that this evocation should be automatic, dissociated from the general activity of the personality at the time.

III

In my lectures on the feeling of reality, I have tried to set up a general scheme in which might be arranged the various aspects assumed by the psychological phenomena and in particular the verbal forms, the reports according to which the feeling of reality, and in consequence the wealth of secondary phenomena, are more or less accentuated in them. At the beginning I should place the psychological phenomena which present in the very highest degree the character of reality ; below these come the phenomena which present it in a less degree. Descending the scale, I should arrive at the phenomena which no longer contain the affirmation of reality, which, in other words, begin to seem unreal to us, and from there take gradual steps downward until the vague and fleeting thought without any reality is reached. This, in brief, is the scheme at which we should arrive :—

1. *The present reality* which applies to material as well as to mental entities and events.
2. *The immediate future* which interests us almost as much as the present, though with somewhat less vividness.
3. *The recent past*, to which is attached the affective memory with the happy and unhappy recollections, illusions (*deceptions*) and regrets.
4. *The ideal* which we do not recognise as real, but which we wish to see realised.
5. *The distant future* which we hope to see realised, but which is too remote to greatly interest us.
6. *The dead or distant past* which is lost in affective character, but whose reality we still maintain as having occurred in time.

7. *The imaginary unreality* in regard to which we take the pre-
caution of denying its reality. The dream, when it is
recognised as such, is one variety of that type.

8. *The idea*, a verbal form whose reality we neither affirm nor
deny.

9. *The thought*, a verbal form in regard to which we do not even
ask the question of reality or unreality.

The reports are associated with one or the other of these groups
in accordance with the strength of the feeling of reality which
accompanies them, that is to say, in the last analysis, in accordance
with the potency and wealth of the secondary acts which surround
them. A report sounds correct to us when it is placed by the
narrator in the proper place, that is to say, where the majority of
men would ordinarily be disposed to place it. On the other hand,
a report sounds incorrect when it is placed by the narrator at an
unusual place, thus causing surprise. A very large number of
mental troubles are nothing but a poor localisation of events
within the compass of this schema. A certain number of patients
are characterised by a peculiar tendency to drop their accounts,
to place them lower than we should have done ourselves under
the same circumstances. Some asthenics doubtless regard certain
events which we should connect with the recent past as having
their place in the distant past, or as imaginary. They present
unreal memories. Some go even farther and transform the
present into a dream or a fancy. Others again resemble the
patient Léon whom we have just discussed and raise their
accounts on the schema : they make out of the bygone past
a recent past, an immediate future or even a present. The
study of these patients is helpful in understanding delirium
and hallucination. It is important to take account of the fact
that these errors in the evaluation of ourselves depend on
complex conditions, the chief feature of which we have tried to
isolate.

These different evaluations of events altogether transform the
conduct of individuals and give birth to different forms and phases
of personality. An individual at a period when he raises his
accounts will be altogether different from what he was during
the period when he would lower them ; and I have seen
patients who in this regard would establish a veritable split of
personality. The subconscious, certain varieties of amnesia,
multiple personality, are often only the results of these modifications.

Dr Morton Prince, who has made some excellent contributions to the study of these variations of personality, will, I hope, be somewhat interested in this short report which it gives me pleasure to add to the more important studies assembled in this volume for the purpose of celebrating his jubilee.

(*Translated by* A.A.R.).

SOME MEDICO-LEGAL EXPERIENCES, WITH COMMENTS AND REFLECTIONS

BY

CHARLES K. MILLS, M.D., Ph.D., Ll.D.

Professor Emeritus of Neurology, University of Pennsylvania

SOME MEDICO-LEGAL EXPERIENCES, WITH COMMENTS AND REFLECTIONS*

BY

CHARLES K. MILLS

How Verdicts are Obtained in Insanity Cases

MANY years ago I was a medical witness in a trial in which the question of insanity was the main issue. A man, the scion of a distinguished family, after certification, had also been found to be insane by an inquisition in lunacy. After consultations with his attorneys, he had decided to traverse this inquisition. *Traverse* is a legal procedure by which the findings of an inquisition can be tried again in a probate or other court before a jury of twelve. The possibility of resorting to a traverse in such cases is one of the evidences of the jealous care with which the rights of the insane are guarded under our Anglo-Saxon system of jurisprudence.

The appellant or traverser had engaged, as his counsels, two of the most eminent attorneys of Philadelphia, one of whom at that time was reputed to be the most eloquent advocate at the Philadelphia bar, and the other was unequalled in his power of making " jury points." The side opposing the traverser had also retained two eminent attorneys.

In addition to lay testimony, five or six well-known physicians testified that the appellant was insane ; that he was the victim of hallucinations of hearing and delusions of suspicion and persecution ; that at times he was dangerous or might become so, and that in his own interest and in that of society it would be best for him to be placed under the restraint of an institution.

Some of the scenes during the trial were highly dramatic, as when, for instance, the oratorical advocate denounced the doctors and others, or when he read extensive citations from the skilful pamphlet which the traverser had written in his own defence. It contained several excellent illustrations of pseudo-logic, especially adduced in explanation of the hostile voices which he said he heard and

* Read before The Philadelphia Psychiatric Society, November 9th, 1923.

which he supposed were the voices of one or more of a band of conspirators against him. He summoned, in defence of his idea that the hostile voices were real, not only the phenomena of the telephone, but an old text-book statement that a ship's sails had been known to convey such sounds or voices one hundred miles across the sea.

At one time during the reading of the traverser's pamphlet, the oratorical advocate, the jury, and even the dignified judge, were all in tears.

The judge's charge was made and proved to be a learned document, whose effect on those in the audience and the jury box was probably much like that sometimes produced by the Delphic oracle on the minds of those who appealed to the mystic shrine. The trial ended by the jury, in a few minutes, rendering a verdict in favour of the traverser, the practical result being that the man was declared to be sane.

After the unfortunate man had been given his legal certificate of perfect sanity, he apparently did not know exactly what to do with himself. One of his counsel, however, as was right and proper, secured for his client an entrance into a well-known boarding house on a thoroughfare somewhat famed for dignified establishments of this kind. In a short time the boarders generally sought other quarters, and our friend the traverser, of his own motion, went back to the hospital from which he had sought release. During the balance of his life he remained voluntarily in an institution for the insane.

I have never forgotten the lessons of this trial, one of which is that it is not wise to gamble beforehand on the verdict in a case in which insanity is the issue. Another lesson is that emotion often plays a large if not the largest part in the decisions of insanity cases.

The Writ of Habeas Corpus in Insanity Cases

Under the law a person alleged to be insane and confined in an institution has the right to appeal to the court through a writ of *habeas corpus*. Occasionally direful results follow the use of this constitutional right.

About a quarter of a century ago I had an instructive experience of this kind. As it was considered that the man alleged to be insane might be dangerous even to those who might examine him, he was placed under arrest and was taken to a magistrate's office, where I made as thorough an examination as was possible, the same process having been gone through by another physician.

Not only his wife, but many others who, through business or place of residence, came in contact with the man had reported their belief that he was dangerously insane. His insanity was of the persecutory sort so often seen. He believed that his neighbours, that those with whom he was concerned in business, and others, were engaged in some sort of a conspiracy to injure or destroy him. He also believed that he was acted on by some unseen agency, probably electricity ; that holes were made in the ceilings of rooms in order that he might be spied upon and that his life was sometimes endangered by his enemies. He was not quite clear about the manner in which his wife entered into the conspiracy, but believed that directly or indirectly she had had something to do with it, and at one time he had told her that he felt he would have to kill her and then commit suicide himself.

At the time of my examination in the magistrate's office, the man was excited and somewhat incoherent in his statements. He was certified to a well-known institution for the insane.

A lawyer asked for and obtained a writ of *habeas corpus*. At this procedure, after hearing considerable testimony, lay and medical, the Court remanded the appellant to the institution for further observation. At the end of two months he was again brought into court.

During his stay in the institution, especially after the hearing of the first writ, he suppressed his delusions, stolidly refusing to talk about matters relating to them, even when hard pressed by those attempting to establish his true mental state. Several well-known alienists who examined him testified that they were not able to find evidence of his delusions, and the judge ordered his discharge. It is difficult to see how he could have done otherwise unless he had taken more fully into consideration the entire history of the case from the beginning.

Very soon after his discharge the man again showed positive signs of alienation of a dangerous character. He was arrested, and it was somewhat difficult to get physicians to certify him because of the action taken by the Court. Eventually, however, he was re-examined and re-certified and sent to a state hospital for the insane. His subsequent history I do not know, except that I believe he continued an inmate of this institution for a long time.

My only comment is that the Court should not only take particular care to inform itself in similar cases of what is apparently the man's immediate condition, but should also review with much thoroughness all known facts.   The Court should also be informed that patients can sometimes suppress their delusions for a long time, or may sometimes have remissions or intermissions in their symptoms.   A patient is not only able at times to suppress his delusions, but he can for a purpose simulate sanity, although he may not be able to continue this procedure for a long time under the pressure of a skilful examination.

As bearing upon the point here discussed, a curious incident occurred recently at the psychopathic wards of the Philadelphia General Hospital.   The physicians of the department were holding a conference to determine the status of some of the patients.   A case was brought in from the waiting room and was questioned regarding his delusions, hallucinations and other facts relating to his insanity, which were well known to members of the staff.   He simply denied that he had any such notions or that he heard voices, etc., and nothing would move him from this position.   Another and still another patient was brought in, who made similar denials. On going to the waiting room, it was found that a young woman who belonged to the dementia præcox group was passing from one patient to another, instructing them to deny everything that was asked them relating to their delusions and hallucinations, encouraging them to do this with the suggestion that in this way they could probably obtain their discharge from the institution.

Not only may an insane man succeed in getting his discharge by suppression of what he has learned to know are regarded as the symptoms of his insanity, but occasionally some strange decisions are given in response to some cleverly presented pleas for discharge under *habeas corpus* proceedings.

A curiosity in this respect was the decision given by a learned judge that a man should be committed to an institution for the insane from six o'clock in the evening until eight o'clock in the morning, and from eight in the morning until six in the evening should be permitted to go where he chose.   Practically the result of the decision was that the man was considered sane by day and insane by night.

Mostly in the Common Pleas Court of Philadelphia a medical witness is allowed to hear the sworn testimony of the trial and give an opinion on this as well as on the results of his examination. For the most part also hypothetical questions are permitted, that is a hypothetical case may be presented to the witness for an opinion.   To one familiar with the subject it would seem that a witness should have access to all the information possible ; and yet, in one of the Courts, it was ruled that a medical witness, like an ordinary witness to facts, was only permitted to express an opinion based upon the results of his own personal examination.   This would seem to defeat the very idea of expert testimony in insanity cases.   A medical witness called to express an opinion with regard to a given case should be permitted to have presented to him all facts relating to such a case which have been included in the sworn testimony.

An Admiralty Case, and the Question of Allowing a Medical Witness to Hear all the Testimony in a Trial

I have had one experience in an Admiralty case.   The Surgeon-General of the Army came to see me, bringing with him an enormous mass of typewritten testimony, which had been taken at different hearings before the Court.   After wading through this mass, I agreed to go to Washington to be a witness.

In those days, and probably at present, although I do not keep myself posted on matters naval and military, a witness before such a Court was not allowed to hear the testimony and follow the course of the trial.   When the proper time arrived he was simply ushered into the dazzling presence of the uniformed members of the Court and his examination proceeded.

I remember how I patiently waited in the ante-room of the Court, where I fortunately met two or three naval medical officers, with whom the time was passed agreeably.   After some time, I was ushered into the presence of the Court.   Presiding at the head of the table was a Rear-Admiral whose fame was nation-wide.   To the right and left of the presiding Admiral and along both sides of the table sat men, most of them noted in the naval history of the Civil War.

I was properly questioned and jolted by the judge-advocate and others of the Court, but on the whole was treated with much courtesy, and was bowed out of the room when my testimony was ended.

One object in introducing this brief and unusual personal experience is to refer to the question of a witness hearing the testimony of other witnesses and personally following the course of a case. In many instances this is a most desirable thing.   In one noted case I sat in the court-room, day after day, for seventeen days ; in another for eleven days, although in both instances the court-room atmosphere, both emotional and material, was far from being sanitary, let alone enjoyable. My object was to get clear light on every feature of the case before testifying, and I reserved the right to withdraw as a witness after hearing all the testimony.

In no way can one's mind be enlightened better with regard to some doubtful question in medicine or law or in both than by hearing the conflict of facts in a trial before a jury.

For the Prestige of the Office

In one of the recently published books about " Tutt and Mr Tutt," a revolting picture is painted of an alleged assistant district attorney, familiarly known as " Billy the Bloodhound." The prosecutor made violent and deceitful efforts to convict an innocent man, apparently to maintain his own reputation as a successful bloodhound and, incidentally, to uphold the prestige of the office in which he was an instrument. As the story goes, the astute and philanthropic Mr Tutt defeated his efforts.

Be it remembered that what is stated in this story relates to the office of the New York city prosecutor, not to that of the Philadelphia office of similar official status. I have had the pleasure to know several members of the staff of the present district attorney, and I do not recall any of the " bloodhound " type. This story, however, seems to me to have some value in recalling the next case of my series in the present paper.

More than thirty-five years ago occurred a trial for homicide famed in the annals of medical jurisprudence in Philadelphia. The accused, some months previously, without provocation, had killed an inoffensive jeweller.

The father of the man on trial was insane and one of his sisters was an epileptic. Together with Dr James Hendrie Lloyd, I examined the prisoner for the attorneys who had been appointed by the Court to defend him, visiting him five times in all. I became thoroughly convinced that he was a delusional lunatic. At the trial a considerable number of witnesses, both medical and lay, including Dr Lloyd and myself, testified to his delusions and insane acts. He believed that his wife was unfaithful to him and wished to drug him to get him out of the way ; that his children were illegitimate ; that he was the victim of the persecution of his friends, relatives, and fellow workmen, and even those with whom he came in contact only occasionally.

No medical evidence was offered in rebuttal. It is fair to infer that the prison doctors and outside physicians who are known to have examined the accused before the trial had reported to the district attorney their belief in his insanity, as they were not called as witnesses by the prosecution.

The insane man was prosecuted relentlessly to a conviction and later was sentenced to death. Evidently, however, some force was at work which withheld the hand of the law in the final act. The sentence of death was never executed and the man remained in prison until he died, becoming more and more delusional and demented.

A member of the bar, with whom I discussed this case, said : " The district attorney evidently knew that this man was insane, but was determined to convict him, probably for what is sometimes spoken of as the prestige of his office."

I believe that it is a man's right, whether he is a prosecuting attorney, a counsel for the defence, or a medical witness, to work either for prestige or money or both, if he can do this honestly. It is in this way that livings are made and reputations are built into very strenuous professions. No man, however, either for prestige or money, should pursue a man to his doom or should use unfair means to save him from the consequences of his just deserts unless he is convinced of the justice of the cause which he is espousing.

The Mental Attitude of Judges in Trials in which Insanity is the Issue

I am not one of those who believe that a judge should sit behind his rostrum like a stuffed image, allowing attorneys and witnesses largely to have their own way. He is there, not only to weigh the evidence and to charge the jury thereon, but to guide the trial through its often tortuous course.

I have been told of one judge that he always placed in easy view a card on which was written " Do not talk." Someone suggested regarding another judge that a card might be placed similarly on which should be written " Do not talk too much."

An incident occurred at the beginning of one of the trials, the details of which I have given, which may be worthy of recall in this connection. When on several occasions during the examination of the accused in prison he was asked to make some statement, he invariably indicated, although sometimes in a half coherent way, that he would tell all about it when he got into Court.

After the trial opened, at an early stage in the proceedings, the prisoner was asked if he had anything to say. He at once arose in the dock and in a jabbering way began to say something about what he had done. The judge, in a loud and somewhat angry voice, shouted to the Court officer who had immediate charge of the dock: " Make that man sit down. We will have no Guiteau business here."

How much this attitude influenced the jury's final decision, I do not know. If the man had been allowed to go on, both his delusions and dementia would have become apparent to every thinking person in the court-room.

The trial of this case had been postponed again and again over a period of weeks and months, and on making inquiry of a member of the bar as to why this was done, he said the prosecutor was waiting until he could get a " hanging judge " to try the case. An attorney for either the prosecution or the defence may prefer to have a certain judge with whose psychology he is familiar, or thinks he is, preside at a case in which he is deeply interested.

Trial to Determine a Man's Mental Condition Before he is Tried for Homicide

When a man who has committed homicide shows marked evidences of insanity as reported by competent investigators, why should he not first be put on trial to determine whether he is sane or insane ? A provision of the law permits this course to be taken. In one of the cases to which I have given much attention in this paper, the counsel for the defence made a vigorous effort when the accused was brought to trial to have a stay of proceedings in order that he first should be tried to determine the question of his sanity or insanity.

The effort was resisted by the district attorney, and the Court decided that the trial for homicide should go on in the usual manner. Although the law allowing the question of insanity to be determined first would appear to be one calculated to further the ends of both mercy and justice, it is unfortunately seldom invoked in the defence of those accused of homicide and alleged to be insane.

False Criteria of Sanity

The question of the criteria of insanity is an old and often discussed subject, but will not be taken up in this paper. It is pretty well covered, as regards homicide, by Sir James FitzJames Stephen's dictum, the " homicide is not criminal if the person by whom it is committed is at the time when he commits it prevented by a disease affecting his mind

(a) From knowing the nature of the act done by him,
(b) From knowing that it is forbidden by law,
(c) From knowing that it is morally wrong,
(d) From controlling his own conduct."

Often the criteria made use of to demonstrate the sanity of an individual under investigation are of the most foolish sort. In the effort to prove that a woman was not insane, for instance, I have seen clever use made of the fact that she could sign her name to cheques and understand what the cheques were for. When one considers that a man (and the argument is equally true for a woman), clearly the victim of insane delusions and hallucinations, cannot only sign cheques and in a general way take care of his estate, but can write entire pamphlets of considerable merit, the folly of the criterion alluded to is quite evident. Besides the case with which I began my series, I might easily produce various instances of men, not only insane, but dangerously insane, who have written not only pamphlets or poems, but books of considerable size and not without literary merit. In certain forms of insanity, the patient may be not only capable of such mental effort, but at least for a time, may be brilliant in his literary output. The ability to write or talk or to conduct business is by no means always an indication of perfect sanity. This is especially true in paranoia and in the manic stage of manic-depressive insanity.

Partial Responsibility in Insanity Cases

The question of the partial responsibility of the insane for criminal acts is one worthy of attention from a body of psychiatrists and medical jurists. The letter of the law seems to recognise no midway position between insanity and sanity in homicide cases, for instance. " Was the individual insane at the time of the commission of the homicide," and " Is he insane now ? " are the questions to which the attention of a jury is necessarily attracted under the statutes and decisions to which attorneys for the defence and for the prosecution are forced to limit their attention. Some uphold the view that it would further the interests of justice to acknowledge the partial responsibility of the insane or some of them for their offences. It is a fact, well known to every alienist, that the insane sometimes are apparently or really conscious of their wrongdoing.

This question of partial responsibility is not one as easily settled as might at first sight appear, and representatives of the law tend to evade the issue. Several instances have come under my observation in which the prosecuting attorney in a homicide case, while knowing that the accused was clearly guilty of premeditated crime, has permitted a verdict of second degree murder, when insanity was adduced as the defence. In a case in which I was consulted but declined to testify, a woman had shot and killed a man whom she declared to have injured her. Unless the woman was insane, the case was clearly one of murder in the first degree. Nevertheless, the district attorney pressed only for murder in the second degree, and the woman was given a long term of imprisonment. In another case, a woman, who was clearly a case of such mental inferiority as to be properly ranked among high-grade imbeciles, was pursued to conviction and hanged.

The Guiteau case has some interest in connection with this question of partial responsibility. I was not a witness during the trial of Guiteau, but received an invitation to be present at his execution and to take part in the post-mortem examination of his brain, owing to the fact that I had written a paper on criminal lunacy in which I had given my views as to the insanity of Guiteau. I have never wavered from my opinion that he was insane, believing that he suffered from a form of constitutional paranoia and that he also acquired syphilis as a result of which he was in an early stage of general paresis. Microscopical examination of blocks taken from his brain and given to three pathologists in different cities, each of whom had no knowedge of the work or views of the others, resulted in reports which indicated that he was a paretic, while the gross examination of his brain showed that its fissural and gyral arrangements were such as are often found in paranoiacs and others exhibiting mental inferiority.

Many of those who believed in the insanity of Guiteau also believed that he should be held accountable for his crime, arguing that he knew exactly what he was doing, and overlooking such criteria of insanity as the knowledge that his crime was morally wrong and that he had not the power to control the act.

The possibility of the occurrence of temporary insanity comes up in connection with this question of partial responsibility. Few alienists will deny that an individual may be guilty of temporary homicidal impulsive or compulsive insanity, but because this very just view is capable of great abuse, others would refuse to acknowledge that temporary insanity is ever a just defence.

The Delusion of Marital Infidelity

The delusion of marital infidelity is one of the most dangerous of all insane delusions and not infrequently results in homicide. Almost the first case of medico-legal importance with which I was connected was based on the existence of a delusion of this ch aracter. The man, before the development of his delusion apparently in good physical and mental health, became possessed by the idea that his wife was unfaithful to him, and, strangely enough, believed that one of her paramours was a man highly distinguished in business and in philanthropy. This insane man seriously wounded his wife and killed his mother-in-law.

The victim of the delusion of marital infidelity is usually a man. Great are the difficulties surrounding the demonstration of the existence of this delusion. It often happens that one suffering from it is able largely to carry on his business or profession. One of the most marked cases that I recall was that of a clergyman ; another victim was a prominent physician ; a third was a man in a high place in the judiciary, and the fourth was a writer and editor.

When a case of this kind comes into court, the attorney representing the man who was asserted to have this delusion often resorts to two lines of questioning, one of which is designed to raise a doubt as to whether or not the person declared to be unfaithful may not be really so, and the other to show that the individual alleged to have this dangerous delusion has not for a long time exhibited any dangerous symptoms—has not, for instance, threatened to kill his wife by shooting or otherwise. Both of these forms of investigation are inadequate and even at times foolish.

The most important point for an alienist or neurologist to keep in mind is that a delusion is not dependent upon a state of facts but upon a state of mind. In the first place, a woman may be entirely faithful to her husband ; secondly, she may be unfaithful,

M

and thirdly, strange as it may appear, she may be unfaithful, having as her paramours one or more of the individuals suspected by her husband, and yet the husband may be the victim of the delusion of marital infidelity.

Recently I examined the transcript of a hearing in a case in which the individual under investigation was accused of having the delusion of marital infidelity. A distinguished physician of this city testified, presumably in support of the idea, that the man accused was really a delusional lunatic. One of the questions asked him was to the effect that if the man's suspicions were well founded would that have made any difference in the conclusions drawn regarding his mental condition. The physician answered that he thought so, if his suspicions had been well founded, but he added very properly that he (the physician) thought that the method by which the man reached his deductions as to marital infidelity showed mental perversion.

A case of real delusional insanity will usually show that a man's mental life exhibits evidences of other delusions than the one in the foreground. If the marital delusional suspects and threatens his wife, it will often be found that he is also insanely suspicious of others.

To prove the existence of the state of mind which is at the basis of a delusion is by no means an easy task. When, however, an alienist or neurologist cannot do this, he is not equal to his job. His lack of knowledge is like that of William Jennings Bryan on the subject of evolution, or of David Lloyd George on the true psychology of the German nation.

SOME MEDICAL ASPECTS OF WITCHCRAFT

BY

E. W. TAYLOR, A.M., M.D.

James Jackson Putnam Professor of Neurology, Harvard Medical School

SOME MEDICAL ASPECTS OF WITCHCRAFT

BY

E. W. TAYLOR

I

As in other matters which have become topics of popular discussion, the term " Witchcraft " has assumed in the lay mind a narrow significance, out of keeping with what it actually represents in human thought. Hysteria, in the field of medicine, has occupied a very similar position. To the man in the street, it still signifies a trifling emotional disturbance, chiefly confined to women, as implied in its name, whereas the modern student finds it quite hopeless to delimit its boundaries or give it adequate definition. The tendency of late years has been to search at a deeper level for causes of disordered function, whether in the physical or mental sphere, with results, which are already showing themselves in broader generalisations and more comprehensive conceptions of both normal and pathological activities. The discovery of a definite etiological factor, such for example, as the tubercle bacillus of Koch, or the spirochæta pallida of Schaudinn, not only throws light on the individual forms of disease, but, much more important, gives us a clear conception of interrelationships. Bone disease and lung disease are brought into a common category, or brain disease (*e.g.*, dementia paralytica) and certain alterations in the skin, into a like unity, through the acceptance of a common principle, which exerts its influence in outwardly devious ways, depending upon the type of tissue attacked. This principle, though naturally with less precision, may be applied to the strange phenomena which have been rather loosely classified as "witchcraft." Until some such basic etiologic factor is supplied, any adequate understanding of the manifold vagaries of the mind in the realm of the supernatural, whether under the name of witchcraft or not, is beyond our reach.

The manifestations of so-called witchcraft, at various periods of the world's history, have varied naturally with the religious feeling of the time, the degree of enlightenment of the people, the social organisation of the country or community involved, and, in fact, with all the factors which make up the complex aggregate which we call society. The common factor of the apparently sporadic outbursts which led to the persecution of witches in Europe and to the tragedy of 1692 in Salem village in this country, and to the minor persecutions under varying names, which have always accompanied civilisation in its halting progress, must lie deep in the constitution of the human mind. This it will be the task of future students of the psychology of history to determine. For the present, and for the purposes of this paper, some light may be thrown on the subject by a necessarily cursory survey of the probable origin and development of the later narrow and opprobrious term, witchcraft, evidently very different in its connotation from the earlier conceptions.

We may suppose, without too great a strain upon the imagination, that the dawn of self- and later of race-consciousness saw the first workings of the principle which later, largely through the influence of the Church, became identified with witchcraft. This idea was the conviction that there were inimical as well as beneficent forces at play in the world, which were capable of influencing directly human beings, and other sentient creatures. The notion of good as opposed to evil, not in a moral sense, but simply as an expression of personal or community welfare, must have been contemporaneous with the earliest dawn of intelligence. The development of magic in its more primitive forms, with the somewhat ominous appearance of the worker of magic—the magician, the conjuror, the necromancer, the soothsayer, and others of like profession—led to an elaborate system of charms and rites and supposedly successful efforts to influence weather, crops, fertility in its various aspects, and all the conditions of life, whether for good or evil. The step to animism was a short one, and the subsequent confusion of religious practices with pure magic and the development of the priestcraft brought about a complexity and confusion in the relations of man to his surroundings through which it is often difficult to trace the connection with the more primitive forms of thought. With the further elaboration of religious conceptions and the consequent withdrawal of the gods from immediate and direct concern in the affairs of man, together with the growth of monotheism, the scene is shifted to a more abstract plane, and the idea of demoniacal possession, conspicuous in the Bible stories,* and actual compact with the evil spirit came into the foregound as the predominant phase of the later developments of the witchcraft conception in its religious setting.

Although our attention will be given especially to some of the more recent and spectacular manifestations of the witchcraft principle,† it should not be forgotten that acceptance of the doctrine in some of its forms has been universal among all peoples of whatsoever grade of culture, and that any proper understanding of its vagaries and excesses must take into account the most fundamental activities of the human mind.

The passage from magic to witchcraft and from priestcraft through kingship to the idea of incarnate gods form a chapter of absorbing interest and importance in the final development of the special offshoot of witchcraft, with which we are now concerned. The point of significance is that what we speak of as witchcraft is merely a transformation of conceptions, which are as old as human thought, and are still in active operation among many of the more primitive races at the present time, particularly in Central Australia and in parts of Africa. Among the enlightened peoples, the increasing abstractness of the conceptions surrounding the gods (or later the single god), served to remove them further and further from immediate relation with human affairs, with the result that magical rites with their accompaniments were relegated to a subordinate place, and the original cleavage between science, represented by magic, and religion, represented first by god-men (incarnations) and later by incorporeal gods, was inaugurated.

Frazer‡ states the matter clearly and, on the whole, convincingly in his emphasis on the essential similarity in principle between " primitive magic " and the later development of what we call " science." As nature and its laws, as then crudely understood, was the object of the magician's study, so, in these later days, the man of science, armed with the accumulated knowledge of the past, is dealing with the same problem and is using the same material. From this point of view the magician, as a man of

* The story of the Gadarene swine (*Luke*, VIII, 27–35, *Matthew*, VIII, 28–33) and many other passages in the New Testament, which have occasioned much theological and lay discussion.

† For an account of the distinction between " witchcraft " and " magic," see G. L. Burr, " New England's Place in the History of Witchcraft " (*Proc. Am. Antiquarian Soc.*, Oct., 1911). No sharp distinction is attempted in this paper.

‡ Frazer, J. G., *The Golden Bough.* This study of Magic and Religion, republished in one volume, Macmillan, 1922, covers exhaustively the relationship of primitive thought to later development in science as well as in religion.

exceptional ability and sagacity beyond his fellows, stands side by side with the modern investigator in the field of knowledge, whom we call by the honourable name of "scientist." The one worked by observation and a process of reasoning which makes small appeal to our modern conception of clear thinking, the other through the formulation and application of what we regard, in our present stage of development, as unchangeable laws. The methods are as widely diverse as the centuries which intervened. The fundamental effort of the mind toward wider knowledge and correct formulation has remained unchanged in principle, whatever the vagaries of its practice in the early centuries of recorded history may have been.

" Thus the analogy between the magical and the scientific conceptions of the world is close. In both of them the succession of events is assumed to be perfectly regular and certain, being determined by immutable laws, the operation of which can be foreseen and calculated precisely ; the elements of caprice, of chance, and of accident are banished from the course of nature. Both of them open up a seemingly boundless vista of possibilities to him who knows the causes of things and can touch the secret springs that set in motion the vast and intricate mechanism of the world. Hence the strong attraction which magic and science alike have exercised on the human mind ; hence the powerful stimulus that both have given to the pursuit of knowledge."*

No doubt the practices of magic, as developed in the later bizarre conceptions of witchcraft, would have died a natural death had it not been for the development of religion, with the bitter and persistent antagonism which was its inevitable consequence. When the early magicians and sorcerers found their predictions false and the conclusion was forced upon them that their rites were often unavailing, it was natural, first, that they should resort to subterfuge and mystery to maintain their prestige and, secondly, that for the accomplishment of this end they should assume priestly and medical functions, which should give to their incantations a superhuman authority. Hence the early association of priest and magician and priest and medicine man† in the same individual. The gradual emergence of religious conceptions from those of a purely magical character and the identification of magic with evil was an entirely natural consequence, and in this may be seen the antagonism between the Church, as later understood, and all

* Frazer, *The Golden Bough*, p. 49.
† This combination, for example, was and doubtless still is found among the American Indians.

magical practices, which was to have so disastrous an effect in the witchcraft persecutions. The counterpart of this antagonism has been amply demonstrated in very recent times by the acrimonious and futile discussion of the so-called conflict between science and revealed religion. It is difficult to realise that Huxley's* masterly essays, published about thirty years ago, met with a storm of criticism and abuse, and that he suffered what in another age would have been actual persecution, and still more astonishing is it that even to-day a vigorous propaganda is on foot to prohibit the teaching of evolution in the schools.

An understanding of the more specific problem about to be discussed demands a liberal interpretation of the background of thought upon which it rests, and a clear recognition of the fact, too often overlooked, that, although methods may change, the springs of action and the search for knowledge are subject to the same pitfalls, now as heretofore.

" If then we consider, on the one hand, the essential similarity of man's chief wants everywhere and at all times, and on the other hand, the wide difference betwen the means he has adopted to satisfy them in different ages, we shall perhaps be disposed to conclude that the movement of the higher thought, so far as we can trace it, has on the whole been from magic through religion to science."†

What broader reaches of thought may be destined to result from present-day conflict of opinion, it is not my purpose to discuss. It is sufficient for our present object to visualise in some degree the phase of knowledge through which we have passed for the purpose of comprehending the concrete topic with which this paper is concerned.

Quite apart from the advent of Christianity, the world was filled with religions, as it still is, having elaborately formulated doctrines and practices. Among these was a cult, which Murray‡ has called the Dianic cult, a form of ritual witchcraft, presumably pre-Christian in origin, embracing the religious observances of persons known in later mediæval times as witches. She emphasises the fact that this " was a definite religion with beliefs, ritual, and organisation as highly developed as that of any other cult in the world."§ The god was incarnate in a human being, male or female,

---

* See especially the volume, *Science and Christian Tradition*, 1893.
† Frazer, *The Golden Bough*, p. 711.
‡ Murray, Margaret A., *The Witch-cult in Western Europe, a Study in Anthropology.* Oxford, Clarendon Press, 1921.
§ Murray, *loc. cit.*, Introduction, p. 12.

or in an animal. It is Murray's belief that the witchcraft of Western Europe had its inception in this cult, rather than in a less systematised form, as commonly thought. Its votaries were widespread and many of them influential in the history of the time. For example, Joan of Arc and her commander Gilles de Rais, both executed after the manner of witches, were presumably, according to Murray, members of the Dianic cult, and there is reason to believe that Joan was regarded as the god incarnate.* The Church of Rome instituted stringent measures for the suppression of the witches as for other heretics, culminating in the bull of Pope Innocent VIII, in 1484, which appears to be an ordinance directed essentially against the supposed power of the witches to influence and prevent fertility, both human and agricultural. With the dawn of Protestantism, the same intolerance towards the witch was shown, and thus by degrees witchcraft and all that it implied came to be regarded as associated only with the power of evil, whose representative was the devil with his cohorts. It therefore became imperative that all who might be in league with the powers of evil should be exterminated as a plain act of Christian piety.† The names of those who escaped the delusion are few and insignificant‡ as compared with those who blindly accepted it and, with it, the obligation for its suppression and final extermination. To name its staunch adherents would be simply to detail the leaders of thought throughout Europe and later in America, a solid phalanx of intellect, for centuries without organised opposition. The explanation lies essentially in the incalculable power of an accepted religious belief. The devil was a very present reality, vouched for by scriptural writing as then interpreted ; he was the personification of evil and its only instigator ; the witches were his agents, and therefore they must die. Accepting the premise, the conclusion was justified, and we must therefore regard the judges and the populace behind them with charity, and even with some degree of sympathy. With such a background, the belief in witchcraft was naturally transplanted to the American colonies. It was by no means

---

* Murray, *The Witch-cult in Western Europe*, Appendix IV, p. 270.

† According to the biblical injunction : If any person be a witch, he or she shall be put to death. " Thou shalt not suffer a witch to live," *Exod.*, XXII, 18 ; " A man also or woman that hath a familiar spirit, or that is a wizard shall surely be put to death," *Levit.*, XX, 27 ; also *Deut.*, XVIII, 10, 11.

‡ Johann Wier, a physician, Reginald Scot, John Webster, Joseph Glanvil, and Balthazar Bekker are some of those who opposed the prevailing beliefs, but with little consistency. See G. L. Kittredge, " Notes on Witchcraft," *Proc. Am. Antiquarian Soc.*, 1907, Vol. XVIII. In this country, Joseph Green, Francis Dane, and Robert Calef may be mentioned.

confined to Salem* as has been at times suggested, but permeated the minds of the leaders of thought everywhere in America, as it had in Europe.

II

It is a somewhat remarkable fact that in the voluminous literature that has grown up about the general subject, little has been written regarding the critical interpretation of the phenomena observed from a medical standpoint.   It is my purpose therefore to attempt a tentative formulation on the basis of the well-reported cases which occurred in Salem village (now Danvers).   It is not altogether to the credit of the medical profession that it failed utterly to recognise the pathological significance of the disorders observed in the bewitched persons and was unable to make a diagnosis on the basis of what medical knowledge it had.   It was in keeping with the accepted doctrine of the time that witchcraft must be in play, and therefore the doctors joined with the ministers and other respected citizens and did their part in propagating the false ideas.   The gifted author of *Religio Medici* was instrumental in the execution of the English witches, Amy Dunny and Rose Cullender, when the learned judge, Sir Matthew Hale, was disposed to leniency, and the activities of Cotton Mather†, who was versed in the medical knowledge of his time, had much to do with the tragic affairs at Salem.   Independence of thought had shown itself in many other fields, but not in this ; in fact, it is only within the

* The unenviable notoriety of Salem, with the charges made against its citizens for the executions of 1692, has been widely discussed, and with considerable vehemence.   During the 17th century, twenty-eight persons were put to death in Massachusetts, of whom twenty were in Salem in a period of one year, nineteen hanged, and one, the redoubtable Giles Corey, " pressed to death," according to the English law, for refusal to plead.   Kittredge is an eloquent apologist for the Puritans and for New England in general (see *Notes on Witchcraft*, and especially the conclusions), whereas in a polemical paper Burr (*loc. cit.*) takes sharp issue with this viewpoint, and incriminates the Calvinists and the Puritans for the later developments in New England.   The whole matter has aroused much difference of opinion, often approaching animosity not only in regard to the general situation, but also in respect to its main actors, among whom the Mathers have been a chief storm-centre.   See Calef, *Salem Witchcraft*, Boston, 1828.   Excellent bibliographical summaries of the literature pertaining to witchcraft in Massachusetts and New England are given by G. H. Moore, *Am. Antiquarian Soc.*, April, 25th 1888, and Justin Winsor, *Proc. idem*, October, 1896.

† Among more recent writers John Fiske, *Witchcraft in Salem Village* (Reprint, Houghton Mifflin and Co., Boston, 1923) finds little to censure in the conduct of Cotton Mather, in contrast to many historians, who see in him an arch-conspirator.   It is certain, at least, that he was not in advance of his time, as might have been expected from one who advocated inoculation for smallpox in those medically benighted times.

last fifty years that a candid discussion of mental phenomena has
not been regarded as a species of heterodoxy within the medical
profession.   It is of some interest in this connection that the first
witch executed in this country, Margaret Jones, of Charlestown,
was reputed to be a physician, whose sole fault appears to have
been that she believed in her own medicines to the exclusion of
those of the regular practitioners.   She was hanged in Boston and,
in justification of the sentence and as proof of her guilt, John
Winthrop, then Governor of Massachusetts, writes that at the hour
of her execution " a great gale in Connecticut blew down many
trees," a damning coincidence.

The conditions of life in the Puritanical settlement at Salem and
its neighbourhood towards the close of the 17th century had been
graphically described by Upham.*   It was a colony of highly
intelligent people, struggling for existence, given to many petty
quarrels, honest and hard-working, in a state of political unrest,
doubtful of their relations with England, and, above all, living in
the fear of God and equally of the devil.   It is difficult for us to
realise their intolerance and the depths of their superstition.   The
difficulties of their life reached a climax when Samuel Parris was
installed as minister of the church at Salem village in 1689.   The
financial situation was troublesome, controversies arose, bitter
animosity broke out with Parris and the church over which he
presided as the storm centre.   Parris had brought with him from
the West Indies, where he had formerly lived, two servants, a man
known as John Indian and a half-breed, Indian and negro, Tituba,
who purported to be John's wife.   To these ignorant and superstitious persons is to be attributed the exciting cause of the tragedy
which followed.   It came about in the following way : Versed as
they were in the folklore and mysteries of the benighted regions
from which they had come, they found willing listeners in the
children—all girls—of their master and others in the town.   These
children ranged from nine to twenty.   Among them, those who
later acquired special notoriety were Ann Putnam, aged twelve,
daughter of a solid citizen, Sergeant Thomas Putnam, and a mother
of unstable mentality, and Mercy Lewis, a servant of seventeen,
in the family of Sergeant Putnam.†   This group of girls has

* Upham (C. W.) : *History of Witchcraft and Salem Village*, Boston, Wiggin
and Lunt, 1867.

† The others were Elizabeth Parris, aged 9, Abigail Williams, 11, Mary
Wolcott and Elizabeth Hubbard, 17, Elizabeth Booth and Susannah Sheldon,
18, Mary Warren and Sarah Churchill, 20.   The ages of most of these so-called
" children " are worthy of note : their intelligence was doubtless at a much
lower level than their years would indicate.

passed into history as " The afflicted children." Under the tutelage of the Indian servants they learned much of trances, magic,
fortune-telling, incantations and the like and apparently were apt
pupils. They soon developed remarkable capacities in these
directions, and came to be regarded as having supernatural powers.
They were visited by the imaginative people of the village and
surrounding towns and naturally came to be the object of a somewhat flattering attention, which must have led to a growing sense
of their own importance and power, both psychological factors of
importance in their later development, and in a measure explanatory of many of their actions. It was a wholly new experience to
the children, and certainly not less so to their wondering and
puzzled elders. Considering the prevailing attitude of the time
toward all things which transcended ordinary observation, it was
inevitable that the idea of some malign external influence should be
accepted as an explanation of the uncanny actions of the children,
and the step was a short one to the assumption that they were
bewitched by certain persons as yet unknown. To this explanation
the children were ready accessories, and the persecutions were
forthwith inaugurated. Accepting the idea that they were
bewitched, they were not slow in announcing by whom this had
been brought about, and named (" cried out upon ") their former
mentor, Tituba, and two harmless and inconspicuous women of
the village, Sarah Good and Sarah Osborn. What followed during
the fateful year of 1692 has been recorded in detail, notably by
Upham.* Our interest lies in the important part taken by the
" afflicted children " in the persecutions and trial of the persons
whom they were chiefly instrumental in condemning to death.
Their responsibility in the matter has been variously interpreted
by commentators and historians. The disorder from which the
children suffered cannot be understood without a constant realisation of the conditions under which they lived and by which they
were surrounded and influenced. To this, general allusion has been
made in the preceding pages. More specifically stated, the main
factors appear to have been as follows : 1. The universal
acceptance of the fact of witchcraft as an integral part of the
religious belief of the time. 2. The character of the community
in which the children were reared. 3. The ignorance of the
children (only two of whom, it is stated by Drake, were able to write
their names), and their consequent increased susceptibility to
external influences.

* Upham, *History of Witchcraft and Salem Village*, Vol. II.

For upwards of fifty years before the Salem outbreak, witchcraft had been a most serious problem in the lives of the American colonists and definite prosecutions began before the middle of the century. It is to be inferred that the subject was widely discussed as one of the most vital issues of the time, and that sermons* and other church observances did much toward influencing the popular mind. With an avidity only now beginning to be understood the children doubtless absorbed a vast amount of knowledge of the black art, distorted by their youth and ignorance into an even more grotesque conception than that held by their elders. Under what we regard as the enlightened attitude of our own time, the susceptibility of children to belief in fairies, in Santa Claus and the doings of the inhabitants of an unseen world, is not only recognised, but at times encouraged as a stimulus to the imagination. The situation was not different with the Salem children, except that, unfortunately for them and their victims, the objects of their imagination were evil spirits capable of inflicting injury upon normal and harmless people. The difference between the fairy and the witch was presumably not so wide in mediæval times as it later came to appear.† It is difficult to picture a more fertile soil for the development of the neurotic disturbance with which the Salem children were affected, with its background of superstition and religious fanaticism, its atmosphere of suspicion, and above all with its abysmal ignorance of natural law. In modern parlance, such children would be exposed and susceptible to suggestion in the highest degree, and if as Coriat‡ has recently suggested, suggestion is a form of medical magic, the stage was prepared for the astonishing performance which was to follow.

Under the tutelage of Tituba and John Indian it is not remarkable that the "afflicted children" should first have been deeply interested and therefore quick to learn the various devices and tricks of hand and mind which they were taught. They doubtless became highly skilful in much that savoured to them of supernatural agency, and with the natural pleasure of children in such acquisition, there was no doubt quickly associated a sense of their growing importance, and their possible relation to the spirits of darkness, in which they implicitly believed. This was the

* An example is the discourse of Rev. Deodat Lawson in March, 1692, which doubtless did much to inflame the populace and hasten the trials which shortly followed. Upham, *loc. cit.*, Vol. II, p. 77.

† Murray, *The Witch-cult in Western Europe*, Introduct., p. 14, and Appendix I, p. 238.

‡ Coriat, I. H., "Suggestion as a Form of Medical Magic," *Jour. of Abn. Psychology and Soc. Psychology*, XVIII, No. 3, 1923.

danger point. It is probable that, had the proper sobering influences been brought to bear upon them, of course impossible at that time, they might have been restored to some degree of sanity. On the contrary, everything was done to precipitate the crisis, and to bring about an hysterical reaction, which removed the children, in part at least, from personal responsibility in the events which were to follow. Inasmuch as the doctors of the time were in profound ignorance of matters relating to the mind, and shared the prevailing belief in witchcraft, it was quite impossible that help should come from that source. The tendency since has been to attribute a diabolical capacity for malicious acts to the unfortunate children, leaving small room for a more charitable interpretation. Hutchinson, writing seventy years after, summarised the matter in these words :

" A little attention must force conviction that the whole was a scene of fraud and imposture begun by young girls who at first perhaps thought of nothing more than being pitied and indulged, and continued by adult persons, who were afraid of being accused themselves. The one and the other, rather than confess their fraud, suffered the lives of so many innocents to be taken away, through the credulity of judges and juries."*

Upham writes as follows :—

" Those girls, by long practice in ' the circle,' and day by day, before astonished and wondering neighbours gathered to witness their distresses, and especially on the more public occasions of the examinations, had acquired consummate boldness and tact. In simulation of passions, sufferings, and physical affections, in sleight of hand, and in the management of voice and feature and attitude, no necromancers have surpassed them. There has seldom been better acting in a theatre than they displayed in the presence of the astonished and horror-stricken rulers, magistrates, ministers, judges, jurors, spectators, and prisoners. No one seems to have dreamed that their actings and sufferings could have been the result of cunning or imposture."†

Drake finds the wickedness of the children almost beyond his power of expression. He says :—

" All things considered, it is one of the most surprising events in history. The smallness of the number of those engaged in it, in its beginning, their youth and position in society, their ability to deceive everybody for so long a time ! In any view that has yet been taken of it, its narrator has found himself baffled to a degree

* Quoted by Winsor, *Proc. Am. Antiqu. Soc.*, p. 21.
† Upham, *History of Witchcraft and Salem Village*, Vol. II, p. 112.

beyond that of any other event in the whole range of history, to account satisfactorily for the conduct of the young females through whose instrumentality it was carried on. It required more devilish ability to deceive, adroitness to blind the understanding and to keep up a consciousness of that ability among themselves, than ever fell to the lot of a like number of imposters in any age of which the writer has ever read ; and he can only say, if there are parallel cases they have not fallen under his observation."*

John Fiske† has discussed the matter judicially and with much fairness in his volume " New France and New England." He discountenances the idea of conspiracy and very properly calls attention to the important fact that the children, like everyone else, believed implicitly in the reality of witchcraft. " It will not do," he says, " to invest those poor girls with a nineteenth-century consciousness. The same delusion that conquered hardened magistrates led them also astray."

Certainly at this late day one need not hesitate to consider malicious conspiracy as a wholly inadequate explanation of the conduct of the " afflicted girls." Collusion there no doubt was, a certain *esprit de corps* which Mistress Ann Putnam and Samuel Parris did much to foster. Doubtless, also, the situation gave ample opportunity for airing and developing trivial and contemptible private animosities. It was natural that retaliation and revenge found therein a ready tool, and that certain of the persons hanged as witches were, primarily at least, the victims of a concerted plan of persecution, with nothing more at its foundation than the fancied satisfaction of a personal grudge. As the trials went on, however, and persons of higher estate than the early victims, for example, Rebecca Nurse and John Burroughs, " were cried out upon," it became apparent that mere retaliation could no longer be considered the compelling motive of the accusing girls or of those with whom they were immediately associated. The pathological aspect of the whole strange spectacle in its later development is apparent, even though it be not capable of complete explanation.

The generally accepted view, therefore, that the girls were the willing tools in the hands of designing persons, among whom were Mistress Putnam, the mother of Ann, and Samuel Parris, whose primary object was to gratify personal or community animosity, is too preposterous an assumption to be considered seriously.

* Drake, *Witchcraft in New England*, Boston, 1869, p. 187.
† Fiske, *Witchcraft in Salem Village*, p. 56 (Reprint).

That it should have gained such wide currency is doubtless due to the fact that up to within a very recent period the phenomena of the disorder, physical and mental, which we now designate hysteria, were so little understood that it was a less strain on the intelligence to conceive a plot of really fiendish ingenuity and completeness than to accept an emotional upheaval of a definitely neurotic character as the explanation of the performances of the accusing children.   It is true that, even at the time of the trials, there was some slight recognition of the neurotic element, but then the explanation was unquestioned, that through the machinations of the devil the children were bewitched, which satisfied all the requirements of the situation.   In general, the much-discussed " afflicted children " have passed through these general phases in popular estimation—first, they were regarded as " bewitched " ; second, by many of the commentators of the last century (e.g., Drake, Upham) as malicious and crafty mischief-makers ; and third, as the victims of an hysterical disorder, carrying in its later development no stigma of responsibility, which owed its peculiar character to the conditions under which it was fostered and elaborated.

Leaving out of consideration the first alternative, which does little more than state the question it is sought to answer, the second and third alternatives are of more present interest, and cannot be sharply separated in reviewing the evidence.   It is not difficult to visualise what took place in " the circle " of impressionable children and young girls, who made up the group at Samuel Parris' house, under the instruction of Tituba and her husband. Like children at any period of time, they delighted in mystery and in extravagant play of the imagination, doubtless gratified to the fullest extent by their increasing proficiency in the apparently occult and supernatural arts, which they were rapidly acquiring. The sombre background of witchcraft, in which the children believed as implicitly as their elders, must have added intensity to the interest of the play which they were more or less unconsciously acting.   The attention which they began to excite and the speculation which their apparently unprovoked and strange acts aroused, inevitably had its effect.   Their sense of importance grew, and with it their feeling of dominance—a principle, no doubt, of much psychological importance in this as in other settings.   It was flattering that they should be looked upon as worthy of the inspection of ministers and doctors, and made the objects of study and speculation.   Under such circumstances it was inevitable—

N

call it suggestion or not—that their gyrations and antics would be intensified and increasingly mystifying to the superstitious, ignorant and bigoted persons who were attempting to determine their basis. It should be borne in mind, at this point, as a matter of no little importance that, with the gratification of exciting attention and its accompanying publicity, there must also have developed a certain fear on the part of the " afflicted children," as they were now called, that possibly they might themselves be regarded as witches and be made to suffer accordingly. If they were not themselves " bewitched," they might well be considered as witches. The matter was determined by the decision in which the doctors, unable to arrive at a diagnosis of so strange a malady, agreed that the children were the victims of the malice of unknown persons by whom they were being afflicted. The children, being asked, gave the names of their supposed tormentors. During the year 1692, the " afflicted children " occupied a position of unique distinction. They were repeatedly called upon to fix guilt upon suspected persons, and they were the chief witnesses in nearly all the trials. Their evidence consisting of fits, convulsive seizures, claims of personal injury, bites and blows, strange attacks of vomiting, and, in fact, the whole category of hysterical manifestations, was accepted as incontrovertible. To the intelligence of the judges of that day such inexplicable occurrences could be due to witchcraft alone. There is a certain similarity in all the trials in that the accused was not allowed to defend himself, the character of the accusations varied little, and the hysterical outbursts of the " afflicted children," constituted proof of guilt.

Among many examples (for the trials have been carefully reported) the following scene at the prosecution of William Hobbs, will suffice by way of illustration :—

" The magistrate commenced proceedings by inquiring of the girls, pointing to the prisoner, ' Hath this man hurt you ? ' Several of them answered ' Yes.' The magistrate, addressing the prisoner, ' What say you ? Are you guilty or not ? '—Answer : ' I can speak in the presence of God safely, as I must look to give account another day, that I am as clear as a new-born babe.'—' Clear of what ? '— ' Of Witchcraft.'—' Have you never hurt these ? '—' No.' Abigail Williams cried out that he ' was going to Mercy Lewis ! ' Whereupon Mercy was seized with a fit. Then Abigail cried out again, ' He is come to Mary Walcott,' and Mary went into her fit. The magistrate, in consternation, appealed to him, ' How can you be clear, when your appearance is thus seen producing such effects before our eyes ? ' Then the children went into fits all together, and ' hallooed ' at the top of their voices, and ' shouted greatly.' The magistrate then brought up the confession of his wife against him, and expostulated with him for not confessing ; the afflicted, in the meanwhile, bringing the whole machinery of their convulsions, shrieks, and uproar to bear against him : but he calmly, and in brief terms, denied it."*

Further hysterical reactions in great number are reported, rolling of the eyes, rigidities, muscular movements corresponding to those made by the accused, and the frequent and immediate relief of violent fits and torments on the part of the girls, through being touched by the accused, on the theory that the " bewitching influence " thereby passed back into the body of the witch.   There are many references to these phenomena in the story of the trials. Their interpretation is the matter of interest.   To the learned men of the day they were proof-positive of witchcraft and led directly to the condemnation of the victims ; to later sceptics of the reality of witchcraft who, however, were still influenced by ideas of unseen evil forces, they were in part mysteries unexplained, but chiefly clever malingering and imposture on the part of the accusing girls and others.   From being regarded as totally irresponsible, by reason of demoniac possession, they came to be regarded as wholly responsible, and have been anathematised correspondingly.

To us the matter presents itself essentially as a medical or a medico-social problem of the utmost complexity, involving for its proper comprehension a study of the background upon which witchcraft itself rests, its relations, broadly considered, to the development of scientific thought and to the growth of philosophic and religious ideals.   The special dramatic outburst which, through a series of apparently fortuitous circumstances, developed at Salem, serves as an example merely of what, under different conditions, has occurred in every part of the world, and will continue to occur, modified only by what we call the progress of civilisation and of liberal thought.   To us the scenes at Salem in 1692, especially the mental condition of the " afflicted children," bear the stamp of " group hysteria," in which suggestion, self-protection, a feeling of domination, in an atmosphere of profound belief in the actuality of witchcraft, played a predominant rôle. The spirit of mischief and maliciousness was certainly subordinate. The elements entering into the composition of so complex a neurosis under conditions so extraordinary are naturally elusive and quite

* Upham, *History of Witchcraft and Salem Village*, Vol. II, p. 131.

beyond the scope of this paper to discuss except in barest outline. The evidence, even somewhat superficially presented, suffices at least to advance our knowledge to a point from which a new attack may be made on the more fundamental problem, and this must evidently be the task of the future. It is somewhat surprising that commentators and historical writers should have so definitely avoided a frank discussion of the obvious medical problems involved, in view especially of the minute analysis of the actual events. Certain allusions are made to hypnotism, to mental disorder of uncertain character, to hysteria in the popular sense, and to various hallucinatory conditions,* but on the whole, those who have been interested in the history and literature of witchcraft have not, with equal zeal, analysed the important medical bearings of the subject. Kittredge finds such discussion out of his province as indicated by his statement: " As to occult or supernormal powers and practices, we may leave their discussion to the psychologists." And yet just here lies one of the most important questions to be faced and solved if possible. Thanks to men like Charcot, Janet, Freud and Prince, a body of exact knowledge has been accumulated, and has been available for many years, which should throw much light into the dark places of the witchcraft problem. We are, therefore, altogether justified in assuming that the descriptions given of the performances of those bewitched, of the sights seen and the sounds heard and the damage done, will find explanation on the basis of demonstrated laws of mental life, discounting always the perverted imaginations of the chief actors in the play. The appearances of imps and familiars so often described were doubtless actual animals or persons, transformed

---

* See Wendell, B., *Were the Salem Witches Guileless ?* (*Hist. Collections Essex Institute*, XXIX, 1892). An ingenious attempt, coloured by personal feeling, to place some of the blame on the witches themselves, on the ground that they had given themselves up to what Wendell regards as the pernicious practice of trance-mediumship. The article is further interesting as showing the lay prejudice existing thirty years ago against hypnotism and all that it was supposed to entail. The possibility of the baleful use of hypnotic methods by certain of the executed witches leads him to make the astonishing query " whether some of the witches may not, after all, in spite of the weakness and falseness of the evidence that hanged them, have deserved their hanging." This, so far as I am aware, is the only modern attempt to place the blame on the victims themselves, a reversion to the attitude of 1692.

Also, Beard (G. M.), *The Psychology of the Salem Witchcraft Excitement of 1692, and its Practical Application to our own Time,* Putnam, New York, 1882. Beard finds a ready explanation for the persecutions in the conditions of " insanity, trance and hysteria," but he fails to get beneath the words to the ideas which they symbolise. His discussion is vehement but uncritical. The comparison of the state of public feeling which prevailed in the witchcraft trials and in that of Guiteau, the assassin of President Garfield, may be read with much interest in the perspective of the intervening fifty years.

at times into satanic forms to satisfy the fear or fancy of the observer, an entirely analogous experience to the effect of fear under ordinary conditions, but naturally exaggerated through the emotional abnormality of the time. The children, ignorant suggestible, important in their own eyes as they were in others, no doubt often fearful lest their disclosures should lead to their own undoing, provided a perfectly normal soil for what appeared to be abnormal reactions. Their acts were purposive in the highest degree and yet involuntarily and often unconsciously performed, call it a splitting of consciousness, or dissociation, subconscious or co-conscious activity, or what one will. Herein lies the secret of the hysterical state, as manifested in the " afflicted children." The defence mechanism naturally lay in the possibility through the fits and other unconventional behaviour of diverting attention from themselves and fixing it upon the convenient person of the accused witch. That this was involuntary, as the paralysis or convulsion of a soldier under the stress of war is involuntary, in the sense of having no conscious relation to the waking intelligence, must be accepted if we are to gain any insight into the workings of the " bewitched " mind. The children, forced into a position in which they were the arbiters of life and death, were consciously aware of the enormity of the crime of witchcraft, and had an ever-present dread, of which they were largely unaware, of being drawn into the fatal net.* The self-preservative instinct was in conflict with a social situation in which they found themselves chief actors, and the result was the production of symptoms, which effected the usual compromise of saving them from being accusers of innocent persons, and at the same time protected them from their own imminent danger of being regarded as witches themselves. This in no way differs in principle from the hysterical reaction of the neurotic soldier,

* It has been generally supposed that, as the excitement grew, many adults in the community, not knowing where the next blow might fall, became accusers as a simple means of self-protection. This presumably was done in many instances with conscious intent, and consequently was not accompanied by hysterical symptoms. The children, on the other hand, according to this view, protected themselves unconsciously from the same danger, through the ordinary mental mechanism of defence, namely, hysterical symptoms, which served to divert suspicion from themselves, at the same time fixing the guilt on another person. Only in this way may be explained the outstanding fact that the elder accusers, with minor exceptions, spread rumours with no manifestations in themselves of violent hysterical symptoms, whereas the children, more impressionable, escaped through the now well recognised unconscious and involuntary defence brought about through hysterical compromise reactions. The elders described events of supposed supernatural character ; the children had fits.

who faces death on the one hand and disgrace on the other, and, unbearable as both situations are, an hysterical compromise without volition on his part is effected which saves him from both alternatives, but at the expense of pronounced neurotic symptoms. The principle is one of wide application.

It requires no effort of the imagination to picture the scene at a Salem witch trial, the judges, the ministers, and people of all degrees crowding into a room much too small to accommodate all who sought admission, the morbidly curious who thronged outside, the usually mystified victim, trying to protest her own innocence while believing whole-heartedly in the existence of witchcraft in others, and finally the " afflicted children " upon whom the final judgment rested, in a state of intense nervous excitement, prepared, at a word or a sign, to pass into an hysterical state. It is, indeed, difficult to imagine a more fitting setting for the development of hysterical reactions, and for this reason it is the more imperative to regard soberly and in the light of recently acquired knowledge, the apparently malicious acts of the children, who are not the least to be pitied among the various actors in the grim tragedy. The worst that may with justice be said of them is that they were ignorant, at the outset perhaps mischievous, like other children, and in the end deluded and overwhelmed by the situation in which they found themselves. The only escape from this dilemma was through hysterical reactions, for which they were in no way responsible. It will be remembered that in 1706, fourteen years later, Ann Putnam, one of the chief actors in 1692, acknowledged that what she supposed true then she had since come to regard as false, and that the devil was her tempter.* Shifting the onus of the proceedings from the accused witches to the devil was apparently to many, at that time and for the succeeding century, a satisfactory explanation, though to our minds a small improvement on the original conception. The devil had lost little of his capacity for evil deeds, but his methods had become more indirect and less concerned with immediate human agents. In this belief intelligent people continued to live, and, we may surmise, many are still doing so in no small measure.

A psychological analysis of the conduct of those actually responsible, if, in fact, they were responsible for the prosecutions,

---

* " . . . though what was said or done by me against any person, I can truly say before God and man, I did it not out of any anger, malice, or ill-will to any person, for I had no such thing against one of them, but what I did was ignorantly, being deluded of Satan." Nevins, *Witchcraft in Salem Village*, Lee and Shepard, Boston, 1892, p. 250.

as conducted in Salem and elsewhere, is a matter as absorbing in interest as that of the " afflicted children." When the reaction came in 1693 it was rather an awakening to the unavailability and fruitlessness of methods employed to suppress witchcraft than a disbelief in its reality. Cotton Mather's half-hearted recantation, and even Judge Sewall's public acknowledgment of his error, was not and could not have been a complete renunciation of their beliefs, since the devil for them was an ever-present reality, after, as before, the year 1692. Chief Justice Stoughton remained obdurate to the end of his life in 1702, and doubtless many others.

It would take us far beyond the scope of this paper to discuss many matters of psychological and medical importance connected with the events which led up to and reached a climax in the persecutions at Salem. Some of these may be alluded to, merely to indicate that a fruitful field of study lies in an adequate survey, from a medical standpoint, of many hitherto only partially explained subjects.

The attitude of the victims themselves is a curious commentary on the general state of mind of the period. Probably, without exception, those who were executed believed in the existence of witchcraft. At least, none denied it even at the supreme moments immediately before their violent deaths. They equally believed themselves wholly innocent of the crimes with which they were charged. It is a remarkable and most noteworthy fact, confirmatory of the incredible belief of the time, that not one among them repudiated the doctrine in its entirety, but died apparently with a sense of the deep justice of the cause for which they were dying, but with natural and vehement protestations of personal innocence. Such a strange conflict may hardly be seen in any other type of persecution. They were not martyrs in the ordinary sense, since they personally died for no moral cause, and they had not the slightest conviction that by this sacrifice they were even remotely helping toward the extermination of a pernicious belief.

The attitude of the judges and others mainly concerned in the prosecutions also offers a problem of speculative interest. The natural sense of justice which these persons presumably had in other affairs of life was for the time wholly submerged. Evidence was accepted at the trials which marked them as the most flagrant travesties on the doctrine of individual rights. No defence was allowed. The accused was prejudged and the outcome was assured. The presumption of innocence until guilt be proved beyond reasonable doubt found no place in the procedure. All this, it would have seemed, must have outraged the sense of fairness of men of recognised integrity of character, but such was not the case. That even so powerful a motive as religious fanaticism should have misled men like the Mathers, one of them the President of Harvard College, Judges Sewall, Stoughton, Richards, Winthrop, Danforth, Governor Phips, and Rev. John Hale, when it conflicted so obviously with the recognised rights of men, in an ordered community, must remain one of the perennial riddles, until perchance some medical philosopher of broad vision may find the solution. One must go far below the surface of ethical or religious theory to reach a proper understanding of this strange psychological phenomenon, no less pathological than the performance of the " afflicted children."

We are on somewhat surer ground when we consider the more specific phenomena which witchcraft, at all periods of history, has brought into prominence. It is not difficult to explain most of them on the basis of present-day knowledge. The imagination, the limits of which are beyond accurate computation, is undoubtedly responsible for a very large number of the appearances and facts described apparently in good faith by many observers, such, for example, as animals of strange character, sundry unexplained noises and supposed apparitions. The animated controversy and discussion regarding spectral evidence is not difficult of explanation on the basis of our understanding of hallucinosis under normal and pathological conditions. The often-repeated details of levitation and strange blows delivered by unseen agents are no doubt partly the result of an imagination excited to such a degree as to be no longer controlled, and partly in the case of apparent personal violence, bites and the like, to self-imposed injury, of which the afflicted person may have had no conscious memory.* In any event, we may safely assume that the various acts of witchcraft are ultimately susceptible of natural explanation, however impossible such explanation may be in individual cases, with the facts now available.

The so-called witches' marks are easier of satisfactory understanding. Admitting, as we do, the power of suggestion to produce anæsthetic areas, the tests of pricking without pain or

---

* The possibility of an explanation of certain cases of *urticaria factitia* on the basis of hysterical amnesia is of interest in this connection.

bleeding* find a ready explanation, constantly observable in any modern neurological clinic. Skin excrescences, small epithelial tumors and other localised affections and particularly the not infrequent supernumerary nipples both in men and women,† which the devil or the familiars were supposed to suck, serve to explain the " little teats," which were unequivocal evidence of the guilt of the person on whom they were found. The trial by water which looms large in the various prosecutions need be mentioned merely as a strange vagary, a form of torture, without medical significance. The often reported vomiting of nails, pins, usually crooked, and various other objects, and the methods by which they were brought to those afflicted is illustrated, for example, in such a statement as the following : "A thing like a bee flew at the face of the younger child ; the child fell into a fit ; and at last vomited up a two-prong nail with a broad head ; affirming that the bee brought this nail and forced it into her mouth."‡ Of course, such statements were implicitly believed and have been reported as facts. How far there was collusion with older and designing persons, how far the victims of these incidents were themselves malingerers, or the dupes of their own imaginations, cannot now be determined. About this it is fruitless to speculate in detail. In general, however, it may be assumed that superstition, trickery, self-deception, and, above all, complicated hysterical reactions, all played a part in the structure of the astonishing product which has descended to us as the intervention of the devil in the affairs of men.

When the whole subject of witchcraft in its medical aspects has been rationalised to the extent of our present ability, there will still remain the foundation-mystery upon which it is built, namely,

---

* Tertullian says, " It is the Devil's custom to mark his, and note that this mark is Insensible, and being prick'd it will not Bleed.   Sometimes, its like a Teate ; sometimes but a blewish spot ; sometimes a Red one ; and sometimes the flesh Sunk ; but the Witches do sometimes cover them."—" There was a notorious Witchfinder in Scotland (no doubt, Matthew Hopkins), that undertook by a Pin, to make an infallible Discovery of suspected persons, whether they were Witches or not, if when the Pin was run an Inch or two into the Body of the accused Party no Blood appeared, nor any sense of Pain, then he declared them to be Witches ; by means hereof my Author tells me no less than 300 persons were Condemned for Witches in that Kingdom."   Cotton Mather, *Wonders of the Invisible World*, pp. 35 and 248, London, 1693 (Reprint, 1862).

† Murray (*The Witch-cult in Western Europe*, p. 90) quotes Bruce as stating that in 315 of both sexes, taken indiscriminately, 7·6 per cent. had supernumerary nipples, and that this abnormality is about twice as frequent in men as in women.   The occasional possibility of milk being excreted through such nipples probably accounts for the idea of giving suck to familiars.

‡ Mather, *loc. cit.*, p. 115.

what lies beyond the reach of the senses, and what is our relation to the "invisible world," a belief in which persists in a large portion of the human race. Whatever our personal belief in this matter may be, we cannot refuse to consider the conviction of many thinking persons, who see no reason to doubt the existence of disembodied spirits having relations with those still living and capable of communication with them. [The story of the Witch of Endor has a strangely modern flavour, (*Samuel* I, 18).] In this we clearly see a continuation of the method of thought and belief which now, in more sublimated form, is replacing the enormity of the witchcraft persecutions of the fourteenth to the eighteenth centuries. Upham, writing in 1869, finds little to choose between the days and methods of active witchcraft and the spiritualism of his time.

" Now it is affirmed by those calling themselves spiritualists that by certain rappings, or other incantations, they can summon into immediate but invisible presence the spirits of the departed, hold conferences with them and draw from them information not derivable from any sources of human knowledge. There is no essential distinction between the old and the new belief and practice. The consequences that resulted from the former would be likely to result from the latter, if it should obtain universal or general credence, be allowed to mix with judicial proceedings, or to any extent affect the rights of person, property or character."*

Kittredge writes :—

" Besides, spiritualism and kindred delusions have taken over, under changed names, many of the phenomena, real and pretended, which would have been explained as due to witchcraft in days gone by."†

Witchcraft, including the earlier magic, as before indicated, cannot be dissociated from the fundamental cravings of the human mind, variously manifested in different periods of history, if the subject is to be studied in a wholly liberal spirit. Tolerance, still far from complete, has replaced gross intolerance, but the fundamental craving remains unchanged. The pursuit of the unknown and mysterious is still the most absorbing occupation of the human mind ; it is well for us in all modesty to be charitable in our estimate of the past that we may escape in a measure the harsh criticism of the future, which must inevitably be our lot. There is no lack of evidence that beliefs widely held to-day will be no less abhorrent to our descendants than the fanaticism of witchcraft is to us.

---

* Upham, *History of Witchcraft and Salem Village*, Vol. II, p. 428.
† Kittredge, *Notes on Witchcraft*, p. 63. See also Wendell, *loc. cit.*

DIVISIONS OF THE SELF AND CO-CONSCIOUSNESS

BY

T. W. MITCHELL, M.D.

Editor of " The British Journal of Medical Psychology " ; formerly President of the (British) Society for Psychical Research

THE SELF AND CO-CONSCIOUSNESS

BY

T. W. MITCHELL

OUR knowledge of mental structure and process has been attained mainly through examination of the experience and behaviour of normal human beings ; and we find that the mind of the normal man presents a semblance of unity and coherence which is lacking in many of those who, for one reason or another, are considered abnormal. The structure of the mind seems liable to disintegration, such unity as has been attained may be broken, and mental process may display aberrancy in various directions.

This disintegration of the mind reveals itself as disorders of the self, as an abrogation of certain faculties or powers which the self ordinarily possesses ; sensations, perceptions, thoughts, feelings, which in mental health form part of normal experience, may no longer enter into consciousness, although their disqualification is not due to any structural defect in the nervous system. Such disintegration of the mind has been commonly referred to as " splitting of consciousness " or " mental dissociation," and in its extreme forms as " double consciousness," " double or multiple personality " or " division of the self."

These disintegrations include all varieties of falling short of the relative unity and continuity which characterise normal experience. They range from the gaps in the field of consciousness discovered in the experience of hysterics to those profound discontinuities in the stream of consciousness known as multiple personalities.

Our knowledge of these states has been obtained mainly from the study of hysteria and hypnotism, and in these days, when the use of hypnotism in therapeutics is discouraged and decried, there is some danger not only that investigation along these lines may come to an end, but that the results so far obtained and the problems which they present may be misunderstood or forgotten. Within recent years new methods of approach to the problems of psychopathology have cut across the old well-worn tracks and have tended to obliterate both the landmarks by which we used to guide ourselves and the clearings we had made in a previously unexplored country. It may be useful, therefore, at the present time, to recall some of the conclusions come to, and some of the problems left unsolved, at the end of what we may call the "hypnotic period."

When Pierre Janet and Morton Prince were carrying on their remarkable investigations on the nature of dissociated states, they had at their command the technique of hypnotic experiment and the knowledge of the phenomena of hypnosis derived from their personal experience and from the labours of many workers in this field from the days of Mesmer down to their own time. In the course of their investigations some novel conceptions of the way the mind works were formulated and used with effect in the interpretation of the astonishing facts revealed in the observation of hypnotised persons and of the spontaneous somnambulisms of hysteria. Both of these investigators were fortunate in encountering persons in whom the peculiarities of behaviour, brought about by hypnotic suggestion, or observed in the so-called automatisms of hysterical somnambulisms, were paralleled or reproduced as relatively permanent phases of their everyday life. These were cases of more or less well-marked double or multiple personality. This form of mental dissociation has been studied at first hand by a comparatively small number of observers, for it is of rare occurrence, and all the records in recent years bear the mark of the influence of the work of Janet and Morton Prince in respect of the phenomena towards which attention has been directed and in the interpretation of the facts which have been observed.

The most far-reaching result of researches in the field of hypnotism, hysteria and multiple personality is the conviction that in these states there is a sort of division or splitting of the mind whereby the existence of a "subconscious" of some kind becomes manifest. This conviction does not necessitate or support the belief that a subconsciousness of the same kind exists in every human being, although this has been very widely held. Perhaps the most noteworthy presentation of this view is that set forth in Frederic Myers's doctrine of the subliminal self—a doctrine based largely, though not exclusively, on data provided by work done in the field of abnormal psychology. But even if we accepted, in whole or in part, Myers's view of the subliminal, we should have to recognise that the subconscious of Janet or the co-conscious of Morton Prince is only a special manifestation of subliminal activity and, so far as the evidence goes, a product of abnormal or psychopathic states. For the subconsciousness of hysteria and of hypnotic experiment has this peculiarity, that it is capable of manifesting as a form of awareness concurrent, though not compresent, with the supraliminal awareness of ordinary waking life ; and this is not a necessary or demonstrable accompaniment of other kinds of subliminal activity.

As has been already indicated, mental dissociation presents itself to us in a great variety of forms, but we may here disregard all the common symptoms of hysteria, such as anæsthesia and paralysis, and confine our attention to those divisions of the self which we meet with in double or multiple personality. All the time, however, we shall have in mind the parallel conditions of hypnotic and hysterical somnambulisms and the incipient forms of secondary personality displayed in fugues or ambulatory automatisms.

We have to consider, then, the opinions most commonly held concerning the nature of secondary personalities and the causes which bring them into being. We speak almost indifferently of double personality, multiple personality, or secondary personality. Sometimes there are only two personalities, the " primary " and the " secondary." Sometimes the division of the self is of such a nature that more than two personalities appear, and these are the cases to which the term " multiple personality " is most appropriately applied. Any one of the new selves, however many there may be, is conveniently referred to as a secondary personality or secondary self.

The most noticeable feature of such divisions of the self is the break in the continuity of memory, for it is on the continuity of memory that the feeling of personal identity is based. When there is no amnesia of one phase by the other, we may hesitate to speak of double personality, notwithstanding the differences of character and conduct which the alternating phases may reveal. Yet from one point of view the change of character is the more important ; and, when there is no amnesia, it is perhaps only because we have no doubt that the " subject of experience " is one and the same throughout the alternating phases that we do not think of the secondary phase as being in any true sense a secondary self. When there is amnesia of one phase by the other, such a doubt may arise, but it is only in those forms of secondary personality which claim co-consciousness that this doubt becomes serious.

The presence or absence of amnesia between the two phases is closely related to the presence or absence of co-consciousness, and all cases of double personality may be divided into two great groups or types, the amnesic and the co-conscious. In the amnesic type one phase, A, alternates with another phase, B, and each phase is amnesic of the other ; A does not know B, and B does not know A. In the co-conscious type, A and B alternate, just as in the amnesic type ; but, although A does not know B, B knows A and remembers all that A has thought or done during its emergent period.

This peculiarity of the memory relations of the two phases in the co-conscious group is due to the secondary phase being a co-conscious personality. When A is "out," in possession of the body, B is co-consciously aware of A's experiences, while, at the same time, it has other and different experiences of its own which are not shared by A. Therefore, when B comes "out," it has no amnesia, for it can recall all the experiences of A. But when A again appears, it has knowledge only of its own former periods of emergence and has no knowledge of those of B. There is amnesia, but it is a one-sided amnesia ; it acts in one direction only.

This is, of course, the ordinary memory relation observed in hypnotic experiment. The hypnotised person has memory of his whole life, including the periods of previous hypnoses ; in the waking state he remembers only his waking life. The hypnotic phase corresponds, in its memory relations at least, to a co-conscious secondary personality. The importance of the distinction between the two types of secondary personality becomes more apparent when we consider the nature and origin of these alternating phases of conscious life.

The common view of the nature of secondary personalities is that they are split-off fragments of the normal self—fragments in the sense of being systems of cognitive dispositions and of emotional and conative tendencies, broken off or dissociated from the " personal consciousness." This view is supported by the records of those cases in which the normal self has been restored by a synthesis of two or more secondary selves. Indeed, everything we know of this type of double personality points to the correctness of this interpretation.

The explanation of co-conscious personalities in terms of dissociation is not so easy and is not so satisfactory. It is not justifiable to speak of a thing being split-off or dissociated from another unless the two things have at some time been joined or associated together. But evidence that co-conscious personalities have, at any time, been integral parts of the normal or primary personality is hard to find ; and it is equally difficult to find records of " cure " in which a co-conscious personality has become assimilated by, or incorporated in, the primary or "personal consciousness." The synthesis which brings about the restoration of the normal self in amnesic cases is a linking-up of memories and an assimilation of tendencies which have been privately owned and separately experienced by each of the secondary selves ; but a co-conscious personality already knows, if it cannot be said to share, the experiences and memories of the primary personality and, in this respect at least, cannot be said to be split-off or dissociated from it. If a mere synthesis of memories were all that is necessary, a co-conscious personality might be considered to be the normal self !

In this connection, however, it must be remembered that, although B knows A's experiences, it knows them as belonging to A. Known by B apparently directly, they yet lack the warmth and intimacy which distinguish all experiences that we call " our own." We seem here to have not merely a dissociation of the contents of the mind, but the appearance of two distinct subjects of experience. Whatever the basis of selfhood may be, we have here a manifestation of two selves in one individual organism, each of which may have, at the same time, a distinct and separate experience—an experience, it may be, of the same object. A may look at an orange and have thoughts and feelings about it. At the same time B co-consciously sees the orange and has thoughts and feelings about it which may be different from those of A. Further, B is aware that A looks at the orange, and aware also of A's thoughts and feelings. How B becomes aware of A's experiences is a problem distinct from the essential problem of co-consciousness, namely, the seeming existence of two subjects of experience related to one bodily organism.

The difficulties inherent in the conception of co-consciousness are so great that many psychologists are prone to deny that true co-consciousness ever occurs. They say either that B's " experience " is not a conscious one or that, if it is, it is not concurrent with A's. Yet this matter ought to be beyond dispute. No one who has made personal observations or experimented with a co-conscious personality can doubt the concomitance of the secondary mental activity, nor can he find any good grounds for believing that it is not a " conscious " activity in the full sense of the word. As Dr Morton Prince has well said, "the evidence for co-consciousness . . . is of precisely the same character as that for the occurrence of consciousness in any other individual but oneself."*

* Morton Prince, *The Unconscious*, p. 158.

O

But we believe this consciousness to be of the same nature as our own, namely, the "experience" of a "subject." It is difficult, therefore, to understand the position taken up by Dr Morton Prince on this very topic which in other respects he has done so much to illuminate. He makes a distinction between "awareness" or "self-awareness" and the mere quality of "consciousness." By "self-awareness" he seems to mean an awareness *by* a self, and he maintains that "consciousness is not synonymous, co-extensive, or identical with self-awareness." He believes that any of the diversified types of conscious processes may become segregated from the main dominant consciousness and function co-consciously, but by functioning co-consciously he means functioning " without the self or ' I ' or anything being aware of the co-conscious process; and without the co-conscious process having any self or self-awareness, or anything, such as an ' experiencer ' that is aware."*

Such a view is only possible if we adopt the epiphenomenalist standpoint and regard consciousness as a mere by-product of neural activity, a sort of phosphorescent glow which may or may not contribute to the experience of some subject, may or may not join up with the more widespread phosphorescence presumably constituting or accompanying the feeling of selfhood. But if the consciousness manifested in co-conscious experiences were of this nature, we should never have known anything about such experiences. We know of them only because they are the experiences of a subject, some self or *ego*, which can tell us about them. All evidence of co-consciousness is evidence of awareness by a self.

Dr Morton Prince was, no doubt, referring more particularly to data derived from the study of abnormal and artificially induced states other than multiple personality, such as hysterical anæsthesia and suggested contractures; and, presumably, he would not deny the " self-awareness " of such a co-consciousness as that exhibited by "Sally." But it seems to me that the whole problem of co-consciousness is bound up with the continuity or gradation of the co-conscious phenomena observed in passing from hysterical anæsthesia to full-blown secondary personality. If the pin-prick on the anæsthetic arm of a hysteric is felt—and there is good evidence that it is—then it is felt by some self ; yet it is not felt by the self that is the "conscious personality" at the moment.

What, then, is this self that is aware in co-conscious experience ?

---

* Proceedings and Papers of the 7th International Congress of Psychology, p. 126.

Is there here a "subject" distinct from that which has the experience of the primary personality ? Some years ago* I endeavoured to reconcile the phenomena of co-consciousness with belief in the unitary nature of man's being, and to show that it may be possible to understand how one and the same "soul" or psyche or subject may be concerned in all states of consciousness occurring in one individual organism, whether these be successive or simultaneous. If, however, this belief is untenable when two streams of consciousness manifest simultaneously, some other hypothesis is necessary if we are not to deny altogether the actuality of co-conscious personalities.

Professor McDougall is one of the few psychologists who have fairly faced the difficulties inherent in the conception of co-consciousness. In a study of Dr Morton Prince's record of the Beauchamp case he set forth the problems presented by the Sally personality.† In his book *Body and Mind* and, later, more explicitly in his presidential address to the Society for Psychical Research in 1920, he maintained that a co-conscious personality must be regarded as a manifestation of a psychic being normally subordinated to the dominant one which forms the conscious self of each of us. He believes we are compelled to recognise that not infrequently a single human organism or person is the seat of more than one stream of conscious knowing, feeling and striving, and that each of such distinct streams is the activity of a unitary self or *ego*. He put the consequences of this view quite plainly when he said‡ : " I who consciously address you am only one among several selves or *egos* which my organism, my person, comprises. I am only the dominant member of a society, an association of similar members . . . But I and my associates are all members of one body ; and, so long as the organism is healthy, we work harmoniously together . . . If I am weak and irresolute . . . one or more of my subordinates gets out of hand, I lose my control, and division of the personality into conflicting systems replaces the normal and harmonious co-operation of all members in one system. And in such extreme cases a revolted subordinate, escaped from the control of the dominant member or monad, may continue his career of insubordination indefinitely, acquiring increased influence over the other members of the society and becoming a serious rival to the normal ruler or dominant. Such

---

* " Some Types of Multiple Personality." *Proceedings, S.P.R.*, 1912 ; and *Medical Psychology and Psychical Research*, 1923.
† *Proceedings, S.P.R.*, Vol. XIX, p. 410.
‡ *Ibid*, Vol. XXXI, pp. 111, 112.

a rebellious member was the famous Sally Beauchamp, and such was, I suggest, the childish phase of the Doris Fischer case."

When Dr McDougall first put forward his views on the nature of co-conscious personalities he believed that "abnormal conditions of two distinct types are commonly confused together under the head of co-consciousness or subconscious activity,* and that a second soul or psyche is necessary in the one type and not in the other. In the one type we cannot refuse to recognise the co-conscious activities "as the activities of an independent synthetic centre, a numerically distinct psychic being . . . In the other type we have to do with a mere insufficiency of synthetic energy of the one centre, from which results a temporary narrowing of the field of attentive consciousness, and the automatic or semi-mechanical functioning of parts of the psycho-physical organisation."†

This view seems open to the criticism that although at the extremes of the series of co-conscious phenomena the conditions do, indeed, seem to be very different, it is impossible to say at what point secondary psychic beings must be assumed. His more recent exposition of his views takes away the point of this criticism ; for he now makes a thorough-going application of the metaphysical doctrine of Leibnitz and Lotze, that "the body is in its real nature an organised system of beings of like nature with the soul" ; and he finds in this conception the most satisfactory solution not only of the facts of co-conscious personality, but also of the automatisms of sleep and hypnosis. Dream images and dream thoughts are for him the reflection, in the passive self of the dreamer, of the thoughts of subordinate members of the psychic hierarchy. In hypnosis, also, the dominant monad is passive and all the phenomena of hypnotic and post-hypnotic suggestion are due to the activity of subordinate psychic beings.

A similar view of the nature of multiple personality has been put forward by Mr Gerald Balfour. In his opinion every distinct stream of consciousness implies a distinct centre of psychical activity or mind, and "a plurality of distinct streams of consciousness in man implies a plurality of minds associated in the human organism."‡ He upholds the Leibnitzian doctrine "that the living creature is a kind of hierarchy of monads arranged in orderly and systematic relations with each other, each reflecting

---

* *Body and Mind*, p. 368.
† *Ibid*, pp. 368–9.
‡ *Proceedings*, *S.P.R.*, Vol. XIX, p. 392.

in its own way the states of consciousness of all the rest."* The *rapport* that is necessary for the harmonious co-operation of all the members of the system is, in Mr Balfour's opinion, of the nature of telepathy—a view which Dr McDougall also accepts.

Thus we have three possible ways of interpreting the facts of co-consciousness, none of which is altogether satisfying. We may try to believe with Dr Morton Prince (and much of Janet's writing carries the same implications) that co-consciousness may exist in the void, " without any self or self-awareness, or anything, such as an 'experiencer' that is aware." Or we may try to understand how the subject of the co-conscious experience may be the same as that of the supraliminal one. Or, lastly, we may feel compelled to fall back on a belief in a multiplicity of psychic beings, connected with one bodily organism and brought into intimate *rapport* with each other telepathically. Strictly speaking, a fourth possibility ought to be referred to. If a separate psychic being is necessary to account for co-consciousness, it may be suggested that this psychic being is an invasion from outside and not a normals constituent of the psycho-physical organism. This is the spiritistic explanation of the secondary personalities of trance-mediumship—the old hypothesis of " spirit possession."

As has been already indicated, the facts of co-conscious personality raise another problem besides those concerning the subject that has the co-conscious experience. It raises the problem of dissociation in so far as this is held to be a splitting-off of some part of the mind which at one time entered into the formation of the " personal consciousness " or " conscious personality." We must distinguish between the use of the term " dissociated " as a description implying merely *not-associated-with* and as a description implying *split-off-from*. We may, if we speak loosely, call Sally a dissociated personality, because she was a separate personality distinct from Miss Beauchamp ; but, as Dr McDougall has pointed out, there is hardly a scrap of evidence to warrant her being described as a split-off personality. At least, there is no evidence that she formed part of the adult Miss Beauchamp before her illness, and there is little evidence that she contributed much to the personality of the Miss Beauchamp restored by Dr Prince's treatment.

The assumption that all secondary personalities are due to fragmentation of an originally whole self has coloured all the hypotheses that have been put forward to account for their formation. The hypothesis for a long time most widely accepted as

* *Proceedings*, *S.P.R.*, Vol. XIX, p. 392.

satisfactorily explaining the occurrence of mental dissociation is that put forward by Janet. He ascribed to it a lowering of mental tension, a lack of synthetic energy and a localisation of the mental insufficiency on one or more functions which in consequence drop out of consciousness. Secondary personalities and their alternations are, in Janet's opinion, due to a kind of oscillation of the mental level which falls and rises suddenly. When the nervous tension falls, some whole state of mental activity becomes dissociated : when the mental level rises again, the normal personality is restored.

In recent years there has been an increasing readiness to abandon this somewhat mechanical explanation and to apply the psychoanalytical conception of mental conflict and repression in explanation of the occurrence of mental dissociation. And this hypothesis is made use of by many who are chary of accepting any other part of Freudian doctrine. But it is only in a very general way that the conception of repression has been applied to the dissociations of multiple personality. Neither Freud himself nor any one of his immediate followers seems to have had the good fortune to study a case of double or multiple personality by the method of psychoanalysis. Moreover, psychoanalysis as a method of psychological investigation is ill-suited to bring into prominence the characteristic features of this condition. It would, we may suppose, rather tend to blur or obliterate them ; whereas the " hypnotic method " not only reveals but tends to accentuate them, sometimes indeed appearing to make more complete the dissociation already existing, and thus give precision of outline to states originally vaguely defined.

The pictures resulting from these two modes of investigating multiple personality may be compared to those represented respectively by cross-sections and longitudinal sections of an object, such as some animal or vegetable tissue under a microscope ; or, to vary the metaphor, the hypnotic method brings into clear relief and preserves the stratification of the mind constituted by the various personalities, while the psychoanalytical method is that of the excavator who digs through the strata and brings to the surface variously-coloured earths which tell him of the existence of a stratification which he cannot directly see.

But, although psychoanalysis has not, up to the present, added much directly to our knowledge of the nature of multiple personality, it has provided us with some valuable conceptions which are applicable here as in all psychopathic states, and it has not been lacking in interesting speculations concerning the mental mechanism underlying some of the observed phenomena.

In so far as the theory of the *libido* is applicable to all hysterical manifestations, it is, of course, applicable to multiple personality, if this is to be regarded as an outcome of hysterical dissociation. So, also, in the conception of mental conflict and repression as a determinant of mental dissociation we have a hypothesis which bears much fruit in the investigation of cases of this kind. But, although repression may be accepted as an adequate explanation of the occurrence of dissociation when some unbearable idea or wish becomes split-off from the conscious self, it does not seem so easy to account for the formation of a fully-developed secondary personality out of the mental material that may thus be dissociated. This has been sometimes accounted for by saying that here, unlike what happens in the minor dissociations underlying ordinary psycho-neurotic states, we have a dissociation of a whole " side of one's character " or of some system of complexes which has been formed in the course of the conscious life of the individual.

Dr Morton Prince has described three such systems which may form the basis of more or less well marked divisions of the self. There are, he says, (1) Subject Systems depending on the various distinct subjects of knowledge or fields of activity which ordinarily form our main interests ; (2) Chronological Systems embracing the experiences of certain periods of our lives ; (3) Disposition or Mood Systems, " sides to one's character," tendencies to which we are prone and to which we may sometimes give way. Of these systems the last is perhaps the most important in relation to divisions of the self. Hardly ever do we meet with pathological dissociation that can be ascribed to a conflict between subject systems or in which the secondary self shows a special predilection for any of the vocational activities or avocational interests of the previously normal self. Chronological systems do not ordinarily appear to play an important part in the structure of the self. The sharply-defined limits of the amnesia sometimes encountered in multiple personality would seem to depend upon affective factors or to be related to traumatic experiences rather than to be evidence of a pre-existing chronological systematisation. Indications of the presence of Disposition or Mood Systems, however, are so commonly seen in everyday life that we must regard this form of systematisation as a normal occurrence ; and the alterations of character which accompany divisions of the self would seem to find their most likely explanation in a morbid exaggeration of dispositions or moods which are in some degree common to all of us.

All recent psychological investigations teach us that we must look to the unconscious for an explanation of these moods. When, then, a secondary personality appears which seems to be an exaggeration of a mood to which the individual was previously liable, we are not justified in saying that the secondary personality has been formed by a *splitting-off from consciousness* of the mood system ; for the mood itself can be explained only by reference to what has been hitherto unconscious. It is rather as if the occurrence of the mood in the everyday conscious life were but a temporary uprush from the unconscious of the activity of a complex there existing. A " mood " personality cannot be explained as being a split-off portion of the normal self ; it is rather the efflorescence of a " personality " already existing in the unconscious.

We are thus led to suppose that when a true change of personality occurs, we are witnessing a " side to one's character " which has been present in its fullness in the unconscious only ; and it has there the attributes, not merely of a mood, but of a secondary self.

How then has such a secondary self come into being ? If we adopt the psychoanalytical view that all unconscious states and tendencies are a result of repression, it is not easy to see how the repression to which the developmental life of everyone is subjected can account for the existence in the unconscious of what may later reveal itself as a secondary personality ; nor is it easy to imagine, even when development has been abnormal and repression presumably abnormal also, that anything corresponding to the secondary personality which may manifest later has ever been assumed in its totality by the " conscious self " and become repressed in mass into the unconscious. We must rather suppose that it has originated and grown in the unconscious and has been kept there by the repressing forces. When, in the unconscious conflict which its presence there engenders, the repressing forces prove too weak, it displaces the normal personality and takes possession of the organism.

So far as can be ascertained from introspection or from observation of the developmental life of others, none of the experiences of life would seem adequate to account for the presence in the unconscious of anything that could give rise to the phenomenon of double personality. Nor, until recently, has psychoanalysis helped us much in our efforts to understand this matter. Freud, however, in one of his latest writings, has thrown out a very interesting suggestion concerning the nature and origin of secondary personalities. In discussing some points connected with the psychoanalytical doctrine of *Identification*, he says : " If these identifications gain ground and become too numerous, too strong and mutually incompatible, we may expect a pathological result. It may end in a disintegration of the *ego*, the separate identifications shutting themselves off on account of their resistances against one another. Possibly the secret of so-called Multiple Personality is that the separate identifications usurp consciousness one after another. Even when it does not reach this point there is the setting-up of conflicts between the different identifications which are causing the disintegration of the *ego*, conflicts which, after all, cannot be described as wholly pathological."*

Jung, also, lays stress on the part played by identification in causing divisions of the self. He says† : " Identification is an estrangement of the subject from himself in favour of an object in which the subject is to a certain extent disguised. . . . Identification is distinguished from imitation by the fact that identification is an unconscious imitation, whereas imitation is a conscious copying." He further says that, just as imitation is an indispensable expedient for the developing personality of youth, so identification may be progressive in so far as " the individual way " is not yet available. "But, whenever a better individual possibility presents itself, identification manifests its pathological character . . . For now it has a dissociating influence, dividing the subject into two mutually estranged personalities."

It is hardly possible to test the value of this hypothesis by examining the records of cases of multiple personality investigated by the " hypnotic method." Observers in the future will have an opportunity of judging whether the conclusions of the analysts are well founded ; and, if they are so, whether identification can be regarded as a constant factor in the genesis of secondary personalities, or one that only sometimes plays a part.

---

* *Das Ich und das Es*, p. 35.
† *Psychological Types*, p. 551.

THE HANDWRITING IN NERVOUS DISEASES, WITH SPECIAL REFERENCE TO THE SIGNATURES OF WILLIAM SHAKESPEARE

BY

CHARLES L. DANA, A.M., M.D., LL.D.

Professor of Nervous Diseases, Cornell University Medical College; Consulting Neurologist to Bellevue Hospital, The Neurological Institute; ex-President of The New York Academy of Medicine

Illustrated

THE HANDWRITING IN NERVOUS DISEASES, WITH SPECIAL REFERENCE TO THE SIGNATURES OF WILLIAM SHAKESPEARE

BY

CHARLES L. DANA

THE object of my studies of handwriting, the results of which are presented here, was to see whether any of the chronic diseases or established toxicities of the nervous system were shown specifically in the handwriting, excluding altogether the mental element both direct and indirect.

Some studies along this line were made by Erlenmeyer in his monograph *Die Schrift* (1905), by Rogner de Fursac, in *Les Écrits et les Dessins dans les Maladies Nerveuses et Mentales* (Paris, 1905), by Bucard, in *La Graphologie et Médecine* (Thèse de Paris, 1905) ; but none of these followed the matter along just the lines that I have done.

One of the things which stimulated this investigation was an interest in the curious and concededly abnormal handwriting of William Shakespeare and my findings are applied to his signatures.

In carrying out my work I have for fifteen years made patients suffering from paralysis agitans, multiple sclerosis, writer's cramp, chronic alcoholism, paresis, tabes, epilepsy, senile deterioration, and various forms of tremor, write their signatures. In many cases, for the special reason suggested above, I made them write also an unfamiliar name, *e.g.*, that of William Shakespeare, and often a long name like Constantinople. My interest sometimes flagged and I have lost some of my material, which consisted of over 200 specimens. Many of these were obtained in the alcoholic and psychiatric wards of Bellevue Hospital, but most of them were from private patients, the signatures being made in my office. My particular collection of " William Shakespeare " signatures was obtained for the purpose of seeing how closely a neuro-psychotic person could approximate some of the characteristics of the dramatist's signature.

I obtained and studied the signatures and specimens of writing in the following cases :—

Paralysis·agitans and encephalitis ...	60
Chronic and convalescent alcoholism ...	14
Paresis	29
Writer's cramp	19
Tabes	5
Multiple sclerosis	5
Petit mal and various types of senility and of organic brain disease (hemiplegia) ...	14
Total	146

In analysing the abnormalities of handwriting due to neural disorders and not to mental states, one finds that there are two quite dominant variants from ordinary script : an ataxia or disorder of form, and a tremor. The former is seen normally in children and in persons who are learning to write or who have been imperfectly educated ; and some of this quality is seen in senility. Tremor, however, does not occur in normal neural conditions. There are several other handwriting variants which I have had to consider. Thus the letters of the script may be very large or very small, and may change in size as the signature is being finished. The letters may be crowded or overspaced or not run together ; the signature may slope up or down and the end of the signature may be blurred. The lines may show unevenness of pressure with blotting and exaggeration of the shaded parts of the lines.

I arranged these variants in the following order :—

Ataxia, including waviness and angularities of line
Tremor
Macro- or micrographia, constant or progressive
Crowding and fusing of letters
Spacing and disuniting of letters (painting the letters)
Sloping of the level
Terminal blurring ; this applying especially to autographs.

These are not the only things possible to find in bad handwriting, but they furnish definite factors for comparative study.

The quality of co-ordinate and orderly movement necessary to normal script can be modified by lesions of the sensory-motor cortex and pyramids which may cause tremor, ataxia, paresis, or rigidities ; by lesions of the caudo-lenticulo-rubral region causing hypertension, tremor, disorder of automatic associated movements ; by cerebellar rubral lesions and by lesions of the afferent nerves, as in tabes.

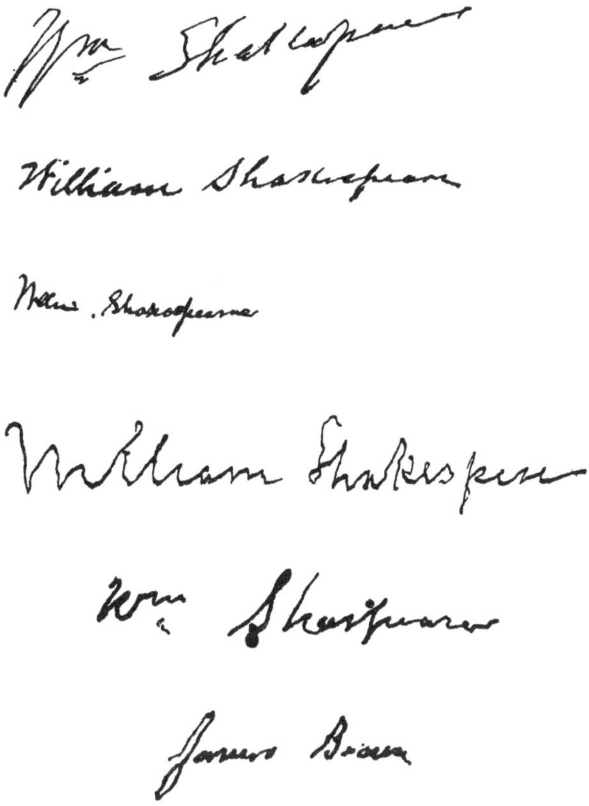

FIG. 1.—Paralysis Agitans.

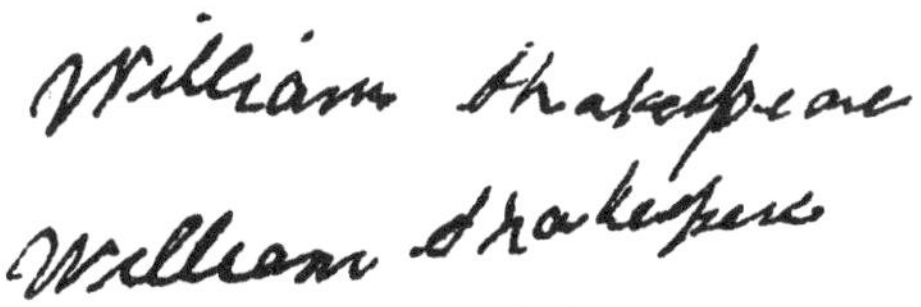

FIG. 2.—Encephalitis lethargica.

Thus we may expect a different handwriting in cortical lesions (paresis), in lenticulo-rubral regions (Parkinson's disease), in the spinocerebellar rubral lesions (writer's cramp, multiple sclerosis), and in the afferent nerves giving deep sensation, as in tabes.

There is a form of bad and formless handwriting, which is largely mental and due partly to carelessness, to vanity, or to a congenital lack of manual dexterity. This is easily recognised as different from the ataxias of a child's signature and those of the graphically uneducated.

After going over my signatures and scripts, I conclude that there are very few nervous diseases or conditions which can be diagnosed by the handwriting alone; among these, paralysis agitans in its somewhat advanced stage stands first; the Parkinsonian types of encephalitis can also be recognised. Tremulousness, lack of terminal finish of the signature, painted lettering and progressive micrographia are the characteristic traits of these conditions; tremor and micrography being especially important (see my *Textbook of Nervous Diseases*, p. 593).

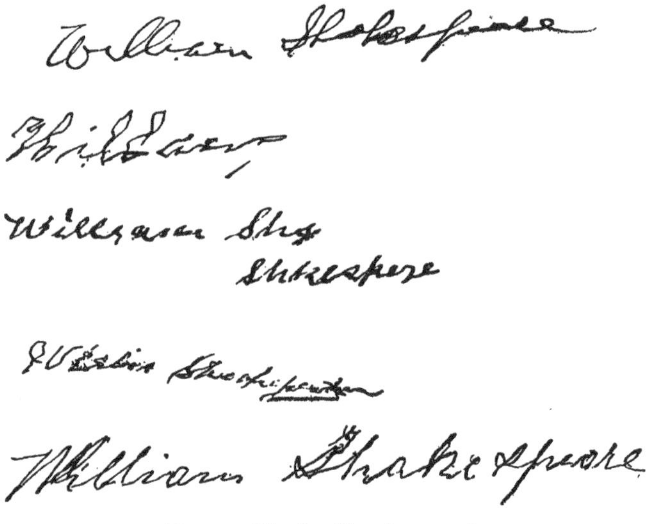

Fig. 3.—Handwriting in paresis.

Paresis can often be recognised by the character of the hand-writing plus the nature of what is written. In this disease one sees ataxia, tremor, irregular level, blots, omission of letters, erasures, etc. It is the character of the written material, however, and not the script that counts most. One thing I rarely observed in paresis, and that was a confusion of the terminal letters. The patient always finished his signature well, as might be expected from a condition in which self-confidence dominates.

The most prevalent element of my signatures in writer's cramp was tremor. It could be observed in almost every case. The tremor is fine, not jerky, and sometimes difficult to note without close study. In writer's cramp, the patient often knows that it is going to be hard to write his signature and so takes special pains to do his best. While writer's cramp cannot be recognised by the signature alone, the study of several lines in which the writing becomes worse and finally breaks down may indicate the disease.

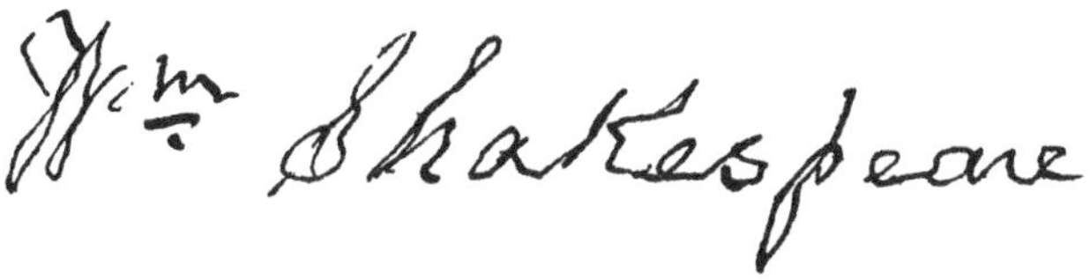

FIG. 4.—Senile tremor.

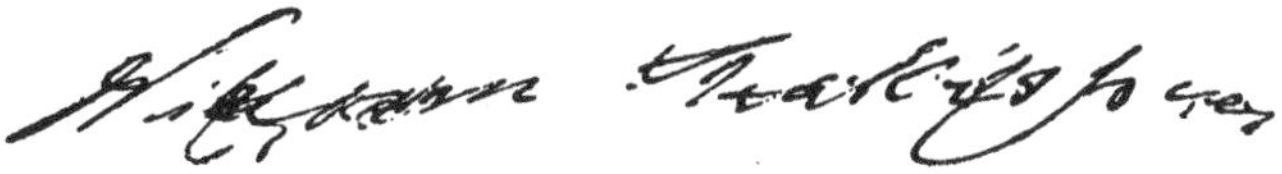

FIG. 5.—Tabes dorsalis.   Arm type.

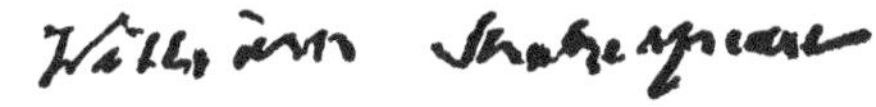

After 3 weeks' drinking.

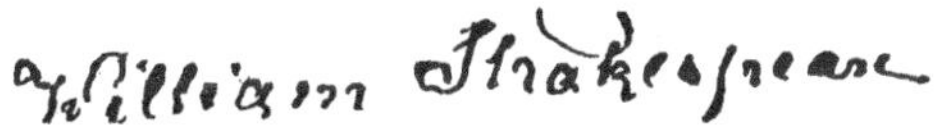

On discharge.

FIG. 6.—Alcoholism.

In multiple sclerosis, the patient's signature is good until the disease definitely involves the arms. Then there is shown some ataxia, but more especially a jerky tremor. In tabes, involving the arms, one gets the worst and most formless of all signatures, due to neural lesion alone.

It is possible to make a diagnosis of epilepsy—or *petit mal*, by the handwriting. This occurred to me with a patient, a man of 40, who had curious motor seizures resembling hysterical attacks. I told him to write his name on the blackboard, and this is what

P

happened. He took the chalk and wrote a tremulous F, then stopped and laid down his chalk ; two or three seconds later he took up the chalk and wrote his name freely and readily. He said he did not know why he made the first tremulous F, or why he did not go on. There was no doubt that it was written in a moment of *petit mal*. It cleared up the diagnosis about which we had been in doubt.

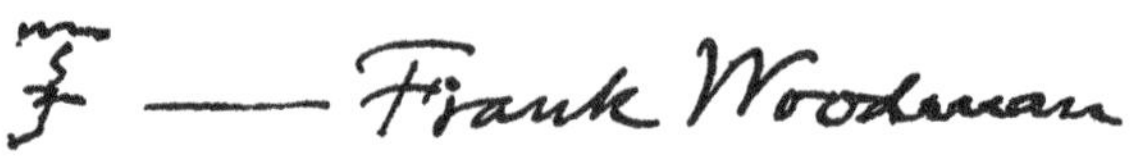

FIG. 7.—Signature started during an attack of *petit mal*.

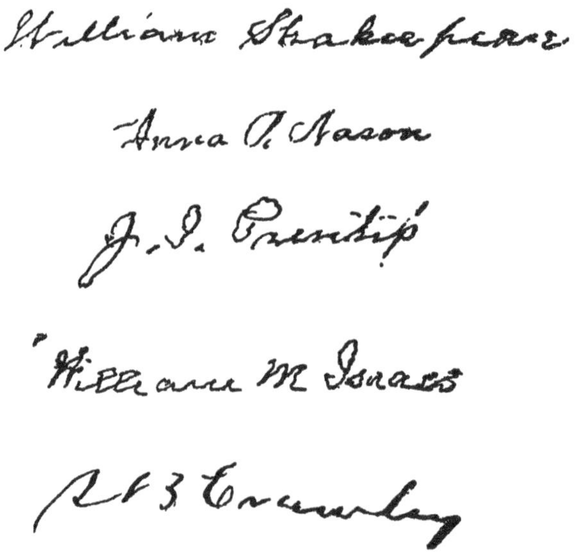

FIG. 8.—Writer's cramp.

Having made these special studies of handwriting, I proceeded to apply them to the signatures of William Shakespeare. I had to be convinced first, and naturally, that Shakespeare's signatures do indicate abnormality.

The problems connected with Shakespeare are hardly less interesting than his dramas, and his handwriting is one of the problems. There are only six veritable signatures of Shakespeare, and no handwriting of his other than these is in existence. These signatures are presented here.   There are three other signatures* that are possibly Shakespeare's, and some high authorities hold that three pages of a certain manuscript play of Sir Thomas More are in Shakespeare's handwriting.†

On the other hand, Sir G. G. Greenwood has written (in 1920) a booklet‡ in which he argues that none of the signatures are those of the great dramatist.

I am not expressing an opinion myself, but there is a general agreement prevailing that the six signatures at least are genuine. The first three were made in connection with the purchase and mortgage of a building about three years before his death.   The last three were the signatures of his will which was drafted in January, 1616, and signed in March.   He died in April, 1616, about a month after he signed the will.

One of his three signatures made on his will has become partially effaced or marred.   But, in 1776, Geo. Stevens traced all the three signatures on the will and they were engraved in 1788.   They were traced and engraved in J. G. Nichol's *Book of Autographs.*   We have now photographic replicas of them all.

The handwriting of Shakespeare's time was a modified inheritance from Anglo-Saxon ancestors and was essentially Gothic, or, as some say, "Old English."   This was the handwriting taught in schools and used by Shakespeare.   Scholars and university-trained men used the cursive Italian script.   The ordinary handwriting of the day was quite good and as legible as is that of to-day (E. Maunde Thompson).

Shakespeare's signatures do not seem to be those of a person with normal control of his handwriting.   The things that can be noted are unequal pressure of the pen, irregularities in the loops and curves, an evidence of a jerky tremor, and a running together and confusion of the letters at the end.   These defects are present in his latest autographs, even if we allow that Shakespeare made contractions in writing his name, as was the custom in those days.

* *Signatures* :
  1. Will, March, 1616.
  2.   „   „   „
  3.   „   „   „
  4. Upon a deposition in a lawsuit, May 11th, 1612.
  5. On a deed and on a mortgage in purchase of Blackfriar's house, March 10th and 11th, 1613.
  6. Florio's translation of Montaigne in British Museum.
  7. Alden's edition of Ovid's *Metamorphoses.*
  8. Plutarch's *Lives.*
  † *Shakespeare's Hand in Sir Thomas More,* by A. W. Pollard and others. (Cambridge University Press, 1923.)
  ‡ *The Handwriting of Shakespeare* (Lane, 1920).

A study of the abnormalities has been made by Sir E. Maunde Thompson (*Shakespeare's Hand in the Play of Sir Thomas More*, p. 57) in great detail and his figures show an apparent progressive deterioration.

This is seen perhaps best in a selection and reproduction of the capital S in five autographs, the first three made 3 years before death, the last two about a month before death, as shown here :—

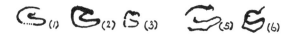

FIG. 10.—The capital letter S of the five Shakespeare signatures. (Thompson.)

The book referred to, *Shakespeare's Hand in the Play of Sir Thomas More*, as already stated, presents arguments to show that three pages in the above play are in Shakespeare's handwriting. The arguments are interesting and are made by eminent Shakespearean scholars and palæontologists. Whether their view is correct or not, does not affect my particular study or point of view, for, if Shakespeare did write the three pages, he did it when he was only twenty-five years old and certainly had no manual neurosis at that time.

One of the contributors to the above work is Sir E. Maunde Thompson, a Shakespearean scholar and palæontologist. He considers that the six Shakespearean signatures made in the last three years of his life are abnormal, and he suggests that Shakespeare had writer's cramp. An ingenious presentation of this view has been made also by Dr R. W. Leftwich (*British Medical Journal*, 1918, p. 542).

After Shakespeare gave up active dramatic work, he lived in Stratford most of the time. He was apparently not suffering from any serious or crippling disease, for he took an active part in local affairs and went occasionally to London ; but in January, 1616, he had a will drawn up, which means that he probably was not well. He did not sign the will, however, until March, and he died a month later.

The question arises, what illness could he have had which affected him for at least three years, which incidentally interfered with his handwriting, and perhaps led to his death ?

The possible diseases which may gradually and later rather seriously affect a man of 50, are Parkinson's disease, which kills in from 8 to 12 years, cerebral arterio-sclerosis with perhaps a moderate degree of right hemiplegia or monoplegia ; tabo-paresis ; chronic alcoholism, complicating arterial sclerosis ; multiple sclerosis ; and pre-senility—with tremor.

I was at first most inclined to think of paralysis agitans ; but a study of the handwriting excludes it. From my studies of abnormal handwriting, I should also exclude paresis, tabes and alcoholism. Alcoholism, as we see it, was comparatively rare in England in Elizabethan days. One can also exclude writer's cramp as a cause of his abnormal writing, in spite of the arguments of Dr Leftwich and Sir E. Maunde Thompson. Writer's cramp is a disease of the nineteenth century and came in with steel pens. It is a disease of clerks and not of brain workers or authors, and develops generally at about the age of 30, very rarely as late as 47. Among 24 private cases, all but four began in the 20's or 30's. Among all the signatures that I have seen or collected, there was none remotely suggesting that of Shakespeare.

I am not able to make a diagnosis of Shakespeare's neural condition. The signatures show a terminal blurring, which indicates fatigue of the automatic mechanism called into play in writing, but one can certainly exclude presumptive troubles like paralysis agitans, alcoholism and writer's cramp. It is a fair supposition, however, that a man who dies at fifty-two and has some trouble with his handwriting, had vascular disease. *A thrombotic condition affecting his left mid-brain and disturbing the automatic association mechanisms of that region would explain his defective signatures.*

THE STATIC AND KINETIC REPRESENTATIONS OF THE EFFERENT NERVOUS SYSTEM IN THE PSYCHO-MOTOR SPHERE

BY

J. RAMSAY HUNT, M.D.

Clinical Professor of Neurology, Columbia University

THE STATIC AND KINETIC REPRESENTATIONS OF THE EFFERENT NERVOUS SYSTEM IN THE PSYCHO-MOTOR SPHERE

BY

J. RAMSAY HUNT

DURING the past few years I have given especial attention to the problem of motility in health and disease and to the neural mechanisms governing its various manifestations. On the basis of these investigations I have formulated a new conception of the efferent nervous system, founded on the existence of separate mechanisms subserving respectively the functions of motion and posture [*see* Bibliography (1)].

The present study concerns the static and kinetic representations of the efferent system in the psychic sphere, and the psychomotor disturbances resulting from disorders of cortical function. This is the realm of purposive acts and movements and includes such disorders of higher motility as apraxia, perseveration and stereo-typed movements and attitudes. Before passing to this subject, however, I will give a brief outline of my views on the dual nature of the efferent system and its bearing on the general question of motility.

According to my theory, the kinetic mechanism consists of a series of systems which are concerned with the production and co-ordination of movement, the static system representing a co-extensive series of neural systems which are concerned with the maintenance and co-ordination of posture. All of the complicated phenomena of motility are dependent upon these twin mechanisms, which function together in harmonious co-operation.

The conception of a static and a kinetic mechanism, functioning together in the interest of motion and posture, finds confirmation in many different fields of research. There is also evidence showing that these two components of motility present a parallelism of structure and function at various levels of the efferent mechanism.

That there is mutual co-operation and harmony in the activity of these two systems is shown by reciprocal innervation, which is represented in the muscular activities of both the vegetative and cerebro-spinal nervous systems. Indeed, reciprocal innervation, as I conceive it, is essentially a harmonious interplay of innervation and denervation between these mutually antagonistic physiological systems.

Not only in the nervous system, but in the muscle fibre itself, there is evidence of a duality of structure and function. Movement is dependent on the fibrillary structure of the muscle fibre and postural fixation on its sarcoplasm and the differentiation of these two substances may be followed through the various stages of muscle development in the evolution of the striated from the nonstriated muscle fibre.

The neural systems of motility, therefore, like those of sensibility, may be resolved into more than one component, subserving different modalities of function, which result from the adaptation of the organism to surrounding physical forces. For the animal body, in its relation to the outer world, is either at rest or in a state of motion, and these two functions, so different in character, are both under the control of separate components of the efferent nervous system and its effector organs.

The cerebellum is, I believe, the essential integrating and correlating mechanism for the control of static function. All of the posture systems pass to the cerebellum for final integration and co-ordination, which is in accord with the nature of the posturing mechanism and its secondary and unconscious rôle in motility. For, while the higher forms of movement are initiated as conscious and voluntary processes, the corresponding postures are secondary, and follow automatically in the path of movement.

In striking contrast to this function, the kinetic mechanism is concerned with the transmission and co-ordination of impulses underlying movement, and represented in the *archæokinetic*, *palæokinetic*, and *neokinetic* systems [*see* Bibliography (2)]. These various physiological levels are in control of reflex, automatic-associated and isolated-synergic types of movement.

In harmony with the duality of function in the central nervous system the striated muscle fibre is also composed of two distinct substances, one subserving a contractile, the other a postural function. The sarcostyle is the contractile portion of the muscle fibre and represents the *myokinetic* mechanism ; the sarcoplasm is a more homogeneous substance and represents the postural or *myostatic* mechanism.

In the disorders of motility, as in normal motility, both the kinetic and static systems participate, although it is possible to indicate one or the other as essentially involved.

Chorea, paramyoclonus multiplex, myokymia and the tremor of paralysis agitans are of kinetic origin. Myotonia, on the other hand, is referable to the static system.

The characteristic symptoms of cerebellar disease, dyssynergia, dysmetria, dysdiadokokinesis and intention tremor indicate a disturbance of posture synergy and are referable to the static system. This subject I have discussed more fully in a special study of cerebellar function [see Bibliography (3)].

The principle of duality of function is also applicable to the vegetative mechanism, which represents the lowest phylogenetic level of the nervous system, the parasympathetic subserving a kinetic and the sympathetic outflow a static function. Here, the unstriped contractile fibre, like the striped variety, is composed of two distinct substances, the fibrillæ and the sarcoplasm, which subserve respectively primitive types of motion and primitive types of posture.

Therefore, in the realm of the vegetative as in the cerebro-spinal system it may be stated, as a general principle, that a disorder of the myostatic component affects postural tone, and a disturbance of the myokinetic system is characterised by a disorder of movement itself.

From this outline of my theory it will appear that the whole efferent nervous system presents a duality of function and structure, each of the great functional levels being characterised by a special type of movement and of posture. Each level is under the control of the higher level so that the efferent system is made up of a series of superimposed mechanisms, which represent a recapitulation of the phylogenetic history of motility.

Psychostatic and Psychokinetic Systems

I will now pass to a consideration of the representations of these two systems in the psychic sphere, for even in this complex realm evidences of a dual function are manifested in the morbid physiology of disease.

In the higher motor activities of the cerebral cortex the simpler elements of motility, both palæokinetic and neokinetic, undergo various combinations and are expressed as purposive acts and postures. This is the field of acquired motility, and one which may be indefinitely expanded with experience and the increasing demands of civilisation. Purposive acts are the natural expression of motility at the psychic level and present every conceivable variation, according to the habits and education of the individual. They represent ideas which are transformed and expressed in action.

In symptomatology a loss of this function is called apraxia, a term signifying an incapacity to execute purposive movements notwithstanding the preservation of muscular power, sensibility and co-ordination. In this disorder the defect is situated in those areas of the cerebral cortex where ideas are formed and expressed as purposive movements and postures.

Among the psychomotor activities of this description may be mentioned such simple acts as lighting a cigarette, closing a door, use of the knife and fork, and indeed all of those arts and crafts which are acquired by training and experience, the imprint of which remains fixed in memory and may be recalled and transformed into their corresponding actions and attitudes. In this sense the idea of an action or of an attitude is dependent for its expression upon a psychokinetic or psychostatic representation, in the same manner that a reflex movement or a synergic movement is dependent upon its corresponding kinetic mechanism.

Two great clinical types of apraxia may be recognised. One is due to a loss of the memories of objects, with a resulting *amnesic apraxia*. The other is dependent upon a loss of the ability to perform the act, the necessary content being undisturbed. This constitutes the *motor apraxia*, and in this sense certain motor disorders of speech and writing may be mentioned as apraxias of a higher order. Motor apraxia is therefore a paralysis of purposive movements and is the analogue in the psychomotor sphere of the other cardinal types of motor paralysis.

Kinetic and Static Perseveration

In apraxia a peculiar manifestation has been described by some writers as perseveration, which appears to have a direct bearing on the question of psychostatic and psychokinetic representation.

Perseveration in motor apraxia may be defined as the continued repetition of a given movement-complex when another act is intended. The repetition does not occur spontaneously but only when some new act is intended and in place of that act. This is a not uncommon symptom and has been termed by Liepmann [see Bibliography (4)] intentional perseveration. Another form of perseveration is that in which the patient continues making a particular movement or movement-complex, showing an inability to inhibit the movement once it has been initiated. Both of these types are well recognised in the symptomatology of nervous and mental disease.

It is interesting to note that perseveration may also occur in the sphere of speech and writing.

In addition to the types which are characterised by a disorder of movement there is another form of perseveration which is related to the posture sphere, and is characterised by a cessation or fixation of movement. In this form the patient comes to a standstill during or at the close of the performance of a given act. This may appear as a local or general manifestation, but in either case there is a fixation in a particular attitude which is maintained almost indefinitely. Cases presenting this symptom have been described by Pick [see Bibliography (5)], Kroll [see Bibliography (6)] and Coriat [see Bibliography (7)].

According to Wilson and Walshe [see Bibliography (8)] the repetition of a given movement in place of another, and the continued repetition of a given movement, when in a normal individual it would cease, should be known as active perseveration, whereas the cessation of action which results in the maintenance of an attitude, either in the middle or at the end of a given movement-complex should be known as passive perseveration. These terms they suggest in preference to clonic and tonic which were used by Liepmann in his description of the same type.

The terms *kinetic* and *static perseveration* may also be used in this connection and are even more descriptive as referring to the specific type of motor representation involved in the disorder.

In Pick's [see Bibliography (5)] study of motor apraxia cases are described which have a special bearing on this problem. One of his patients, asked to take a drink out of a jug on the table, put his lips and face into the mouth of the jug and remained so practically without moving. Another patient, asked to light a candle, held the match alight in her right hand, in the neighbourhood of the wick, quite immobile, until the match burned her fingers. These are examples of static perseveration. There is a premature postural fixation of a purposive movement before the purpose of the movement has been carried out.

In kinetic perseveration the patient continues uninterruptedly making a particular movement or movement-complex. Liepmann's patient, for instance, having begun to write certain words was unable to stop, and continued scribbling in senseless repetition. Campbell's [see Bibliography (9)] patient " continued to shake hands for an unusual length of time." A patient observed by Wilson, writing her name " Winnie," wrote Winninninninn . . indefinitely. A patient of Breukink, peeling potatoes, went on peeling indefinitely, apparently unable to cease.

Both of these forms therefore represent a cortical disorder of motility and are dependent on the release of static and kinetic representations at this level of the nervous system. One is a kinetic perseveration and the other a static perseveration, and both are referable to an organic disorder of the efferent system in the psychic sphere.

Psychokinetic and Psychostatic Manifestations of Hysteria

Among the various paroxysmal crises of major hysteria psychostatic and psychokinetic types of reaction may be recognised.

The classical types of hysterical disorders of motility :—convulsions, chorea, myoclonus, and tremor are all examples of the release of kinetic representations. These motor phenomena are all of psychogenic origin and are initiated by unconscious mental mechanisms or dissociations of cortical function. They often simulate very closely other kinetic manifestations which originate in lower motor mechanisms.

Disorders of the posture mechanism may also occur in major hysteria, an important example of which is catalepsy ; this may be partial or general and is characterised by a peculiar stiffness of the musculature and a waxy resistance on making passive movements. This is the *flexibilitas cerea* which fixes the limb in posture as soon as movement ceases and which may persist for a long period of time. A certain resemblance between myotonia and catalepsy may be mentioned and is of special interest, as both of these symptoms, I believe, are referable to the static system.

Stereotyped Movements and Attitudes in Dementia Præcox

In other disorders of cortical function, the occurrence of kinetic and static types of reaction are also evident in the symptomatology.

In dementia præcox, with its widespread disorder of psychic functions many peculiar disturbances of motility are described. Where there is a disturbance of the static mechanism, there is permanent fixation of certain muscles in various postures or attitudes, which may persist for weeks, months or even years. In the kinetic sphere there occur the various stereotyped movements which are so common in the catatonic form of this disorder. These movements may be repeated countless times over long periods.

According to Kraepelin [see Bibliography (11)] "stereotypy is a persistent fixation of certain muscle groups or a repetition of the same movement; in the first case the patients, in spite of all external influences, may retain the same attitude for weeks, months or years, with scarcely any change.   They may stand in the same posture, often a very uncomfortable one, or kneel on a certain spot.   The facial expression is stiff and mask-like, and the winking reflex diminished or obliterated.

"Stereotyped movements are naturally much more varied in character.   Among these may be mentioned the somersault, rhythmical clapping, making the sign of the cross, jumping, falling, rolling and creeping on the ground.   Bizarre arm movements, pulling the clothing and hair, bowing, balancing, rocking movements and grinding of the teeth.   These movements may be repeated numberless times for weeks and months.   It is almost impossible to stop them and they sometimes cause injury.

" In the terminal stage of catatonia one encounters occasionally a form of stereotypy which only faintly resembles those just described.   This form is characterised by regular rhythmical movements, especially balancing and swinging of the body, biting and nodding movements of the head."   According to Kraepelin, such symptoms are always the sign of a serious loss of volitional power and one is reminded of the rhythmical movements of certain animals, and it is possible that such movements are the expression of lower representations in our nervous system, which by the destruction of higher activities attain an independent expression in the sphere of motility.

Concluding Remarks

In the foregoing pages I have considered briefly the posture and motion components of the efferent system, their underlying neural mechanisms and their relation to symptomatology.

In the central nervous system of man, four great physiological divisions of the efferent mechanism may be recognised, which correspond to the evolutionary epochs in the development of motility. These are represented by reflex, the automatic-associated, isolated-synergic and purposive types of movements.

In the psychic sphere, as at the other levels, there are evidences of the dual nature of the efferent system. In this realm mental processes and movements are associated in innumerable combinations. This is a vast domain where motility ranges with intellect in the manifold activities presented by the life of man, and where purposive movements are but the functional homologues of reflex and synergic movements of lower levels.

BIBLIOGRAPHY

(1) Hunt (Ramsay) :
   a. The Dual Nature of the Efferent Nervous System. A Further Study of the Static and Kinetic Systems, their Function and Symptomatology. *Archives of Neurol. and Psych.*, July, 1923, Vol. x, p. 37
   b. The Static and Kinetic Systems of Motility. *Archives of Neurol. and Psych.*, October, 1920, Vol. IV, p. 353
   c. The Static or Posture System and its Relation to Postural Hypertonic States of the Skeletal Muscles, Spasticity, Rigidity and Tonic Spasm. *Neurological Bulletin*, June, 1921, Vol. III, No. 6, p. 207

(2) Hunt (Ramsay) :
   a. Progressive Atrophy of the Globus Pallidus (Primary Atrophy of the Pallidal System) : a System Disease of the Paralysis Agitans Type, Characterised by Atrophy of the Motor Cells of the Corpus Striatum. *Brain*, 1917, Vol. XL, Part 1, p. 58
   b. Primary Atrophy of the Pallidal System : a Contribution to the Nature and Pathology of Paralysis Agitans. *Archives of Intern. Med.*, November, 1918, Vol. XXII, p. 647

(3) Hunt (Ramsay) :
   Dyssynergia Cerebellaris Myoclonica (Primary Atrophy of the Dentate System) : a Contribution to the Pathology and Symptomatology of the Cerebellum. *Brain*, 1921, Vol. XLIV, p. 490

(4) Liepmann :
Ueber Störungen des Handelns bei Gehirn-Kranken, Berlin, 1905

(5) Pick :
Studien über motorische Ataxie, Leipzig and Wien, 1905

(6) Kroll :
Beiträge zum Studium der Apraxie. Zeitsch. f. d. ges. Neur. u. Psych., 1910, Bd. 11, S. 315

(7) Coriat :
The Psychopathology of Apraxia. Amer. Journ. of Psych., 1911, XXII, p. 65

(8) Wilson and Walshe :
The Phenomena of Tonic Innervation and its Relation to Motor Apraxia. Brain, 1914, XXXVII, p. 199

(9) Campbell· (MacFie) :
Agraphia in a Case of Frontal Tumor. Review of Neur. and Psych., 1911, IX, p. 289

(10) Breukink :
Ueber Patienten mit Perseveration und asymbolischen und aphasischen. Erscheinungen. Journ. f. Psych. u. Neur., 1907, IX, p. 113

(11) Kraepelin :
Stéréotypie : Psychiatrie, Vol. 1, 1909, p. 389

THE DEVELOPMENT OF PSYCHOPATHOLOGY
AS A BRANCH OF SCIENCE

BY

BERNARD HART, M.D.

Fellow of University College, London; Physician in Psychological Medicine, University College Hospital, London ; Lecturer in Psychiatry, University College Hospital Medical School

THE DEVELOPMENT OF PSYCHOPATHOLOGY
AS A BRANCH OF SCIENCE

BY

BERNARD HART

THE aim of this paper is to describe, in summary fashion, the history of psychopathology as a branch of science, and to consider how far it has succeeded in establishing its claim to an assured position within the fold of science.

The extent and boundaries of the path we desire to traverse will be made clearer if some preliminary words are devoted to the precise meaning of the terms in which the subject of inquiry has been defined. Psychopathology is to be understood, not as a mere description of mental symptoms, but as an endeavour to *explain* disorder or certain disorders in terms of psychological processes. Its difference from a mere description of mental symptoms is of the same order as that which exists between clinical medicine on the one hand, and on the other hand that explanation of the phenomena of clinical medicine in terms of causal processes which constitutes pathology. "Explain" is used here in the sense in which it constitutes the goal of the method of science. Science is not a compilation of facts, but a method of dealing with our experience. It consists in (1) the recording and classification of phenomenal experience, (2) the finding of formulæ which will serve to resume that experience. This latter part involves the construction of concepts or "laws" which will embrace the phenomena we have observed, and enable us to predict the occurrence of further phenomena, the validity of the "law" being tested by its capacity to fulfil these two conditions. The function of the scientific law and its relationship to the phenomena with which it is concerned may be exemplified by chemical phenomena and the atomic theory, physical phenomena and the law of gravitation, the phenomena of light and heat and the ether theory. It should be observed that these laws are not found or observed by the investigator, they are constructed by him to explain what he has

231

found or observed. The aim of science is to understand and control our phenomenal experience, and the validity of the concepts it constructs is determined by the extent to which they satisfy this aim. Each branch of science claims the right to construct its own concepts, provided that they are constructed according to the rules of scientific method.

That portion of our experience which is constituted by the behaviour of living organisms has been attacked by several branches of science, each regarding the phenomena from its own standpoint, and interpreting them in terms of its own concepts. Biology, for example, interprets the phenomena of living organisms in terms of life process and biological laws, physiology in terms of nervous energy, reflex action and so forth, chemistry in terms of the interaction of chemical compounds. Some of the phenomena are capable of explanation by the concepts of more than one branch of science, some can be more intelligibly and usefully explained by the concepts of one branch than by those of another, some are at present capable of explanation by the concepts of one branch only. The hope is always before us that the concepts of one branch may ultimately be reduced to the concepts of another, especially when the latter are concepts of a wider validity. There is a reasonable hope, for example, that the concepts of nervous energy and reflex action may ultimately be reduced to the wider concepts of chemistry and physics. But to a large extent such a reduction is a goal of the future, and for the present each branch must be content to explain whatever phenomena it can in terms of its own concepts, having always in view the essential aim of all science, the understanding and control of our experience by the fashioning of scientifically constructed " laws."

Can psychology claim a place as one of the branches of science capable of usefully explaining the phenomena of living organisms ? For a long time this claim was denied, and psychology was treated as an alien with no right of entry into the fold of science, because it dealt with non-material and non-spatial objects which the crude philosophy of the nineteenth-century scientist regarded as necessarily incapable of scientific treatment, and even as " epiphenomenal " and unreal. So soon as it was realised, however, that science is not defined by the nature of the objects with which it deals, but by the method of investigation applied to those objects, and that its field comprises the whole field of our experience, then the right of psychology to contribute its quota to the explanation of the phenomena presented by living organisms could no longer be gainsaid. Moreover, psychology could claim the right to interpret the phenomena in psychological terms, and to construct psychological concepts in order to explain those phenomena. The only condition, but one rigidly to be observed, was that the concepts must be constructed according to the method of science, that is to say, they must be based on carefully observed experience, they must serve to resume that experience, and they must be verifiable by an appeal to experience.

How far psychology has attempted to carry out this task in the elucidation of certain disorders of the human organism, how far it has succeeded, and what limitations have been found to beset its path, these are the problems which form the subject of this paper.

There are certain disorders in which the clinical phenomena have a dominantly psychological character, and are only capable of being adequately described in psychological terms. These are the psychoses, comprising the various types of insanity. This sphere would seem to be the most obvious one to attack by a psychological method, and it might have been thought that psychopathology would have found here its most suitable material and its best chance of successful results. Actually, however, the historical development of psychopathology has taken a different road. The first great advances were made in a field where the most prominent phenomena were not mental at all, the field of hysteria with its anæsthesias, paralyses, and other disturbances of an apparently physical kind. Physiology had previously attempted to explain hysteria by its conception of " functional nervous disorder," but this conception failed to satisfy the canons by which every scientific conception must stand or fall. It was not based on observed experience, but merely on a theoretical assumption designed to bring hysteria into line with organic diseases. It did not enable the investigator to understand the phenomena with which he had to deal, it did not enable him to predict their course and occurrence nor to control their course and occurrence, and it could not be verified by any appeal to experience. It was, in fact, useless, in the sense that a scientific conception, being a weapon with which we hope to achieve our end, is useless if it does not help us towards that end. The way was clear, therefore, for a fresh attempt to explain hysteria, and the foundation of a psychopathological conception was laid by Charcot when he proposed the view that certain hysterical phenomena were due to "ideas." The avenue thus opened was explored by one of Charcot's pupils, Pierre Janet. He investigated the various phenomena of hysteria and found that they were capable of being interpreted in precise psychological terms, and finally he succeeded in formulating a conception which served to explain, in part at any rate, the nature of those phenomena. This conception will be best understood by describing the steps of Janet's researches with regard to one group of hysterical phenomena, functional anæsthesia, and we shall do this in some detail because it provides an excellent example of the employment by psychopathology of a method which conforms strictly to the method of science. In the first place, it was found that the anæsthesias, although they did not correspond in their distribution to the distribution of any section of the nervous system, did have a distribution which corresponded to something. The familiar glove anæsthesias, for example, ending in sharp lines at the level of the wrist, had a distribution inexplicable by any lesion of the nervous system, but their distribution corresponded precisely to the patient's idea of his own hand. That is to say, the incidence of the symptom was plainly determined by a factor of a psychological order, and it would therefore be profitable to seek for a psychological conception in order to explain it. Secondly, these anæsthesias exhibited a curious paradoxical character. Patients suffering from extensive anæsthesias involving a whole limb or half the body rarely appeared to sustain any accidental injury to the anæsthetic part, whereas in patients with relatively far smaller organic anæsthesias, syringo-myelics for example, such injuries frequently occurred. It would seem, indeed, that the hysterical patient must be able to feel with his anæsthetic limb in order to evade the accidents which would otherwise inevitably befall it. Similarly, patients with hysterical amblyopia of such a degree that the field of vision was reduced to a single point were able to play at ball, a performance obviously impossible unless the greater part of the retina were capable of receiving visual impressions. This paradoxical character was, perhaps, exemplified most clearly by the case of a boy who, after being in a fire, developed hysterical phenomena consisting, on the one hand, in the occurrence of hysterical fits whenever the patient saw a flame, and, on the other hand, in an amblyopia whereby the visual field was restricted to 30°. If the boy were tested with a perimeter he was unable to see the paper disc until it had travelled along the perimeter arm to the 30° radius. If, however, a lighted match were substituted for the disc of paper, then immediately it reached the limits of normal vision a fit occurred. Quite clearly, therefore, the patient was able to see over the whole field of normal vision, and equally clearly, he was blind to everything outside 30°.

The conception which Janet constructed to explain these phenomena was the conception of " dissociation of consciousness." He presumed that consciousness, instead of pursuing its course as a single homogeneous stream, was capable of being split into two or more independent currents, so that the consciousness belonging to one current would be unaware of, and unable to control, that belonging to another contemporaneous current. Hysterical anæsthesia was then explicable as the result of such a dissociation, the sensations from the anæsthetic area not being non-existent, but diverted into a current separated from the main stream of consciousness. Although thus cut off and therefore incapable of being perceived by the main stream, they could influence the motor apparatus, and thereby produce just those phenomena which had been observed, the avoidance of injury by the hemi-anæsthetic and the fits in the blind boy. The conception of dissociation therefore served to explain the observed phenomena, and it could, moreover, be experimentally verified. The patient could be hypnotised, for example, and access being thereby obtained to the dissociated portion, the actual existence of the sensations belonging to the anæsthetic area could be conclusively established.

Functional paralyses could be similarly explained, and the conception of dissociation was found to be applicable to a wide range of hysterical phenomena, including amnesias, somnambulisms, and double personality. Janet's work was confirmed and amplified by a number of subsequent investigators, in particular by the extensive and important researches of Dr Morton Prince, and the value of dissociation as an explanatory concept has now been established beyond question. Certain difficulties appear in applying it to some of the phenomena with which we have to deal, but these are due rather to misapprehension of the nature of the concept than to defects in the concept itself. For example, in many cases of hypnotic somnambulism the hypnotic consciousness is aware of the whole range of the patient's experience, whereas the personal consciousness has no knowledge of the experience belonging to the hypnotic consciousness. This one-sided and non-reciprocal lack of awareness may seem difficult to explain by dissociation, which would appear necessarily to involve a break between the two streams of consciousness, equally untraversable in whichever direction it might be attempted, whereas in the example we have cited the break is impassable when viewed from the side of the personal consciousness, and traversable with ease when viewed from the side of the hypnotic consciousness. The difficulty is, however, dependent upon a misconception of the nature of dissociation, and an abuse of the spatial metaphor in which it has been defined. Dissociation, of course, does not imply an actual separation in space, and from the nature of the phenomena with which it is concerned it obviously can have no real spatial significance whatever. The dissociation is a functional dissociation, an " out of gear " relationship, and if this is understood the existence of a non-reciprocal dissociation ceases to be inexplicable. The spatial metaphor, in which psychological concepts are often expressed, is valid and useful so long as its real nature is carefully kept in mind, but it leads easily to abuse and untrustworthy deductions.*

Dissociation may be regarded as the first-fruit of psychopathology. It was a conception built up by a strictly scientific method, it illuminated a vast field of phenomena which had hitherto baffled every attempt at explanation, and it opened up the way to therapeutic possibilities in which that control of phenomenal experience which is the ultimate goal of science was abundantly satisfied. Dissociation, however, only takes us a certain distance in the understanding of the phenomena with which we are dealing, and a further step is clearly required to answer the question, " Why does dissociation take place ? " This further step was attempted by Freud, but before considering the immensely important concepts which he has introduced, it will be desirable briefly to trace out a path of development in psychopathology parallel to that traversed by Janet.

Psychopathology had approached the problem of hysteria with the aid of another conception, that of " suggestion." This conception had had a long historical development including in its course the observation of certain phenomena by Mesmer, ascribed by him to " animal magnetism," the observation and induction of similar phenomena by the hypnotists, and the ascription of these phenomena by Bernheim to " suggestion."

---

* This danger, for example, has particularly to be kept in mind in estimating the value of the Freudian psychology with its extensive use of a complicated, spatial terminology in the conceptions of the conscious, pre-conscious, and unconscious.

Suggestion has since been investigated from many aspects, down to the work of Coué at the present time, and it has been invoked by Babinski as the essential and finally sufficient explanation of the phenomena of hysteria. The conception involved may be crudely described as the principle that the introduction of an idea, or, more properly, a conviction, into the mind of an individual, will tend to produce certain definite results in that individual. These results may be pathological, as in the production of hysterical symptoms, indifferent as in the countless examples of suggestion which we see in everyday life, or remedial as in the practice of suggestion as a therapeutic measure. The conception is clearly a psychological conception, and it has proved its value beyond all question as a weapon in the hands of the practising physician. It is, moreover, a valid conception when examined by the test of its conformity to the rules of scientific method. But it is a conception so vague, and so general in its application to mental processes, that it does not help us far in an understanding of the particular problems presented by disease. Babinski's use of it as a sufficient explanation of hysteria is clearly inadequate, and does not constitute more than a first step in the understanding of that disorder. We want to know why suggestion is so potent in this individual patient, and why certain suggestions are immediately effective in him, while others fail entirely.

We find, indeed, that in this case, as in the conception of dissociation, we have been helped to travel a certain distance, but that the need of a further advance is imperatively felt. The stage in the development of psychopathology to which these conceptions belong is comparable to that existing in the history of astronomy at the time of Kepler. Kepler had shown that the planets move in ellipses round the sun, but he could not explain why they did so. This latter achievement was the work of Newton with his formulation of the law of gravity. Newton's step was based on the conception that the phenomena observed were the result of certain hypothetical forces, interacting in accordance with certain precisely definable laws. It thus added a *dynamic* conception as a means of understanding the observed sequence of phenomena. The corresponding step in the construction of a psychological conception capable of taking us beyond the level reached by dissociation and suggestion clearly required a similar advance to a dynamic point of view, and this was, as a matter of fact, the advance which was actually attempted at the stage of the history of psychopathology which we are now describing.

This advance was made by Freud, and it constitutes a landmark of the first importance in the development of psychopathology. It marks the essential point of transition from the arid days of the academic psychology with its meticulous introspective description of mental processes, to the vigorous conceptual and dynamic method of attack which characterises all growing science. Space does not permit of a detailed description of the growth of this dynamic conception, and the general lines of Freud's teaching are now so well known that it is unnecessary to recapitulate them here. It will be profitable, however, to emphasise those broad features which mark the place of Freud's work in the line of historical development which we are considering, and from this point of view the essential principles underlying Freud's conceptions may be sketched as follows. The series of phenomena which constitute conscious life and behaviour are the result of the interaction of a number of psychological " forces," acting according to precise psychological " laws."* Two or more forces may work harmoniously together or they may conflict with one another. In the latter case an attempt at adjustment occurs, and certain of these attempted adjustments are of such a kind that morbid phenomena are produced, these morbid phenomena constituting the symptoms observed in certain forms of disorder.

Freud has built upon these basic principles a very elaborate structure, and in it are incorporated many further concepts, amongst which two may be selected for special mention. These are the conception of the Unconscious, and the Sex Theories. Both have been subjected to vigorous attack, partly on grounds which are inadequate and misleading, and it is necessary to deal with these inadequate criticisms before passing on to the problem which is our immediate concern here, the conformity of Freud's teachings to the canons of scientific method.

The conception of the unconscious, formulated by Freud in order to explain the facts of consciousness and behaviour, has been attacked on the ground that it is philosophically untenable and intrinsically absurd. It has been held that mental phenomena must be conscious or non-existent, and that the notion of unconscious mental processes therefore involves an inherent contradiction. This objection rests upon a confusion between phenomena and concepts, and a misapprehension of the function of a scientific

---

* A parallel, and in many essential respects identical dynamic principle has been reached by other psychologists, in particular by McDougall in his *Introduction to Social Psychology*.

concept. The conception of the unconscious has been formulated to explain the observed phenomena, and its validity is no more dependent on its existence as a phenomenal fact, than the validity of a weightless, frictionless ether as a weapon of scientific explanation is dependent upon its phenomenal existence. In both cases the validity of the concept is measured by its utility in resuming, explaining, and enabling us to control the observed phenomena.

Freud's sex theories have been attacked, sometimes explicitly, but more often implicitly, on ethical grounds. Objections of this kind have, of course, no place or relevancy in positive science, and only need to be mentioned in order that they may be at once dismissed.

Freud claims that his doctrines have been built up entirely on an empirical basis, by the observation of the facts of consciousness and behaviour, and the legitimate formulation of concepts to explain those observed facts. There seems good reason to accept, moreover, the frequently made statement that most observers who have investigated these facts by Freud's method have arrived at similar results and have confirmed Freud's teaching. It would seem, also, that Freud's concepts are constructed in a form which is unimpeachable according to the canons of the method of science, and that, if they are based upon observed facts, they satisfy all the requirements of those canons. It is, however, precisely the relation of psychoanalytic doctrine to the observed facts which requires careful investigation and consideration, and there is some reason to question whether the claim that the doctrines are directly based on facts of observation is legitimate. It is true that the doctrines are based on " facts," but these facts are not directly observed—they are reached by the employment of a peculiar method, the method of psychoanalysis. This method intervenes, as it were, between the actual facts of observation and the prepared facts upon which the concepts are based, and it is of such a character that the possibility of distortion cannot with certainty be excluded. The preconceptions of the analyst and of the patient, the deductions made by either or both from the material which rises into consciousness, the stage at which a series of associations is taken to have reached a significant point, all these may be influenced by disturbing factors, and unfortunately the influences at work are, at any rate so far as our present knowledge goes, of an incalculable character. It is at least clear that the " facts " of observation, upon which the Freudian conceptions are based, are of a very different type to those to which we are accustomed in other branches of science. An essential rule of scientific method is that in the construction of concepts and theories a frequent appeal to experience or experiment must be possible, and when made should yield results consonant with the concept or theory in question. In other words, our course in the regions of conceptual thinking, where it is possible to wander unconstrainedly in almost every direction, must be constantly guided and checked by stepping frequently on to the solid ground of phenomenal experience. We have seen that, in the evaluation of Freudian psychology, this appeal is not available in the sense in which it is available in other branches of science. There is an appeal to experience, but this experience is a specially " prepared " experience.

It is necessary to point out, however, that the defect which has been described is not peculiar to the Freudian methods, but is to some extent inherent in all psychological research. It constitutes, indeed, as Drever has shown, the essential weakness of all psychological method. In psychology the only objective facts are behaviour facts, and in order to deal with them by the psychological method we require to go behind these facts to the subjective experience underlying them, and thereby to find a new series of facts on which the concepts are ultimately to be constructed. For this reason psychology seems doomed always to occupy an invidious position in the scientific hierarchy, and hence explanation of a particular series of phenomena by the concepts of another branch of science is always likely to be accepted in preference to a psychological explanation if both are available.* Nevertheless, the defect under consideration is more glaringly apparent in the Freudian theories than in other instances of psychological method, in that the process of " going behind " the facts to establish a second series of facts is more extensive and complicated, and takes one further and further from an appeal to phenomenal experience as we are led into the depths of the " unconscious." In such relatively simple conceptions as Janet's " dissociation," on the other hand, the amount of inferential deduction beyond objectively ascertainable facts is very slight ; an appeal to phenomenal experience can be made at almost every step, and the objections on the score of scientific method are therefore correspondingly small.

* J. Drever—*Instinct in Man*. Cambridge University Press. 2nd edition, 1921. Chap. I.

Confirmation of the criticism just put forward is furnished by comparing the widely divergent conceptions reached by different investigators in the analytic field, those, for example, put forward by Freud, Jung and Rivers. In all these different schools of thought the weapons of research are forged of much the same metal, and in not very dissimilar patterns, and yet the results obtained by their use are extraordinarily divergent. Moreover, in face of this divergence we can make no confident decision between the conflicting claims, because the test of appeal to phenomenal experience, the test by which a similar situation in other branches of science is generally speedily resolved, cannot be adequately and satisfactorily applied.

An attempt may now be made to summarise the position reached by our review of the development of psychopathology. Psychology has clearly established its right to deal with the phenomena of human behaviour, and to formulate psychological concepts which will serve to explain those phenomena, provided that they are constructed according to the rule of scientific method. It has to be recognised that psychology is at a disadvantage in that its method is of a character which presents inherent difficulties to the complete satisfaction of those rules, and this disadvantage is equally apparent in the section of psychology constituted by psychopathology. Nevertheless, many of the simpler conceptions of psychopathology, such as dissociation, fail to satisfy the canons of science by so small a margin that it can safely be neglected. In other conceptions, however, particularly those of the analytic schools, the margin is so large that the doctrines of these schools cannot be said to have yet attained the standard which science demands. Yet the islands of rock which dot the sea of analytic speculation are so fertile and so suggestive of further solid ground extending far around them, that we cannot but feel that ultimately much of that sea will one day be turned into cultivated ground, and that the weapons of analytic research will be shown to be worthy of admission into the accredited armoury of science. The opinion may be ventured that the real need of the moment is the careful examination, testing, and perfecting of those weapons, rather than the fashioning of further structures by their aid.

THE SUBCONSCIOUS, THE UNCONSCIOUS, AND THE CO-CONSCIOUS

BY

KNIGHT DUNLAP, A.M., Ph.D.
Professor of Experimental Psychology, Johns Hopkins University

R

SUBCONSCIOUS, UNCONSCIOUS, CO-CONSCIOUS

BY

KNIGHT DUNLAP

THE concept of subconscious processes has been developed in the theories and interpretations of many psychologists. The doctrine of " the unconscious " or the " unconscious mind " (the two terms have not always the same meaning) came into psychology through the philosophers, and has been taken up by Freud and his disciples as the foundation of the " new psychology." The conception of " co-consciousness," although vaguely involved in many of the theories concerning the " subconscious " and the " unconscious," we owe primarily to Morton Prince, and it has been an exceedingly valuable contribution towards the clearing up of a much confused field.

The three terms—subconscious, unconscious, and co-conscious—are used interchangeably by loose writers. Especially are the first two frequently interchanged. Hence it is necessary to insist at this point that concepts are important primarily, and that names are of secondary importance. We shall apply these three names to the three distinct concepts, and what we shall say about each concept must not be confused with what might be said about another concept called by the same name.

While these concepts might be discussed without reference to any general theory of psychology, it is much clearer to conduct the discussion in terms of a definite theory. We shall adopt, therefore, the reaction-hypothesis, which is rapidly coming to be the accepted basis for psychology. Further, we shall employ the distinction between the process of *being conscious*, or *aware*, on the one hand, and the *content*, or *that of which* one is aware, on the other, a distinction for which the author has been contending for some years, and which is well emphasised by Ginsberg,* as a means of avoiding needless confusion.

The concept of subconscious processes is nothing more than the admission that the consciousness involved in our reactions

* *The Psychology of Society*, p. 53.

245

varies in degree, from the " focal " or highly " attentive " on the one hand, to the " marginal " or " fringe " consciousness on the other. Difference in respect to degree (vividness) may obtain between the consciousness at one moment and the consciousness at the next ; and also, in any given moment, between the consciousness of different details in the content. We need not enter into the discussion whether the gradation in degree is of a continuous sort, or whether there are three, five, or more distinct " grades " between " focus " and " margin." The occurrence of the " marginal " degree of subconsciousness, in other words, is tacitly or explicitly admitted by modern psychology.

That subconscious processes are important, not only as modifying the total conscious pattern of the moment, but also as profoundly influencing succeeding processes, both conscious and non-conscious, is also generally admitted. The detail of the reaction-hypothesis which ascribes consciousness and its degrees to the integration of the total nervous system, and the variations in completeness of integration, is of high importance in the explanation of the efficacy of subconscious process, but it is not necessary to enter into the discussion of that explanation. The admission of the facts is sufficient.

The adoption of the conception of subconscious processes does not commit us to any of the various doctrines of the " unconscious mind " or of " co-consciousness," unless we commit an obvious logical fallacy and assume that, since the names of two concepts are confused, the concepts are the same. Both of these other concepts must be analysed, and their relations to fundamental facts and theories of psychology shown.

If we may use the term " personality " for the *system of conscious processes* in an organism, rather than for the outward expression of such processes, the " behaviour," as observable by another individual (both usages being, of course, permissible, if not confused), we may say that there are cases in which it appears as if two (or perhaps more) " personalities " are involved in one and the same total organism. Such cases are those which Dr Prince has investigated.

Now, from the point of view of the reaction-hypothesis, there is no reason to doubt, *a priori*, that such cases of " double personality " may occur, and Dr Prince's observations certainly establish a probability, even if some psychologists may deny that it is more than probability. But we must distinguish here between various possible forms of double personality.

Over and above the specific integrations of the nervous system, and hence of specific phases of personality, we are forced to recognise that there are systematic tendencies to integration in each individual, and that these tendencies are not only emotional, but ideational. The individual tends to fall into certain emotional states upon certain stimulation : he also tends to think of certain things, and to remember certain types of things, under certain circumstances. And these integrative tendencies vary from day to day, and even over shorter periods.

The interrelation of " instinct " and " habit " in these tendencies need not concern us here. Both " instinct " and " habit " are " tendencies " in the sense in which we here use the term, and are, according to our general psychological hypothesis, determined by the actual status of the nervous system at given moments. Changes in the nervous status, and hence in the " tendencies," are assumed to be brought about by nutritional processes to some extent, but to a greater extent by the successive operations of the nervous system under various stimulation. The *status* of the nervous system at a given moment is the basis of the tendency to react in this or that way upon a given stimulus pattern : but in so reacting it may modify its own status, and hence modify its reaction tendencies.

Between some of the cases of alternating personality (such as the classic case of Ansel Bourne) and the modifications of personality which are constantly occurring in all of us, there seems to be no essential difference except in the degrees of modification suffered. In no such case is it necessary to assume that there are *two* personalities co-existing : that the integrations of the nervous mechanism form two simultaneous systems, but rather, that the two " personalities " depend upon systematically different integrations of the mechanism at different times. So far as we know, the whole nervous system may be acting in both cases, and acting as integratedly in one as in the other ; but the system acts differently in the two cases, and in the most normal man the system, however well integrated, is acting differently at different moments.

Yet, on the other hand, it may be true, as I understand Dr Prince to hold, that *in some cases* there are actually two personalities co-existing in the same organism, and, therefore, the nervous mechanism, instead of being integrated into a single system, is integrated into two systems, between which the connections are less close than the connections within them.

Now, this conception offers no theoretical difficulties to our modern psychobiological theories.   That a few million nerve cells might be able to combine into two systems, instead of one, our theories certainly do not deny !   Further, that these integrations may vary from time to time, one now including elements (such as the cells controlling the speech mechanism), which at another time are included by the other, is not excluded by our fundamental hypothesis.   Nor can we see any reasons why *both* of these systems might not be " conscious " at the same time : that is, might give rise to highly integrated complex reactions—therefore, conscious reactions.   We accept, therefore, the hypothesis of co-consciousness as an important one, to be held distinctly in view in the interpretation of the phenomenon of personality, and to be accepted whenever it shall be experimentally demonstrated, or when we find phenomena which cannot be explained without it.

There are, however, several points which must regulate our use of this hypothesis at the present time.

1. If shown to apply to certain pathological cases, it would not necessarily be shown to be applicable to normal cases.   The general tendency of the nervous system *seems* to be to integrate into a *single* system, and our general psychological interpretation of learning and habit formation is based on this assumption.   We would, therefore, unless we abandon much of our present psychology, be forced to conclude that co-consciousness is an exception, pathological like Siamese twins, due to a failure of normal processes and tendencies.   The existence of cases of co-consciousness would then be no proof of the assumption of a secondary " mind " or " consciousness " in normal individuals.

2. Proceeding on the general principles essential to science, we should not adopt this hypothesis as explaining any cases, unless the ordinary hypotheses of psychology are obviously incompetent to explain them.   And without wishing to be dogmatic on the point, I must confess that it seems to me that the same prosaic principles which explain the average individual's manifold personality change, and the change of Ansel Bourne, explain also the change in other cases just as well as the hypothesis of co-consciousness does.   But, of course, I speak here only from second-hand acquaintance with the case, and should not wish to set my opinion against that of first-hand experts of such recognised scientific ability as Dr Prince.

3. We must remember that our general psychobiological hypothesis includes no details as to the exact quantitative relation between conscious vividness and neural integration.   We assume

that with more complete integration, there is higher vividness. But what level of integration must be attained before *any* consciousness occurs? In particular, is it necessary, in order to have conscious reaction, that certain specific neural tracts must always participate in the reaction? Or is it necessary to have in every case so large a part of the mechanism involved that the remaining parts, however well integrated into a nervous system, would be " below the threshold " of conscious activity? We do not know the answers to these questions yet : but it is not impossible that we shall some day find out.

There need be no confusion between the concept of the subconscious and that of the co-conscious. It is obvious that, if we accept the former, it applies to the latter also : each of two co-conscious personalities might have subconscious processes, just as might a single personality.

When we turn from the scientific hypotheses of the subconscious and the co-conscious to the theories of " unconscious mind," we enter a region strikingly like that which, on some of the theories, the " unconscious mind " itself is supposed to be. A realm of shadows, dim lights, and confusion : a realm in which statements are vague, and meanings difficult to locate. A realm, in short, in which more importance is given to the vague suggestion of words and phrases than to their exact meaning. Professor James has summed this up by calling the alleged psychology of the unconscious a " tumbling ground for whimsies."

There seem to be several types of psychological phenomena which have suggested to various philosophers doctrines of " unconscious mind," and it is well to take these up in turn.

1. Psychology is obliged to take into consideration *more* than conscious (or than conscious and subconscious) reactions. Assuming for the moment that there actually are *non*-conscious reactions, that is, reactions not involving consciousness, our fundamental psychobiological hypothesis includes the assumption that all reactions, both conscious and non-conscious, are causally connected; that conscious reactions influence not only other conscious reactions, but non-conscious reactions as well ; and that the reverse is true. For we assume that all reactions are dependent upon the same general mechanism, under the same general laws.

Now, if we define " mind " in terms of conscious reaction, it is obvious that psychology is vitally interested in more than mind. We might (and should, perhaps) extend the definition of mind to include this farther region. But what we do, actually, is to call it the *domain of merely physiological reaction* : or more briefly, the *physiological*. There would be no real objection to calling it " unconscious mind," if the word *un*conscious were always understood as exactly equivalent to *not* conscious. Unfortunately, few, if any, of the partisans of " unconscious mind " are willing to make the identification.

2.. The individual may carry on certain conscious activities at one time : then desist from them for a shorter or longer period, and then again carry on these activities in much the same form. Thus, I learn to play billiards : then, a year later, I may again be able to play nearly as well, without relearning the game. Again, I think of some problem : perhaps worry about it, for a time. Then I forget it, but a long time afterwards I again think about it.

Furthermore, the activities which I have ceased to carry on affect other activities carried on in the meantime. Having played billiards, I control my hand movements in some other ways better. Having thought out a problem, I may solve other problems more efficiently. Having worried over something, I may be thereafter in a state of emotional excitation or depression which affects all my activities.

Now, such causal relations are well known, and are fully in accord with the fundamental principles of psychology. We find that they are provided for in our general psychobiological reaction-theory. In all of these phenomena the same laws of activity of the nervous system are involved. The differing details under differing circumstances are, of course, matters for experimental investigation.

To persons who observe some of these phenomena without noticing the others, and who are ignorant of psychology, the causal sequences are as marvellous as are the causal sequences of lightning and thunder to the savage. And as the savage constructs mystic powers to explain the phenomena of nature, the metaphysician constructs a mystic principle to explain these phenomena of mind. And the " unconscious mind " is nowadays seized upon by these theorists as the mystic explanation.

In some theories, developed on this simple basis, the " unconscious mind " remains as vague as the nature-divinities of the savage. It is just " something " which somehow explains. The phenomena appear mysterious : and the name " unconscious mind " is sufficiently paradoxical and mysterious to satisfy. The old showman's term " the what-is-it ? " would do as well, but perhaps it does not sound " scientific " enough.

Other adherents to the doctrine of " unconscious mind " as the explanation of the (to them) mysterious sequences of mind, attempt to analyse the mystery somewhat by resorting to the old confusion between conscious activity and the content of consciousness. Selecting only certain conscious activities, such as remembering, or worrying, and ignoring the vast range of co-ordinated reactions, they confuse these activities, under the terms " ideas," " thoughts," " wishes," etc., with the objects *of which* the idea, thought or wish is, because the same terms are applied to both. These conscious processes are then conceived not as activities, but as *things*, and what is really the reoccurrence of an *activity* is treated as if it were the reappearance of a *thing*.

You " have a thought " to-day, and again to-morrow : it is " in your mind " at those two times, but where was it in the meantime ? Why, in the " unconscious mind, of course." You have been worrying about a certain matter, and still your activities show the results of the worry : you are not *really* worrying about it now ; therefore you must be worrying about it in your " unconscious mind " !

It is obvious that of the two types of theorists, the first, who make the " unconscious mind " a mysterious force, and let it go at that, are nearer to scientific method than are those of the second type. For science has its beginning in the recognition of something needing to be explained. And there would be no objection to the labelling of this hiatus in explanation " the unconscious mind " or " the what-is-it ? " if the application of these names did not lead the applier to ignore the fact that psychology has already found explanatory principles for these phenomena. There is no objection to the explanation of lightning and thunder as the work of Jove, if the explanation does not shut one's eyes to the explanation which physics has supplied : and there would be no objection to the designating of the causal relation in the mind as " the unconscious mind," or " the dæmon," if one understood that the names explained nothing, and did not let them stand in the way of the actual explanations.

This second basis of the " unconscious mind " theory, it is clear, is not the mere distinction between conscious reaction and non-conscious (physiological) reaction which constitutes the basis first discussed, but is relatively independent of that distinction. It is the fact that there are *causal relations* in mind : that the activities of to-day are modified by those of yesterday and last year. This, of course, is well known to, and explained by, the psychologist, to whom it is amusing to see these relations subsumed under the term "unconscious mind," and the mere phrase offered as if it were an explanation.

3. Another psychological fact which has apparently impressed some of the " unconscious " theorisers, is the fact that *connections* between conscious processes are not themselves *conscious*. Here again the non-psychologist has been impressed because he has noticed only a few striking cases of the rule, and has not made extensive observations.

Two successive ideas, for example, may be connected by " association." This connection, however, is not " conscious " in any sense of the term, but is a matter primarily of causal sequence, which psychology explains by the principle of activity of the nervous system. It is true that subsequently we may reflect upon the sequence, and make it a *content* for further conscious activity, but it is the activities which are conscious, not the causal connections. This uniform fact, that the direct connections between conscious activities are not themselves conscious, has seemed mysterious to those who are not versed in psychology, and has been to them another seeming indication of an occult " unconscious mind " which makes the connection. Here again the term really should be " nervous system."

4. Very frequently the fact that the consciousness involved in a reaction is often not conscious " of " the object or occurrence which stimulates the reactor has been confusedly described as " unconscious perception " or in some other terms has been drawn into the concepts of " unconscious mind." Thus, we are told, the individual " unconsciously " perceives the disparity of the two pictures in a stereoscope, and therefore " consciously " perceives depth. This form of confused explanation has been in vogue for several hundred years, but makes no appeal to the psychologist. The actual facts are that, in such cases, certain details of the stimulating object are not perceived at all : but they are effective, along with other details, in the stimulus pattern, in causing conscious activity in which *something else* is perceived. And psychology has no difficulty in explaining how this condition is brought about by the usual principle of habit and integrative action. The introduction of the term " unconscious " here adds nothing to the explanation, except confusion.

From a consideration of these four sources of the " unconscious mind " doctrine, it is obvious that the concept of " unconscious mind " is superfluous in psychology and that, although it may not mislead the psychologist, it very much misleads the non-psychologist who constructs large psychological theories, and helps to keep him and his readers in ignorance of the actual psychological explanations. The psychologist sees that " unconscious mind " is, in some cases, merely another term for *activity of the nervous system* : for *causal connections* between conscious reactions in others ; and in still other cases a mere term of negation, as when " unconscious perception " means merely " no perception." But the person without knowledge of the psychological principle of explanation, of course, does not know what principles his term " unconscious mind " really obscures, and fancies that it is an " explanation."

The doctrine of the " unconscious mind " is obviously one of the modern types of a very old system : the " faculty " psychology. It must not be confused with the hypotheses of subconscious or co-conscious, which really belong to modern psychology.

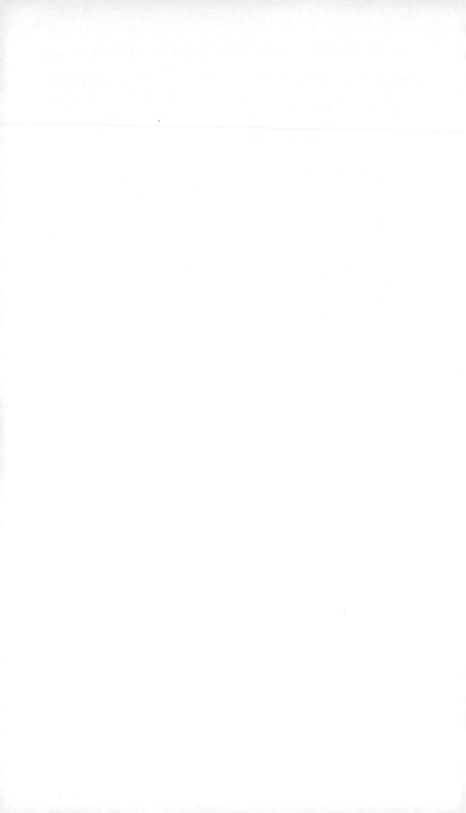

THE ASSOCIATION OF PSYCHO-NEUROSIS WITH MENTAL DEFICIENCY

BY

CHARLES S. MYERS, C.B.E., M.A., M.D., D.Sc., F.R.S.

Director, National Institute of Industrial Psychology; formerly University Reader in Experimental Psychology, Cambridge.

THE ASSOCIATION OF PSYCHO-NEUROSIS WITH MENTAL DEFICIENCY

BY

CHARLES S. MYERS

In this paper I wish to present an account of two school children which have come under my observation during the past five years, in which mental defect was associated with psycho-neurotic symptoms. For much of the information which I am able to give I have been dependent on, and wish to express my gratitude to, Miss Peyton, the Head Mistress of the School for Mental Defectives in which the boys were being educated, and Miss L. G. Fildes, who carried out the tests described in the paper.

The first case, A.B., was admitted to the School in January, 1915, then aged 8 years 2 months. When tested four years later, in May, 1919, by the Stanford-Binet tests, his intelligence quotient proved to be 52, his mental age being 6 years 6 months ; *i.e.*, there was a retardation of about six years. He had an apparently normal brother at work. A fatal accident befell his father, a heavy drinker, two months before the boy's birth. His mother, a cook in service, stated that until two years old he was boarded out with an aunt, that he began to talk normally while he was with his aunt, but that afterwards he was transferred to another woman's care, where he " lost his speech " after being shut up in a dark cupboard.

When admitted to the School for Mental Defectives, his speech was very imperfect ; and although he had previously attended school he could do no school work. He left this School shortly after I saw him, by which time his speech had improved enormously and he had learnt to carry out some coarse handwork. He could also read and write the alphabet and many small words. His behaviour and speech were marked by complete absence of continuous attention. He was always restless and anxious to do something, but was perpetually distracted by any passing occurrence. Through such inattention he was wholly incapable of learning at school, except under individual instruction. In his talk, which was incessant, he repeated himself constantly and showed little restraint or selection in the words he used. He could sing extremely well and was distinctly musical. He was mischievous, cheerful, happy, excitable and suggestible, clever at mimicking others, but he readily lost control over bodily movements, speech and laughter. He explained his wild behaviour by the words " me happy." He exhibited no distrust of strangers.

In the absence of external excitement, however, he showed certain dominant interests. Some of them had reference to recent passing events, *e.g.*, his birthday, Christmas, etc. ; these controlled much of his speech and conduct. One interest, however, was permanent. Almost any topic, if pursued, would lead to the subject of death, birth, God, Satan and angels. Thus, when Miss Fildes asked him in an experiment to give an association in response to the word " goat," he replied : " Can milk him—get milk out of him—only butt you like a cow. Oh ! when a cow toss you you come down bang and are dead. God knows, don't He ? I know how God looks [shows this with foot stretching out, hand over eyes]. Satan—God's best angel—naughty—if Satan made you naughty he put you in the burning fire. No good—ought to be in fire himself."

Again, in the middle of solving a jig-saw puzzle, he remarked : " How did God get you down here when He made you ? Funny how He got you down. Come down small. Mr S.'s baby not growed to boy yet. Been here long time I think. Do you come down hole ? I seen them at funeral put box into hole. Make hole deep—*this* big—oh ! deeper than this floor. Man put cord round box and put it down slow—not fast—might break it. How do God get box up ? I think it go along and He pull it up by cord —angels carry it to heaven. How do He make you ? Do you be an angel when you get to God ? I seen Him when He make me— ugh ! great big man. Do you remember when He make you ? Funny how He get you to earth," etc.

These instances are typical of a constant form of speech, whenever free speech was allowed ; and there is evidence that the same topic was a favourite one when he talked to other boys. A dream of his recorded is one of " black things sitting on the end of the bed, which had come to take him."

We were able to get from him his distinct recollection of being taken one day, when he was about three years old, by the woman with whom he had been boarded, to a funeral. He saw the coffin put into the ground and he was told that the coffin lid was screwed down over the body, and that if the body happened to be too large it was squeezed and forced into the coffin. Unfortunately, as I have said, the boy left the School shortly after we began to observe him, since a certain educational Body desired to transfer him to its own School. But from the facts here described the psycho-neurotic condition of the boy is obvious.

The second case I am able to record in fuller detail. C.D. is now in his eighteenth year and has been in the School for eight years. When first admitted, he refused to speak to anyone and nothing would induce him to smile. He repelled all advances towards friendliness and remained in this state for about three months. Shortly after admission he began to show great interest in the bedrooms belonging to the staff of the school, expressing a wish to " help clean them " ; and late one night he was discovered peeping through the keyhole of the cook's bedroom while she was undressing. When asked why he was doing this, he replied, " I wanted to see what clothes she wore." He was overheard telling another boy the nature and names of women's underwear.

C.D. lived at home until he was admitted to the School. His father, when he visits the boy, is generally under the influence of drink. The father's version of his son's early childhood is that the mother treated him very cruelly, throwing him downstairs and often injuring him. The mother died (or went away) when the boy was about three years old and another woman took her place who left before the boy was admitted to the School.

The boy is reported by the Head Mistress of the School to be now much less anti-social than before, but to be still morose and reticent. He is selfish and hoards everything on which he can lay his hands. He works in the garden and kitchen now and is generally amenable to reason under good management. He is a good worker and gives valuable service when not " upset."

The following determinations of his intelligence were made by Miss Fildes :—

Date of Examination	Age	Mental Age	Intelligence Quotient
8. 10. 20	14 yrs. 10 mos.	7 yrs. 8 mos.	52
27. 4. 21	15 yrs. 4 mos.	7 yrs. 8 mos.	50
25. 10. 21	15 yrs. 10 mos.	7 yrs. 10 mos.	49

In 1922 our attention became more closely directed to him

s

chiefly because of the results of some 400 free associations to which Miss Fildes had subjected him, 50 words at a time, on four different occasions, during November and December of the previous year. Each different series of fifty words was repeated a second time at each sitting. His average reaction time was about five seconds, therein agreeing with those of 18 other boys tested at the school during the same months. But the number of his " senseless " associations was more than three times as great. The striking feature of his senseless replies was that a large number of them, about 20 per cent. of the total number of associations returned, referred to women's articles of clothing, or to objects connected therewith, as may be seen from the tables.*

The sequences—drawers, petticoat, bloomers; frock, skirt, coat; drawers, windows, bodice, bloomers, drawers, blouse, frock, stockings, shoes—are noticeable. Likewise such sequences as nose, eyes; teeth, mouth; teeth, eyes, nose, hair, occur among his replies. It will also be observed that the reaction times for these words are not different from those for " sensible " replies.

Classification of the above 400 Associations

Type of Association	1st response		2nd response	
	Number	Aver. time	Number	Aver. time
Co-ordination ...	38	4·8	42	3·1
Predication ...	12	6·4	10	3·9
Causal Dependence	0	—	0	—
Co-existence ...	9	6·2	12	5·3
Identity	1	4·0	2	3·0
Motor Speech ...	4	4·0	8	4·0
Sound	1	6·0	1	4·0
Mediate	0	—	—	—
Senseless ...	135	5·1	124	5·3
Fail	0	—	1	28·0

The average percentage of senseless responses among eighteen other mentally defective boys tested with the same associations is 20 per cent., as against about 67 per cent. in this case. Much the commonest form of senseless response, in the majority of cases, is the name of an object present. Normal children above the age of seven years seldom give senseless responses.

*EDITORIAL NOTE.—For technical reasons it was found necessary to omit the tables which illustrate very well the point made here, viz., the recurrence of response words dealing with objects of female attire.

Taking the results of the same eighteen boys :—

1. The average reaction time is about as long and is very variable. (Average time = 5·60 seconds.)

2. Only 48 per cent. of the whole number of reactions are repeated on the second response.

3. There is a great deal of repetition in the responses. On the average, each boy uses only seventy different words for each hundred responses.

I saw him first on March 1st, 1922. He then appeared a dull, loutish youth, somewhat shy and reticent. His general conduct was otherwise not abnormal, save for an occasional jerkiness of the head. He appeared to remember nothing of his mother, save by hearsay that she beat him and starved him. He recalled an occasion when two men living in an adjoining room terrified him by letting a collie dog into his bedroom which climbed on to his bed. He admitted that thoughts of women's clothes often intruded into his daily work. The word " petticoat " proved to evoke in him an image of a certain lady who frequently visited the School (he revealed her name after great pressure had been put upon him) going to the lavatory and lifting up a white petticoat. He said that " stockings " evoked an image of one of the members of the school staff (her name was also revealed only after persuasion) putting on her black stockings. These were incidents, no doubt, he had actually witnessed by surreptitious peeping.

He proved to be quite ignorant of the nature of sexual connection, believing that babies were brought into the world by angels who carried them under their wings.

After some difficulty he was induced to pass into a dreamy hypnoidal state, in which I succeeded in reviving memories of his mother. He recalled seeing her pass urine. " It was nice," he observed. The word " stockings " now revived an occasion of being in bed with his mother and seeing her get up, sit on the bed and put on her stockings. He spontaneously recalled seeing his father being " on top of his mother and playing about."

On waking, he recalled all that he had just said, and he observed that he had never been able to recall these scenes before. He said that he dreamed occasionally of seeing " a woman's number one," but that it was of no particular woman.

Thereupon I attempted to explain to him the reasons for the intrusion into his thoughts of ideas of women's underwear, and he was given some notion of the nature of sexual differences and functions.

A few days afterwards the Head Mistress asked what we had been doing with the boy, as he was showing so much improvement in general demeanour and behaviour and was now so much more tractable. She wrote recently, " his mental attitude was wonderfully improved after you had talked to him." Miss Fildes noted, in July last, " his general attitude and response certainly improved, and I think the improvement is, on the whole, maintained."

When I saw him again in May, 1922, he said that the intrusion of the thoughts of women's underwear, etc., had entirely ceased, that he had no dreams of a woman's private parts and that he felt, as he expressed it, " more sensible." He appeared far brighter and more responsive.

Two months later—nearly five months after the psychoanalytic interview with the boy—the Stanford-Binet tests were re-applied. The results of this and the two previous tests are as follow :—

Date of Examination	Age	Mental Age	Intelligence Quotient
27. 4. 21	15 yrs. 4 mos.	7 yrs. 8 mos.	50
25. 10. 21	15 yrs. 10 mos.	7 yrs. 10 mos.	49
27. 6. 22	16 yrs. 6 mos.	8 yrs. 7 mos.	52

The improvement indicated in the last examination is especially well-marked, comparing it with the earlier ones. In the course of eight months his mental age advanced nine months—a somewhat unusual occurrence in a defective of his age, the more ordinary condition being a gradual lowering of the intelligence quotient. It is, perhaps, more unusual in his case, seeing that he advanced only two months in mental age during the preceding year. There was no indication in the results of the tests that this improvement in intelligence had taken place along any particular line. But the boy was unquestionably improving. For on three occasions in May, 1923, repetition of the association tests evoked reaction words or responses which might be normally expected of a boy of his mental age. They were obtained by the same experimenter. Nothing had been said to him about the type of response so commonly returned by him on the previous occasions.

The sitting on May 12th took place in the morning before work, that on May 16th in the afternoon after he had been working from 7 a.m. and when he might be presumed to be tired. The sitting on May 25th was at 9 a.m., when the boy had been upset by some household disturbance and had been crying for some time.

Despite these circumstances, favourable to loss of higher control, there is not a single reference in his 300 replies to women's articles of clothing ; indeed, there is not a single instance even of a " senseless " response. The reaction time has also fallen to about $2\frac{3}{4}$ seconds. The associations may be thus classified :—

Classification of the above 150 Associations (first responses only)

Type of Association.	May 12, 1923		May 16, 1923		May 25, 1923	
	No.	Aver. Time	No.	Aver. Time	No.	Aver. Time
Co-ordination ...	18	2·3	25	2·56	25	2·3
Predication ...	10	7·3	6	4·1	11	2·4
Causal Dependence	1	4·0	0	—	0	—
Co-existence ...	18	3·4	13	3·1	7	2·2
Identity	0	—	0	—	2	2·5
Motor Speech ...	1	2·0	1	1·0	1	2·0
Sound	2	2·0	4	2·5	3	4·0
Mediate	0	—	0	—	0	—
Senseless	0	—	1	2·0	1	14·0
Fail	0	—	0	—	0	—

No mention has yet been made of the experiments in free continuous, or serial, association which were carried out on the boy in November, 1921, and in January, 1923. Here is a list of 70 successive words returned by him in ten minutes on November 8th, 1921 :—

Bloomers, petticoat, drawers, night-gown, skirt, frock, shoes, stockings, eyes, nose, teeth, smell, glasses, fire, coal, flowers, hat, coat, clothes, books, hands, legs, feet, stockings, shoes, bloomers, coal, chair, hair, comb, dog, cat, rat, picture-frame, book-stand, pen, ink, coal, wood, stone, glass, stand, handkerchief, lavatory, watch, bed, chamber, paper, coat, petticoat, drawers, bloomers, skirt, frock, stockings, legs, hair, eyes, teeth, nose, trees, glass, stone, house, number two, paper, table, laughing, leaving the room, fire, cardboard.

It will be observed that nearly 40 per cent. of these words refer to articles of women's clothing, excretions, etc. This test was repeated on May 25th, 1923, with the following result :—

Hair, eyes, teeth, nose, coat, skirt, frock, petticoat, drawers, bloomers, stockings, feet, shoes, chamber, lavatory, dog, rat, trees, field, books, glasses, combs, stays, chair, paper, chemise, rubber, rule, cup, tale, knife, pen, ink, water, bed, nightgown, watch, window, chair, bedroom, cup, skirt, legs, coat, drawers, bloomers, petticoat, stockings, shoes, feet, petticoat, stays, chemise, hair, comb, spectacles, eyes, teeth, nose, water, boat, ink, chamber, lavatory, match, glass, coat, book, rule, rubber, money, pin, coat, fire, coal, bucket, wood, skirt, petticoat, shoes, stockings, bloomers, case, chamber, bedroom, lavatory, table, chair, house, curtain, carpet, cardboard, box, can, puzzle, matches, pictures, window, skirt, petticoat.

These words were returned more speedily than before ; but their character is unchanged, despite the fact that the ordinary association test applied on the same day failed to reveal even a single instance of reference to articles of female clothing, or the like. The following series of responses were then obtained from him :—

Series 1 : Serial association   *25th May*, 1923

Horse, cow, skirt, petticoat, drawers, bloomers, stockings, shoes, coat, frock, hair, eyes, teeth, nose, glasses, stays, chemise, table, paper, bedroom, nightgown, watch, pictures, stove, carpet, chair, puzzle, picture, house, looking-glass. (Time=2 min. 8 sec.)

Series 2 : Told to give any words which " dog " made him think of

Dog, cat, horse, cow, pigs, chickens, rat, mouse, peacock, pheasant, duck, gander, geese, turkeys, frogs, toads, pigeon, rabbit, hares, mole, birds, eagle, stag, dog, snake, stoat, weasel, cat, butterfly, worm. (Time=3 min. 28 sec.)

Series 3 : To give words suggested by " motor "

Motor-car, bike, motor-car, motor-bike, motor-lorry, train, railway, trucks, motor-scooter, bus, charabanc, trams, steam-roller, cart. (Time=3 min.)

Series 4 : To give names of objects in the room

Fire, chimney, stove, coalbucket, shovel, table, papers, books, matches, box, typewriter, case, jug, pictures, cupboard, drawers, vases, bookcase, books, poker, oilcan, glass, windows, looking-glass, curtain, chair, coat, box, watch, pen, carpet, floor, door, electric light, paper clip, pencil, ink, walls, ceiling. (Time=3 min. 30 sec.)

Series 5 : Serial association

Trees, skirt, coat, petticoat, bloomers, drawers, stockings, shoes, hair, eyes, teeth, nose, chemise, stays, bedroom, nightgown, chamber, lavatory, trees, house, table, jump, grass, window, drawers, ink, pen, watch, glasses, stove, pencil, paper, wire, books, motor, skirt, shoes, chair, electric light, post-office, comb, brush, carpet, ceiling, frock, skirt, coat, drawers, bloomers, petticoat, shoes, stockings, stays, chemise, case, typewriter, table, vase, chair, lamp, garden, trees, shed, pen, ink, fire, glass, window, paper, pencil, box, garden, plants, comb, brush, box, motor, oilcan, puzzle, matches, coat, cap, act, rain, field, town, country, walk, play, shops, wheelbarrow, table, books, typewriter, bookcase, chair, trees, shop, sweets. (Time=8 min. 39 sec.)

Throughout these tests of May, 1923, he showed remarkable improvement in his attitude towards the experiments and his general behaviour has continued to improve, although he is still always easily " upset," whereupon he becomes difficult to manage.

[Since this was written, however, he has left the School, as he was getting too old for it and had, on one occasion, attempted to embrace one of the matrons.]

Conclusion

In these two cases we see the influence (a) of the emotion of fear; (b) of infantile "sexual" feeling; (c) of interest and curiosity, associated with thoughts (i) on the before- and after-life, and (ii) on sexual differences and women's underwear. In the first case the original experience—the funeral—was not repressed ; in the second—seeing his mother in her bedroom—it was readily recoverable in the hypnoidal state. In the first case it was associated with a defective development of attention, flight of ideas, loquacity, openness to strangers, cheerfulness and mischievousness ; in the other it was associated with taciturnity, moroseness, selfishness and hoarding. In the latter, removal of the repression and brief " re-education " induced an appreciable improvement in intelligence and especially in his ability to make the best use of his mental powers.

In both cases the all-distracting " complex " was practically undisguised. Its affect led in both cases to constant intrusion of the theme into the current of everyday thought ; in the first case to constant inquiry, and in the second case to peeping through keyholes in order, apparently, to gratify curiosity.

Psycho-therapeutic treatment was attempted in the second case, and led to very definite intellectual and moral improvement.

In normal children such themes would most likely have been repressed or disguised, and the associated impulses more or less controlled. But in the mentally defective child, criticism and control must prove far less potent. Thus, in her instruction of such children in reading, Miss Fildes has reached the conclusion that their inability to read is often due to their uncritical, uncontrolled acceptance of the idea that they are unable to read.

It is suggested that not only is the mentally defective state thus responsible for the development and persistence of the psychoneurotic condition, but that the latter reacts in turn on the slowly-developing mind of the mentally defective child, aggravating his mental deficiency, and responsible perhaps for the often continued childishness of his later behaviour. It seems unlikely that mental deficiency is ever directly and solely due to a psycho-neurosis; but I feel convinced that certain cases of mental deficiency, and especially that many cases of mental backwardness, can be enormously improved—above all, in early life—by attention being paid to any concomitant psycho-neurotic disturbance, thereby permitting of the full development of such intelligence as lies dormant. The undesirable surroundings in which many such children spend the first years of their life are only too favourable for the later appearance of psycho-neurotic symptoms.

PROFESSOR FREUD'S GROUP PSYCHOLOGY AND HIS THEORY OF SUGGESTION

BY

Wm. McDOUGALL. M.B., D.Sc., F.R.S.
Professor of Psychology, Harvard University

PROFESSOR FREUD'S GROUP PSYCHOLOGY AND HIS THEORY OF SUGGESTION

BY

WILLIAM McDOUGALL

It is matter for rejoicing that the great leader of the psycho-analytic movement has of late years turned his attention to some of the deepest problems of social psychology. In so doing he brings his theories of human nature, built up through the study of individuals, to the test of their usefulness in wider fields, fields in which students who cannot claim to be psychoanalysts by profession may hope to weigh and to criticise them on a footing of equality. We are grateful to Professor Freud because, in thus coming out into the open, he grants us a taste of

" That stern joy which warriors feel
In foemen worthy of their steel."

In an earlier article I have examined one of Professor Freud's contributions to Social Psychology.* In this place I propose to examine a more recent contribution, one which aims to go to the very roots of Group Psychology, namely, " Group Psychology and the Analysis of the Ego."†

Professor Freud begins by pointing out that many writers on Social Psychology have been content to found much of their construction on the postulate of a " social instinct " in man.

" But we may perhaps venture to object that it seems difficult to attribute to the factor of number a significance so great as to make it capable by itself of arousing in our mental life a new instinct that is otherwise not brought into play. Our expectation is, therefore, directed toward two other possibilities ; that the social instinct may not be a primitive one and insusceptible of dissection, and that it may be possible to discover the beginnings of its development in a narrower circle, such as that of the family."

Having thus defined his goal, Professor Freud proceeds to

---

* A Review of *Totem and Taboo* in *Mind*, 1920.
† A translation of *Massenpsychologie und Ich-Analyse*, published by The International Psychoanalytical Press, 1922.

examine the views of some other writers on the fundamentals of Group Psychology, more especially those of M. le Bon and of myself. He accepts le Bon's assertion that participation in the life of a " psychological group" profoundly modifies the thinking, feeling, and acting of the individual ; and he asks :

" What, then, is a group ?   How does it acquire the capacity for exercising such a decisive influence over the mental life of the individual ?   And what is the nature of the mental change which it forces upon the individual ?   It is the task of a theoretical Group Psychology to answer these three questions."

Freud finds himself in substantial agreement with le Bon in respect of the peculiarities of the individual in the group.

" When individuals come together in a group, all their individual inhibitions fall away and all the cruel, brutal and destructive instincts, which lie dormant in individuals as relics of a primitive epoch, are stirred up to find free gratification."

And

" The apparently new characteristics which he [the individual] then displays are, in fact, the manifestations of this unconscious, in which all that is evil in the human mind is contained as a pre-disposition.   We can find no difficulty in understanding the disappearance of conscience or of a sense of responsibility in these circumstances.   It has long been our contention that ' dread of society (Sociale Angst) ' is the essence of what is called conscience."

The captious critic might here interpose to ask—Why should conscience, if it is simply dread of society, disappear or cease to function just when a man is most thickly surrounded by the fellow members of society ?

Also, without captiousness, we may fairly ask for more definition of " all the cruel, brutal and destructive instincts " which constitute the predisposition of all that is evil in the human mind.

In his later writings Professor Freud no longer has been content to postulate a single instinct, the sexual, but makes reference to a considerable array of instincts.   These references excite in me the liveliest curiosity ; a curiosity which seems doomed to remain unsatisfied.   For my part, although since childhood I have been familiar with references, in sermons and popular addresses, to " cruel, brutal and destructive instincts, which lie dormant in individuals as relics of a primitive epoch," I have always been sceptical as to the existence of such instincts in the human species ;

and the more I have studied the problems of instinct, the more has this scepticism hardened toward flat disbelief.

Perhaps it is unreasonable to demand consistency from so great a pioneer as Professor Freud : yet I will venture to point out that in another recent work (*Reflections on War and Death*) Freud has asserted what I believe to be a truer doctrine :

" Psychological or, strictly speaking, psycho-analytical investigation, proves that . . . the deepest character of man consists of impulses of an elemental kind which are similar in all human beings, the aim of which is the gratification of certain primitive needs.   These impulses are in themselves *neither good nor evil.*"

Freud accepts le Bon's assertion of increased suggestibility of the crowd-member, rightly points out that le Bon leaves this fact entirely unexplained, and marks it down as a fundamental problem to be dealt with.   He notes also, as two other important problems brought out by le Bon's descriptive account of crowds, the contagion of emotions and the prestige of leaders.

Freud (unlike le Bon, Sighele, Schallmeyer, Trotter, Martin, and most of the other writers who have dwelt upon the defects and ferocities of the crowd) is not blind to the fundamental paradox of group psychology, the paradox on which I have insisted in my *Group Mind*, namely, that, while immersion in the crowd commonly degrades the individual below his normal level, yet it is only by participation in group life that any man achieves his humanity and rises above the level of animal life : for, passing on to give in Chapter III an excellent, though incomplete and brief, *résumé* of my views, he recognises this paradox as another fundamental problem.   In my *Group Mind* I maintained that the solution of this problem is to be found in the organisation of the group ; that, in proportion as a group becomes organised, it gets rid of the peculiar defects and weaknesses of the crowd and becomes capable of higher modes of functioning and, under the better forms of organisation, capable of raising its members rather than degrading them.   But Freud seems to reject my explanation by organisation, for he writes :

" It seems to us that the condition which McDougall designates as the ' organisation ' of a group can with more justification be described in another way.   The problem consists in how to procure for the group precisely those features which were characteristic of the individual and which are extinguished in him by the formation of the group.   For the individual, outside the primitive group, possessed his own continuity, his self-consciousness, his traditions and customs, his own particular functions and position, and kept apart from his rivals. Owing to his entry into an ' unorganised ' group, he had lost this distinctiveness for a time."

But this is merely a restatement of the problem ; it suggests no alternative solution of it. Curiously enough, Freud, having recognised this problem and having implied that he has some alternative solution for it, passes on and does not, in the course of this book, return to it. He closes his reference to it with the following cryptic comment :

" If we thus recognise that the aim of the group is to equip the group with the attributes of the individual, we shall be reminded of a valuable remark of Trotter to the effect that the tendency towards the formation of groups is biologically a continuation of the multicellular character of all the higher organisations."

In this chapter Freud mentions also the principle I have invoked for the explanation of the intensified emotional reactions of crowds. He writes :

" The manner in which individuals are thus carried away by a common impulse is explained by McDougall by means of what he calls the ' principle of direct induction of emotion by way of the primitive sympathetic response,' that is, by means of the emotional contagion with which we are already familiar."

Now, le Bon, fully recognising the fact and the importance of emotional contagion in crowds, had treated it as one manifestation of suggestion. I, on the other hand, had treated it as a fundamental phenomenon, distinct from all the phenomena of suggestion and requiring a different explanation or theory. That explanation I had supplied in the theory of primitive passive sympathy or direct induction of emotion. In this I had been anticipated in some measure by Malebranche, as Dr Drever has pointed out, but by no other writer. The theory is bound up with my view of the relation of the primary emotions to the instincts, and stands or falls with that view. The theory is based on a large array of facts of behaviour of the gregarious animals ; namely, that among such animals the display of any instinctive emotional reaction by one member of the species is apt to provoke similar instinctive emotional reactions in all other members of the species that perceive these reactions ; as when the behaviour of fear in one member of a flock provokes fear behaviour in other members. For the explanation of these facts, my theory assumes that each of the major instincts is so organised on its perceptual side that the expressions of the same instinct in other individuals of the species are effective provocatives of the instinct in the perceiving animal. And it postulates a similar special perceptual organisation of the major instincts of the species *Homo sapiens*. Freud, in saying of my theory, " that is, by means of the emotional contagion with which we are already familiar," reduces my explanation to a mere restatement of the facts in generalised form.

It is true that we are all familiar with the facts of emotional contagion. The question is—have we any theory adequate to the explanation of them? The fact or phenomenon is one of the most fundamental with which a theoretical Group Psychology has to grapple. I have endeavoured to progress from the purely descriptive stage, represented by le Bon, to a theoretical explanation of the fact. Freud entirely overlooks my theory, in saying that I explain the fact " by means of the emotional contagion with which we are already familiar." I protest that I do not suffer from any such delusion as is here attributed to me by Professor Freud ; the delusion, namely, that, in describing a large array of phenomena in general terms, I in any sense explain them. My theory of primitive passive sympathy is a perfectly definite and plausible theory for the explanation of the facts of emotional contagion ; it is not a mere restatement of the facts in general terms. Let me illustrate the point by reference to laughter. Laughter is notoriously contagious. But why and how ? We do not explain the fact by saying that it is a case of the emotional contagion with which we are already familiar. In saying that, we merely classify it with a wider group of similar phenomena. My theory is that the laughter instinct* (like most of the major instincts of man) is so innately organised on its receptive or perceptual side that the auditory and the visual perception of laughter excite the laughter instinct. If we seek any deeper or further explanation, we may plausibly suppose that these special perceptual adaptations of the instincts of the gregarious species have been produced in the course of evolution, because they secure, among the members of any group, that emotional and impulsive congruity which is a principal foundation-stone of all group-life, animal and human. There is no rival theory in the field, so far as I know. Freud does not further deal with the problem, beyond implying that he agrees with le Bon in regarding emotional contagion as one of the manifestations " so often covered by the enigmatic word ' suggestion '." And he proceeds in the following

* *Cf.* my theory of laughter in *Outline of Psychology*, p. 165.

chapter to deal with the enigma of suggestion. In fact, the rest of the book is devoted to the elaboration of a theory of suggestion. He begins by insisting again on

" the fundamental fact of Group Psychology—the two theses as to the intensification of the emotions and the inhibition of the intellect in primitive groups. Our interest is now directed to discovering the psychological explanation of this mental change which is experienced by the individual in a group."

" It is clear," says Freud, " that rational factors . . . do not cover the observable phenomena. Beyond this, what we are offered as an explanation by authorities upon Sociology and Group Psychology is always the same, even though it is given various names, and that is—the magic word ' suggestion.' Tarde calls it ' imitation ' ; but we cannot help agreeing with a writer who protests that imitation comes under the concept of suggestion, and is in fact one of its results. Le Bon traces back all the puzzling features of social phenomena to two factors : the mutual suggestion of individuals and the prestige of leaders. But prestige, again, is only recognisable by its capacity for evoking suggestion. McDougall for a moment gives us an impression that his principle of ' primitive induction of emotion ' might enable us to do without the assumption of suggestion. But on further consideration we are forced to perceive that this principle says no more than the familiar assertions about ' imitation ' or ' contagion,' except for a decided stress upon the emotional factor."

Now, if Professor Freud had done me the honour to read my *Introduction to Social Psychology* (a thing which, so far as I can judge, neither he nor any one of his many disciples has ever done), instead of reading only my *Group Mind* (which is explicitly founded upon the other book and is essentially an attempt to apply to the problems of group psychology the principles arrived at in the earlier work), he would have seen that I distinguish clearly between suggestion and emotional contagion, and, further, that I have there propounded, not only a theory of emotional contagion, but also a distinct theory of suggestion. He would then not have committed the error of saying that there has been, during thirty years, no change in the situation as regards suggestion and that

" there has been no explanation of the nature of suggestion, that is, of the conditions under which influence without adequate logical foundation takes place."

Since Freud has thus entirely overlooked my theory of suggestion, I beg leave to restate it here, in order that the reader may compare it with the very complicated theory which is the main substance of Freud's book. My theory sets out from the fact of observation that, among animals of gregarious species, we commonly find relations of dominance and submission ; we see some members of a herd or flock submitting tamely and quietly to the dominance, the leadership, the self-assertion of other members. This submission does not always or commonly seem to imply fear. Yet it is unquestionably instinctive. I have argued, therefore, that such behaviour is the expression of a distinct and specific instinct of submission : an instinct which is apt to be evoked by the aggressive or self-assertive behaviour of other, especially larger and older, members of the group, and whose goal or function it is to secure harmony within the group by prompting the junior and weaker members of it to submit to the leadership of others, to follow them, to "knuckle under to them" without protest, to accept their slightest word as law, to feel humble or lowly in their presence and to adopt lowly or "crestfallen" attitudes before them. My theory maintains that the human species also is endowed with this instinct of submission ; and that, with the development of language and intellect, verbal indications of the attitudes of the strong become very important means of evoking and directing this submissive impulse ; that this impulse, the emotional conative tendency of this instinct, is the main conative factor at work in all instances of true suggestion, whether waking or hypnotic. Further, that, in human societies, reputation for power of any sort becomes a very important factor in evoking this impulse, supplementing and, in fact, largely supplanting, the bodily evidences of superior powers which, on the animal plane, are the principal excitants of this impulse ; such reputation constituting the essence of all that we call prestige, the power of using suggestion, of compelling bodily and mental obedience or docility, without evoking fear. My theory maintains that, if the human species were not gregarious, and if its native constitution did not comprise also this special submissive instinct, human beings would not be suggestible ; and, therefore, the social life of man would be profoundly other than it is.*

* I say that this instinct of submission is evidenced by the animals of many gregarious species. But I maintain that it is distinct from the gregarious instinct itself ; that there are species of animals which have the gregarious instinct, but lack the submissive instinct ; just as there are men who are strongly gregarious, but in whom the submissive instinct operates very little, if at all ; that is to say, I maintain that the gregarious and the submissive tendencies are independent variables and, therefore, cannot be properly ascribed to the same instinct. In this I dissent strongly from the teaching of Mr Wilfred Trotter, who, throughout his famous little book on *Instincts of the Herd in Peace and War*, assumes without question that all the phenomena commonly classed under the head of suggestion are sufficiently explained by invoking the " herd instinct."

T

Freud and his disciples make frequent reference to ego-instincts ; but they have never, so far as I know, attempted to define these postulated ego-instincts. I imagine that, if they would undertake to attempt to define them, it would appear that these ego-instincts are identical with what I have attempted to distinguish and define as two distinct instincts, the instincts of self-assertion and of submission. But Freud does not seek in the ego-instincts the explanation of suggestion. Rather his theory of suggestion is very much more complex. I will try to sketch it briefly and fairly.

Freud's theory of suggestion derives all the phenomena of suggestion from his " libido." " ' Libido ' is an expression taken from the theory of the emotions. We call by that name the energy (regarded as a quantitative magnitude, though not at present actually measurable) of those instincts which have to do with all that may be comprised under the word ' love '."

Then comes a passage, in which Freud seeks to justify once more his acceptance of the popular usage of the word " love " as evidence of the essential unity of all manifestations to which the word " love " can with any propriety be applied, including, besides sexual attraction or lust, " on the one hand, self-love, and on the other love for parents and children, friendship and love for humanity in general, and also devotion to concrete objects and to abstract ideas." He goes on to say : " We will try our fortune, then, with the supposition that love relationships (or, to use a more neutral expression, emotional ties) also constitute the essence of the group mind." He adds : " Let us remember that the authorities made no mention of any such relations. What would correspond to them is evidently concealed behind the shelter, the screen, of suggestion."

Freud then proceeds to the study of highly-organised groups and especially churches and armies ; for, as he says, " the most interesting examples of such structures are churches—communities of believers—and armies." He finds common to them one essential feature, namely, " the same illusion holds good of there being a head—in the Catholic Church, Christ ; in any army its Commander-in-Chief—who loves all the individuals in the group with an equal love. Everything depends upon this illusion ; if it were to be dropped, then both Church and army would dissolve, so far as external force permitted them to." To all the members of the Church, Christ is " their father surrogate " ; and to all the members of an army, the Commander-in-Chief is their father surrogate. In the latter case the relation is multiplied by the official hierarchy :

" Every Captain is, as it were, the Commander-in-Chief and the father of his company, and so is every non-commissioned officer of his section.
" It is to be noticed that in these two artificial groups each individual is bound by libidinal ties on the one hand to the leader . . . and on the other hand to the other members of the group . . . It would appear as though we were on the right road toward an explanation of the principal phenomenon of Group Psychology—the individual's lack of freedom in the group. If each individual is bound in two directions by such an intense emotional tie, we shall find no difficulty in attributing to that circumstance the alteration and limitation which have been observed in his personality."

Precisely ! *If* the individual is so bound, and, given the protean nature of the *libido*, anything may follow, any phenomena of group life may with a little ingenuity be attributed to these alleged libidinous ties. But the question remains—Are these ties really there in all groups ? Are they really the fundamental factors of all group life ? Or are they merely asserted to be there by Professor Freud, in order to make Group Psychology a mere annex of his psychoanalytic system ?

Freud finds in the panic evidence of the truth of his view. He would distinguish between collective fear and true panic. He writes :

" The contention that dread in a group is increased to enormous proportions by means of induction (contagion) is not in the least contradicted by these remarks. McDougall's view meets the case entirely when the danger is a really great one and when the group has no strong emotional ties—conditions which are fulfilled, for instance, when a fire breaks out in a theatre or a place of amusement."*

But he contends that in a body of troops panic may break out under conditions no more threatening than others which they

---

* Freud's theory compels him to make this distinction between collective fear and the true panic; for he can hardly ask us to believe that *all* the members of every theatre audience are bound together by strong libidinous ties, nor can he hope to persuade us that *all* the members of every such audience are dominated by a common father surrogate special to the occasion. Yet every such assembly is liable to collective fear. It is, perhaps, worth while to point out that Freud makes no attempt to show that there is any difference between the phenomena of the collective fear and of the panic ; as there surely should be, if these are two distinct and differently conditioned manifestations.

have encountered without disorder; and that in these cases the essential condition of this, the true, panic, as distinguished from mere collective fear, is the death of the leader.

Now, if this new theory of the panic is true, there must have occurred during the late war a multitude of such panics; and we might fairly demand that Freud should support his theory by the citation of one or two authentic accounts of such panics induced by the death of leaders. But we find no such citations. In place of them we are offered in evidence only a scene from a play; or rather not even from a play, but from a parody of a play.

" The typical occasion of the outbreak of a panic is very much as it is represented in Nestroy's parody of Hebbel's play about Judith and Holofernes—a soldier cries out : ' The General has lost his head ! ' and thereupon all the Assyrians take to flight."

Freud adds :

" Anyone who, like McDougall, describes a panic as one of the plainest functions of the ' group mind,' arrives at the paradoxical position that this group mind does away with itself in one of its most striking manifestations."

In answer to this, I would point out that I do not ascribe a group mind to a crowd, nor do I regard a panic as a function of the group mind ; the panic is rather a function of an instinct operating in an unorganised group. I admit that the death of a leader may contribute to bring about a panic ; but I submit that the grounds of this are sufficiently obvious, that it requires no far-fetched theories for its explanation. The reasoning of Freud's paragraphs, following those in which he treats of panic, shows that his theory requires that, on the death of the leader, the group shall break out, not into panic, but into an orgy of mutual murder. For, he tells us, it is only the libidinous ties between the leader and the members and those between the members (which latter *somehow* are derivative from the former) which keep in check our narcissism ; and narcissism is ruthless murderous self-seeking. That this, rather than panic, is the consequence of the death of the leader logically demanded by Freud's theory is clearly shown by his next section, which deals with the religious group.

" The dissolution of a religious group is not so easy *to observe* " (italics mine). And so here also Freud turns to literature and finds his evidence in a story which, if not a parody of a story, is little more, namely, the notorious sensational novel *When It Was Dark*.

This novel, which achieved a great popular success, is offered us as evidence, because it was recommended by the Bishop of London, and because " it gave a clever and, as it seems to me, a convincing picture of such a possibility and its consequences." The whole passage deserves citation :

" The novel, which is supposed to relate to the present day, tells how a conspiracy of enemies to the figure of Christ and of the Christian faith succeeds in arranging for a sepulchre to be discovered in Jerusalem. In this sepulchre is an inscription, in which Joseph of Arimathea confesses that for reasons of piety he secretly removed the body of Christ from its grave on the third day after its entomb- ment and buried it in this spot. The resurrection of Christ and his divine nature are by this means disposed of, and the result of this archæological discovery is a convulsion in European civilisation and an extraordinary increase in all crimes and acts of violence, which only ceases when the forgers' plot has been revealed. The phenomenon which accompanies the dissolution that is here sup- posed to overtake a religious group *is not dread*, for which the occasion is wanting. Instead of it, ruthless and hostile impulses toward other people make their appearance, which, owing to the equal love of Christ, they had previously been unable to do."*

In the next chapter Freud briefly recognises the existence of leaderless groups. These, which might be supposed to offer some serious difficulty to a theory which makes the leader the centre of all group-ties, he brushes lightly aside with the suggestion that an idea, an abstraction, or even a common wish, may serve as a substitute for a leader, as an object or centre for our libidinous impulses.

Having arrived at the view that libidinous ties are constitutive of every group, Freud very properly turns to being-in-love in the ordinary sense of the words, in order to study the phenomena more intimately ; and here he finds "identification" to be the centre of interest. " Identification is the earliest and original form of emotional tie." It culminates in the cannibal, who,

" as we know, has remained at this standpoint ; he has a devour- ing affection for his enemies and only devours people of whom he is fond."

There follows an intricate discussion of love, in the course of which the *ego* and the ego-ideal and other entities spring back and forth be-

* It happens that I have some slight acquaintance with the author of this precious story, and I venture to think that he would be immensely tickled to know that his successful effort to boil the domestic pot is now seriously cited as evidence in support of a scientific theory.

tween the self and the object, the object becoming the self and the self the object, in a manner so puzzling to any but a hardened believer that I can make out of it only the following : Freud recognises, as I have done, two principal factors in normal sexual love, sensuality or lust on the one hand, tenderness on the other : but, whereas I have identified these two factors of sexual love with the impulse of the sex instinct and the impulse of the parental or protective instinct, respectively, Freud feels himself bound to derive both of them from the sexual *libido*. He describes the tender factor as a part of the sexual impulse inhibited in its aim. By what influence this part is supposed to be inhibited is not very clear. Nor is it clear why, being inhibited, its nature should be transformed into its opposite. The natural result of obstruction to the sexual instinct would seem to be, as in all other cases, anger, as we see in animals. However, granting this transformation into tenderness of one-half of the libido, we then have sexual love consisting essentially in one-half of the sexual libido working toward its sexual goal, but restrained by the other half, which, by inhibition, has been transformed into its opposite, tenderness. How much simpler to recognise that parental love is primarily the expression of a special instinct independent of and quite different from the sexual instinct ; and to see in sexual love the play of these two impulses reciprocally modifying one another, and modified still further in most cases by other equally independent tendencies !

Freud seeks further light on love from hypnosis :

" From being in love to hypnosis is evidently only a short step—the hypnotic relation is the devotion of someone in love to an unlimited degree, but with sexual satisfaction excluded . . . But, on the other hand, we may also say that the hypnotic relation is (if the expression is permissible) a group formation with two members . . . Hypnosis is distinguished from a group formation by this limitation of number, just as it is distinguished from being in love by the absence of directly sexual tendencies. In this respect it occupies a middle position between the two."

Hypnosis contains, then, the key to the crowd. The reader at this point in the book begins to think he is near the end of his journey. A group is a crowd hypnotised by its leader ; and to be hypnotised is to be in love, to have one's sexual libido fixated upon the hypnotiser in two halves, one half inhibited, the other half uninhibited. The group is a crowd in love with its leader ; and suggestibility

is a consequence of being in love. But the explanation of suggestion is not so simple.

" There is still a great deal in it which we must recognise as
unexplained and mystical. It contains an additional element of
paralysis derived from the relation between someone with superior
power and someone who is without power and helpless."

So the indefatigable Freud sets off on another tack to find the grounds
of this further unexplained and mystical element in suggestion. He
begins by examining Mr Trotter's view, which finds the explanation
of all suggestion in the herd instinct. He rejects this view on the
grounds, first, that " it can be made at all events probable that the
herd instinct is not irreducible, that it is not primary in the same
sense as the instinct of self-preservation and the sexual instinct."
Secondly, on the ground that it explains the group, without assigning
an essential place or function to a leader ; and Freud has already
asserted that the leader is the essential key to the group. Freud
then makes the following astonishing *tour de force*, and brings
us back to the original position from which he set out.

" *Gemeingeist, esprit de corps*, ' group spirit,' etc., does not
belie its derivation from what was originally envy . . . Social
justice means that we deny ourselves many things so that others
may have to do without them as well, or, what is the same thing,
may not be able to ask for them. This demand for equality is the
root of social conscience and the sense of duty."*

But what then is envy, which is thus identified with a demand
for equality and as the root of all the social virtues ? Is envy the
expression of some special instinct ? No, its explanation is to be
found in the fact that man is not, as Trotter asserts, a herd animal,
but " rather a horde animal, an individual creature in a horde led
by a chief." Now, the characteristics of a crowd imply regression
of its members " to a primitive mental activity, of just such a sort
as we should be inclined to ascribe to the primal horde. Thus the
group appears to us as a revival of the primal horde. Just as
primitive man virtually survives in every individual, so the primal
horde may arise once more out of any random crowd."

* The reader should notice here that, according to this strange doctrine,
the group spirit and social justice alike are founded in, or are expressions of,
an attitude considerably meaner and more despicable than that of the dog in
the manger ! The dog in the manger says—" You shall not eat, because I
cannot eat!" According to Freud, the socially just man's attitude essentially
is—" I will not eat, in order that I may have the pleasure of preventing you
from eating."

Thus the long trail leads back to " Totem and Taboo " and the horde father. This primal superman "had prevented his sons from satisfying their directly sexual tendencies ; he forced them into abstinence and consequently into the emotional ties with him and with one another which could arise out of those of their tendencies that were inhibited in their sexual aim. He forced them, so to speak, into group psychology. His sexual jealousy and intolerance became in the last resort the causes of group psychology." Now we see why, in the opening chapter, Freud wrote of *the illusion* that is the prime condition of all group-life, the illusion on the part of the members that they are equally loved by the leader. For the primal horde father does not love his sons ; he is merely consumed and motivated by sexual jealousy against them. " The illusion that the leader loves all of the individuals equally and justly . . . is simply an idealistic remodelling of the state of affairs in the primal horde, where all of the sons knew that they were equally persecuted by the primal father, and feared him equally " ; and where the primal father, by forbidding them all sexual gratification, forced them to love him and to love one another. This is described as a process of " recasting upon which all social duties are built up."

This same recasting process explains " what is still incomprehensible and mysterious in group formations—all that lies hidden behind the enigmatic words 'hypnosis' and 'suggestion.'"

" Let us recall that hypnosis has something positively uncanny about it ; but the characteristic of uncanniness suggests something old and familiar that has undergone repression. Let us consider how hypnosis is induced. The hypnotist asserts that he is in possession of a mysterious power which robs the subject of his own will, or, which is the same thing, the subject believes it of him. This mysterious power . . . must be the same that is looked upon by primitive people as the source of taboo, the same that emanates from kings and chieftains, and makes it dangerous to approach them (mana). The hypnotist, then, is supposed to be in possession of this power ; and how does he manifest it ? By telling the subject to look him in the eyes ; his most typical method of hypnotising is by his look. But it is precisely the sight of the chieftain that is dangerous and unbearable for primitive people, just as later that of the Godhead is for mortals."

" By the measures that he takes, then, the hypnotist awakens in the subject a portion of his archaic inheritance which had also made him compliant toward his parents . . . What is thus awakened is the idea of a paramount and dangerous personality, toward whom only a passive-masochistic attitude is possible, toward whom one's will has to be surrendered . . . the uncanny and coercive characteristics of group formations, which are shown in their suggestion phenomena, may therefore with justice be traced back to the fact of their origin from the primal horde. The leader of the group is still the dreaded primal father ; the group still wishes to be governed by unrestricted force ; it has an extreme passion for authority ; in le Bon's phrase, it has a thirst for obedience.* The primal father is the group ideal, which governs the ego in the place of the ego-ideal. Hypnotism has a good claim to being described as a group of two ; there remains as a definition for suggestion . . . a conviction which is not based upon perception and reasoning but upon an erotic tie."

Further :

" we have come to the conclusion that suggestion is a partial manifestation of the state of hypnosis, and that hypnosis is solidly founded upon a predisposition which has survived in the unconscious from the early history of the human family."

Here we have come to the end of the long and tortuous trail, and have found as the root of all social psychology an ancient predisposition impressed upon the race (or rather upon the male half of it) by its experiences during the period of life in the primal horde under the dominance of a brutal horde father; this predisposition makes men desire to be persecuted, makes them love those that persecute them and at the same time love their fellow victims of persecution. The remainder of the book restates some of the positions reached and deals with some other hardly related problems.

Let me try to summarise the complex theory as fairly as possible in a few lines. The main factor in group life is suggestion. The fundamental problem of Group Psychology, therefore, is the nature of suggestion. Suggestion is always of the same nature as the suggestion of hypnosis ; and the study of hypnosis shows that suggestion depends upon a peculiar emotional attitude of the patient to the hypnotiser. This attitude results from the re-animation (by regression) of an atavistic survival, an attitude acquired by the race during the long period in which men lived in the primal horde, a horde dominated by a brutal horde-leader fiercely jealous of his sexual rights over all the women. This

* How or why the persecuted sons of the primal horde father acquire a passion for being persecuted is nowhere explained. Even if we accept Freud's dictum that to " persecute a man and to force him to deny himself all sexual gratification is the surest way to earn his love," it is not obvious that the victim will at the same time develop a passionate desire to be persecuted, or that he will transmit this desire to his remote descendants.

horde-leader forced all his fellow-males to repress their sexual urgings ; their repressed libido then became fixated on him, so that they loved him, and falsely believed that he loved them, at the same time that they feared him for his brutal domination and plotted to slay him. When any man lives as a member of a group and is subject to group influences, when he accepts the traditional morality and develops the virtues of the good and patriotic citizen, it is because some leader throws him back from his hard-won individuality, forces upon him an atavistic regression to the complex attitude proper toward the leader of the primitive horde, so that he becomes suggestible toward him ; but the part of the leader may be played by an abstract idea, or even by a wish or aspiration held in common by a number of individuals.

What verdict shall be given upon this theory ? First, it may be said, if there were no other explanations of the facts of group life, we should have to entertain it seriously. But, as I have endeavoured to show, other simpler, less extravagant, explanations are possible and are at least as adequate.

Secondly, the theory, if accepted with all the peculiar Freudian assumptions upon which it is based, leaves or rather raises many obscure problems. For example, it leaves the leaderless group unexplained ; for we can hardly take seriously the assertion that an abstract idea or a wish may play the rôle assigned to the leader in forcing regression to the atavistic attitude. It leaves untouched the fact that women are at least as suggestible as men, and probably on the whole more so ; we shall have to invent some other story to account for their suggestibility. It leaves very obscure the suggestibility of the members of a group toward one another. Here I would especially cite such instances as the famous spread of the rumour of Russian troops passing through England in the autumn of 1914. It is impossible to point in such instances to a leader. We must be content to suppose this to be an instance where a wish played the rôle of leader. But is not this equivalent to rejecting the theory *in toto* ? Further, it does not explain the primary fact of contagion of emotion, so fundamental to all group-life. And it does not explain how a leader attains leadership ; how he manages to force regression upon his followers and to constitute himself a leader.

Finally, it reduces all the social life of men, including all team-work, all patriotism, all moral self-control and discipline, all self-sacrifice for the good of the community, to the working of an atavistic regression, to a return to the behaviour proper to the (very hypothetical) remote age in which the violence of a bully, armed with a club and prompted by sexual jealousy, was the only controlling force in human society. It makes sexual jealousy and envy the roots of all the nobler manifestations of human life. Yet it leaves these roots themselves unexplained. Why jealousy? Why envy? If the sexual impulse, the fear of death, and the urge for food, were the whole of the instinctive endowment of primitive man, why should not the primal horde have enjoyed a delightful promiscuity? On that plane one woman can serve many men. We should expect sexual jealousy, if anywhere, only among the women.

My verdict is " not proven and wildly improbable." If we positively knew, if by any supernatural unchallengeable authority we were assured, that all the phenomena of human life, all the modes of human activity, had been derived from sexuality, and must be explained as manifestations of the sexual libido, we might be induced to say that Professor Freud's theory of suggestion and his theory of social phenomena in general was a most ingenious and praiseworthy effort to solve an insoluble problem.

But we have no such guarantee. The only authority we have for accepting this as the necessary and sole permissible line of speculation, for regarding our explanations of social phenomena as necessarily confined within the limits of the sexual libido, is the authority of Professor Freud and of his devoted disciples. I, for one, shall continue to try to avoid the spell of the primal horde father and to use what intellect I have, untrammelled by arbitrary limitations.

PSYCHOLOGICAL TYPES

BY

C. G. JUNG, M.D., LL.D.
Formerly of the University of Zürich

PSYCHOLOGICAL TYPES*

C. G. JUNG

OF ancient origin, indeed, are the attempts to solve the problem of types. It has been sought, on the one hand, to bring together into definite categories the manifold differences of human individuals, and on the other to break through the apparent uniformity of all men by a sharper characterisation of certain typical differences. Without caring to go too deeply into the history of the development of such attempts, I would like to call attention to the fact that the oldest categories known to us have originated with physicians, most especially with Claudius Galen, the Greek physician who lived in the second century after Christ. He distinguished four fundamental temperaments, the sanguine, phlegmatic, choleric and melancholic. But the basic idea of this differentiation harks back to the fifth century before Christ, to the teachings of Hippocrates, who described the human body as composed of the four elements, air, water, fire and earth. Corresponding to the elements there were to be found in the living body, blood, phlegm, yellow and black bile ; and it was Galen's idea that by reason of the unequal admixture of these four factors, men could be separated into four different classes. Those in whom blood predominated were sanguine ; those having relatively more phlegm were designated as phlegmatic ; when yellow bile prevailed the temperament was choleric ; and those under the sway of black bile were melancholic. As our modern speech attests, these differentiations of temperament have become immortal, although their naïveté as psychological theory has long since been apparent.

Without a doubt Galen deserves the credit of having created a psychological classification of human individuals which has endured for two thousand years, a classification which rests upon perceptible differences of emotionality or affectivity. It is interesting to note that the first effort toward a classification of

---

* Paper read at the International Congress of Education.

289

types concerns itself with the emotional behaviour of men, manifestly because it is the play of emotion involved which forms the most frequent and obviously striking feature of any behaviour.

But it is not in the least to be supposed that affect is the only thing characteristic of mankind ; one can expect characteristic data from other functions as well, it being only necessary for us to perceive and observe the other functions with the same clearness we lend to affect. In the earlier centuries, when the concept " psychology " as we employ it to-day was, so to speak, entirely lacking, the other psychological functions were veiled in darkness, just as to-day they appear to the great majority of people as scarcely discernible subtleties. Affects reveal themselves readily to superficial observation and the unpsychological man, that is, *he to whom his neighbour's psyche is not a problem*, contents himself with such an observation. It suffices him to observe affects in others, but if he sees none, then the other person becomes invisible to him, because, aside from affects, it is impossible for him to read anything in another's consciousness. In one word, he is blind to the other functions.

The primary condition which permits us to discover in our fellow-men functions other than affects, is obtained when we ourselves pass from an unproblematical into a problematical condition of consciousness. By " unproblematical," as I use it here, I mean the instinctive attitude toward life, as exemplified by the primitive, while by " problematical " I understand a state of mind in which the easy, " taking-things-for-granted " attitude has passed over into one in which a certain amount of psychological tension exists. In this latter state our neighbour steps out of his invisibility and becomes a factor with which we have to grapple consciously. Resuming the thread of the argument, in so far as we judge others only by affects, we show that our chief and perhaps only criterion is affect. That means, then, that this criterion is valid also for our own psychology, which is equivalent to saying that our psychological judgment altogether has no objectivity nor independence, but is a slave to affect. This is, in fact, a truth which holds good for the majority of people, and upon this fact rests the psychological possibility of a murderous war and its ever-probable recurrence, optimistic blindness to the contrary notwithstanding. It must be so as long as a man judges those on the " other side " by his own affect or emotion. I call such a state of consciousness unproblematical because manifestly it itself has never been looked upon as a problem ; there is no sense of inadequacy or maladaptation to the facts involved. It only becomes a problem when doubt arises as to whether the affect, that is, one's own affect, offers a satisfactory basis for forming psychological judgments. We cannot deny the fact that we ourselves are always inclined to justify ourselves to anyone who wishes to hold us responsible for an emotional act, by saying that we acted only on the spur of feeling, and that we are not generally nor always as we were in that moment. When it concerns ourselves we are glad to explain affect as an exceptional condition of lessened accountability, but we are loathe to make this allowance for others. But even if it is only an effort not altogether admirable, perhaps, towards exculpating the beloved *ego*, still, in the feeling of justification that such an excuse brings, there lies a positive element, namely, the attempt to separate oneself from one's own affect, and thereby also to distinguish one's fellow-man from his affect condition. And even if my excuse is only a subterfuge, still, it is an effort to cast a doubt on the validity of affect as the sole index of personality, and an effort furthermore, to make myself aware of other psychological functions which are just as characteristic of the self as the affect, if not, indeed, even more so. Whoever judges us by our affect is readily accused by us of lack of understanding, or, worse still, of being unjust. But that puts us under the obligation of not judging others by affect.

The primitive, unpsychological man, looking upon affect in himself and others as the only essential criterion, in order to avoid the act of false judgment, must develop in himself a problematical condition of consciousness, that is to say, he must reach a condition in which, together with the affect, yet other factors are recognised as valid. In this problematical condition a paradoxical judgment is formed, that is, one says, " I am this affect, and I am not that affect." This antithesis forces a splitting of the *ego*, or rather, a splitting of the psychological material which makes up the *ego*. In that I recognise myself just as much in my affect as in something else that is not my affect. I differentiate between an affect factor and other psychological factors, and in doing this I force the affect to descend from its original heights of unlimited power and make it take its place as one psychological function among others.

Only after having gone through such a process and after acquiring thereby the power to discriminate between various psychological factors in himself, is a man placed in a position to summon other criteria than affect in his psychological judgment of others. In

U

this way only can there develop a really objective psychological critique.

That which we call "psychology" to-day is a science which is possible only on the basis of certain historical and moral conditions, conditions which have been created by Christian education covering nearly two thousand years. A saying such, for example, as "Judge not that ye be not judged," has through its religious connotation created the possibility of a volition which, in the last resort, strives toward a simple objectivity of judgment. And this objectivity not being merely an attitude of disinterestedness toward others, but resting as it does on the fact that we wish others to benefit by the fundamental principles by which we excuse ourselves, this objectivity then is the basic condition leading us to a just evaluation of our fellow men. You wonder, perhaps, why I dwell so emphatically on the point of objectivity, but you will cease to wonder if ever you seek to classify people in practice. A man of outspoken sanguine temperament will tell you that taken fundamentally he is deeply melancholic; "a choleric," that his only fault consists in his having always been too "phlegmatic." But a division of people in whose validity I alone believe is about as helpful as a universal church in which I am the sole member. We must, therefore, find criteria which are accepted as binding not only by the judging subject but also by the judged object.

Quite in contrast to the old classification according to temperaments, the problem of a new division of types begins with the express convention, neither to allow oneself to be judged by affect, nor so to judge others, for no one can or will finally declare himself identical with his affect. Using affect as the point of departure, therefore, there can never be brought about a general reciprocal understanding such as science represents. We must then look about us for those factors which we call upon when we excuse ourselves because of an emotional act. We say perhaps "Granted that I have said this or that in a state of affect, naturally that was an exaggeration and I had no evil intentions. As a matter of fact, what I really think is thus and so, etc." A very naughty child, having caused his mother painful anxiety, may say, "I didn't intend to do it. I didn't intend to hurt you, I love you very much." Such explanations bespeak the existence of a personality other than that appearing in affect. In both cases the affect personality appears as something inferior which has spread over and clouded the real *ego*. However, the personality revealed in such an affect is often a higher and a better one, whose heights unfortunately one cannot attain. There are well-known instances of generosity, altruism, sacrifice and similar " beautiful gestures," for which, as an ironical observer might spitefully remark, one does not care to be held responsible—perhaps a reason why so many people do so little good.

But in both cases the affect obtains as an exceptional condition whose qualities are either presented as invalid for the " real " personality, or else not convincingly connected with it as lasting attributes. What is this " real " personality then ? Manifestly it is partly that which one distinguishes in oneself as separate from affect, and partly that of which one is stripped by the judgment of others as non-essential. Since it is impossible to deny that the condition of affect belongs to the *ego*, it follows that the *ego* is the same in affect as in the so-called " real " condition, although in a different attitude toward the existing psychological facts. In affect the *ego* is unfree, driven, in a state of compulsion. Over against this, the normal state is understood as a condition of free choice, of disposability of one's physical forces ; in other words, the condition of affect is unproblematical while the normal condition is problematical, recognising as it does the existence of a problem to be resolved and, at the same time, containing the possibility of a free choice of action in regard to the problem. In this latter condition an understanding can be effected because in this condition, and in it alone, is to be found the possibility of the recognition of motives and self-knowledge. Discrimination is indispensable to knowledge. But discrimination means the splitting up of the content of consciousness into distinguishable factors. Therefore, if we wish to define the individuality of a man in terms that will satisfy not only our judgment but also that of the judged object, then we must make our point of departure that condition or that attitude, which is felt by the object to be a conscious, normal state of mind. Therefore also, we must concern ourselves chiefly with conscious motives while we abstract from the situation our own arbitrary interpretations.

If we proceed in such a way we shall discover after a time that, in spite of a great variety of motives and tendencies, certain groups of individuals, characterised by an obvious conformity in their manner of motivation, can be separated from one another. For example, we shall come upon individuals who find themselves actuated in all their conclusions, apperceptions, feelings, affects and actions, chiefly through external factors, or at least the emphasis is laid on the latter whether causal or final motives are in question. I shall give some illustrations of what I mean. St. Augustine says, "I would not believe in the Evangels if the authority of the Church did not compel me." A daughter says, " I could not think something that would be displeasing to my father." A certain person finds a modern piece of music beautiful because everybody else professes to find it beautiful. Cases are not infrequent in which a man has married in a way pleasing to his parents, but very much against his own interests. There are people who can make themselves absurd in order to amuse others, in fact they may even prefer to make butts of themselves rather than remain unnoticed. Many people have in all their reactions but one consideration in mind, namely, what others think of them. Someone has said, " One need not be ashamed of something nobody knows about." There are those who can only realise happiness when it excites the envy of others; there are individuals who wish for troubles and even make them for themselves in order to enjoy the sympathy of their fellow men.

Such examples could easily be multiplied indefinitely. They point to a psychological peculiarity which is to be sharply distinguished from another attitude determined, in contradistinction to the former, chiefly by inner or subjective factors. Such a person says, " I know I could give my father the greatest pleasure if I did such and such, but none the less I have a different idea about it " ; or, " I see that the weather is vile but none the less I shall carry out the plan I made yesterday." Such a man does not travel for pleasure, but in order to carry into action a preconceived idea. A man may say, " Apparently my book is incomprehensible, but it is perfectly clear to me." One can also hear it declared, as a man once actually did say, " The whole world believes I could do something, but I know absolutely that I can do nothing." Such a man can be so ashamed of himself as not to dare to mix with people. Among persons such as these are to be found those individuals who can only experience happiness when they are sure that no one knows anything about it, and to these people, a thing is disagreeable just because it is pleasing to everybody else. Good is sought as far as possible where no one would think it could be found. At every step the agreement of the subject must be obtained and without it nothing can be undertaken or carried out. Such a one would say to Augustine, " I would believe in the Evangels if the authority of the Church did not coerce me to it." His constant effort is toward showing that everything he does is on his own decision and from his own conviction, never because influenced by anyone, nor for the purpose of catering to any person or opinion. This attitude then characterises a second group of individuals who derive their motives almost exclusively from the subject, from the inner necessities.

Finally, there is a third group in which one can hardly say whether the motivation is derived from within or without. This group is the most numerous, and embraces the less differentiated normal man who is normal partly because he brings to focus no exaggerations, and partly because he is not under the necessity of exaggerating. The normal man, according to definition, is influenced in equal measure from within and without. He makes up, as has been said, the widely inclusive middle group, on the one side of which appear those individuals who are chiefly determined in their motivation by their outer object and, on the other, those who respond in the majority of cases to the demands of the subject. I have designated the first group as *extraverts*, the latter as *introverts*. These terms scarcely need special elucidation, since, from what has been said, they are self-explanatory.

Although there are without a doubt individuals in whom one can recognise the type at a first glance, for the most part this is by no means the case. As a rule only careful observation and a weighing of the evidence permits a sure classification. Clear and simple though the fundamental principle of the two opposing attitudes may be, nevertheless their concrete reality is complicated and obscure, for every individual is an exception to the rule. Therefore, one can never give a description of a type, no matter how complete, which applies to more than one individual despite the fact that thousands might, in a certain sense, be strikingly described thereby. Conformity is one side of a man, uniqueness is the other. The individual soul is not explained by classification, yet at the same time, through the understanding of the psychological types, a way is opened to a better understanding of human psychology in general. The differentiation of the types begins often very early, so early that in certain cases one must speak of it as being innate. The earliest mark of extraversion in a child is his quick adaptation to the environment, and the extraordinary attention he gives to objects and especially to his impress upon them. Shyness of objects is slight ; the child moves and lives in and with them. He makes quick perceptions, but in a haphazard way. Apparently he develops more quickly than an introverted child, since he has less inhibition and, as a rule, no fear. Apparently, too, he feels no barrier between himself and objects and therefore can play with them freely and learn through them. He gladly pushes his undertakings to an extreme and risks himself in the endeavour. Whatever is unknown appears alluring.

Reversing the picture, one of the earliest marks of introversion in a child is a reflective, thoughtful manner, a pronounced shyness, even anxiety toward unknown objects. Very early there appears also a tendency toward self-assertion in relation to the object, and efforts to master the latter. Whatever is unknown is regarded with mistrust. Outside influence is, in the main, met with emphatic resistance. The child wants his own way and under no circumstances does he wish to submit to a strange rule which he cannot understand. When he asks questions, it is not so much out of curiosity or desire for sensation, but because he wants names, meanings and explanations that offer him a subjective assurance over against the object. I have seen an introverted child who made her first efforts to walk only after she was familiar with all the things in the room with which she might come in contact. Thus very early in an introverted child can be noted the characteristic defensive attitude which the adult introvert shows toward the object, just as in the case of the extraverted child one can observe very early a marked assurance and enterprise, and a blissful trustfulness in his relations with objects. This then is the basic characteristic of the extraverted attitude : the psychic life is displayed, so to speak, outside the individual in objects and relationships to objects. In especially marked cases there occurs a sort of blindness for one's own individuality. In contrast with this, the introvert always conducts himself toward the object as if the latter possessed a superior power over him against which he had to steady himself.

It is a sad but none the less uncommonly frequent fact that the two types are constantly conflicting with one another. This is a fact which will immediately come to the notice of anyone who investigates the problem. It originates from the circumstance that the psychic values are localised diagonally opposite each other. The introvert sees everything which is of any value to him in the subject ; the extravert, on the other hand, sees it in the object, but this dependence upon the object seems to the introvert a state of great inferiority, while to the extravert the inferiority condition lies in an unmitigated subjectivity, and he is able to see nothing in such an attitude save infantile autoerotism.

There is small wonder then, that the two types combat one another, a fact, however, which in the majority of cases does not prevent a man from marrying a woman of the opposite type. Such marriages are very valuable as psychological symbioses so long as the partners do not seek to be " psychologically " understood by one another. But such a phase belongs to the normal, developmental phenomena of every marriage in which the couple has either the necessary leisure or the necessary urge to development, or both indeed, together with the needful amount of courage to risk breaking up the marital peace. If, as was said, circumstances favour it, this phase enters quite automatically into the lives of both types, and for the following reasons : the type is a one-sidedness of development ; the one develops only his outer, and neglects his inner relationship, while the other grows subjectively only and remains at a standstill with respect to external factors. But in time there arises a necessity for the individual to develop that which previously he has neglected. The development occurs in the form of a differentiation of certain functions, and because of their importance for the type problem, I must now take up the question of these functions.

The conscious psyche is an adaptation—or orientation—apparatus, consisting of a number of psychic functions. As such fundamental functions one can designate *sensation, thinking, feeling* and *intuition*. Under the heading *sensation*, I wish to include all apperception by means of sense organs ; by *thinking* I understand the function of intellectual cognition and the forming of logical conclusions ; *feeling* is a function of subjective evaluation, and *intuition* I hold to be apperception by an unconscious method, or the perception of an unconscious content.

These four fundamental functions appear to me, as far as my experience reaches, to be sufficient to express and represent the ways and means of conscious orientation. For a complete orientation of consciousness all the functions should co-operate equally ; thinking should make cognition and the forming of judgments possible ; feeling should say to us how and in what way a thing is important or unimportant for us ; sensation by means of sight, hearing, taste, etc., should enable us to perceive concrete reality ; and finally intuition should permit us to guess the more or less hidden possibilities and backgrounds of a situation, because these hidden factors also belong to a complete picture of a given moment. But in reality it is seldom or never that these fundamental functions are uniformly developed and correspondingly under voluntary control. As a rule one or the other function is in the foreground, while the others remain in the background quite undifferentiated.

Thus there are many people who restrict themselves chiefly to a simple perception of concrete reality, without reflecting much about it or taking into account the feeling values involved. They bother themselves little about the possibilities which lie hidden in a situation. Such people I describe as "sensation" types. Others are exclusively influenced by what they think and simply cannot adapt themselves to a situation which they cannot comprehend intellectually. I designate such people "thinking" types. Again, there are others who are guided in everything wholly by their feelings. They merely ask themselves if something is pleasant or the reverse, and orientate themselves by their feeling impressions. These are the "feeling" types. Finally, "intuitives" concern themselves neither with ideas nor with feeling reactions, nor yet with the reality of things, but give themselves up wholly to the lure of possibilities and abandon every situation where no further possibilities are scented.

These types then present a different kind of one-sidedness, but one which is complicated in a peculiar way with the generally extraverted and introverted attitudes. Just on account of this complication I was forced to mention the existence of these function types, and bearing it in mind, let us return to the question outlined above, *viz.*, the one-sidedness of the extraverted and introverted attitudes. This one-sidedness would indeed lead to a complete loss of balance if it were not psychically compensated by an unconscious counterposition. The investigation of the unconscious has revealed the fact, for example, that in the case of an introvert, together with his conscious attitude, there is an unconscious extraverted attitude which automatically compensates his conscious one-sidedness.

Confronted with a given individual, one can, of course, surmise intuitively the existence of an introverted or an extraverted attitude in general, but an exact scientific investigation cannot content itself with an intuition, but must turn to the actual material presented. It is then revealed that no person is simply extraverted or introverted, but that he is so in the form of certain functions. Let us take, for example, an intellectual type ; most of the conscious material which he offers for observation consists of thoughts, conclusions, deliberations, as well as actions, affects, feelings and perceptions of an intellectual nature, or at least directly dependent *on intellectual premises*. We must interpret the essence of his general attitude from the peculiarity of this material. The material offered by a feeling type will be of a different kind, that

is, feelings and emotional contents of all sorts, thoughts, deliberations and perceptions dependent *upon emotional premises*. Therefore, only by reason of the peculiar nature of his feelings shall we
be in a position to say whether this individual belongs to this or
that general type. For this reason I must again mention the
function types, because in individual cases, the extraverted and
introverted attitudes can never be demonstrated as existing *per se*,
but appear as the characteristics of the dominating conscious
functions. Similarly, there is no attitude *per se* of the unconscious,
but only typically modified forms of unconscious functions, and
only through the investigation of the unconscious functions and
their peculiarities can the unconscious attitude be scientifically
determined.

One can scarcely speak of typical unconscious functions, although
in the economics of the psyche one should attribute a function to
the unconscious. I think it is wise to express oneself cautiously
in this respect, and therefore I would rather not assert more than
this, namely that the unconscious, as far as we can now see, has a
compensatory function in relation to the conscious. As to what
the unconscious is, in and for itself, it is idle to speculate. It is
according to its nature, beyond our knowing. We merely postulate
its existence on the basis of its so-called products such as dreams
and the like. It is an assured finding of scientific experience that
dreams, for example, almost invariably have a content which can
act as an essential corrective of the conscious attitude. From this
comes the justification of speaking of a compensatory function of
the unconscious.

Together with this general function in relation to the conscious,
the unconscious contains also functions which under other circumstances can become conscious as well. The thinking type, for
example, must necessarily always suppress and exclude feeling,
since nothing disturbs thinking so much as feeling, and conversely,
the emotional man must avoid thinking as far as possible, since
nothing is more disastrous to feeling than thinking. Suppressed
functions fall to the unconscious. Just as among the four sons
of Horus only one had a human head, so with the four fundamental
functions, only one, as a rule, is fully conscious and so differentiated
that it is free and subject to the direction of the will, while the
remaining three functions are partly or wholly unconscious. By
this "unconsciousness" I do not in the least mean that an intellectual, for example, would be unconscious of feeling. He knows his
feelings very well in so far as he has any power of introspection, but

he gives them no value and allows them no influence. They manifest themselves against his intention ; they are spontaneous, finally taking to themselves the validity consciousness denies. They are activated by unconscious stimulation, forming, indeed, something like a counter-personality whose existence can only be divined through the analysis of the products of the unconscious.

If a function is in no sense under control, if it is felt as a disturbance of the conscious function, if now it comes forward whimsically, now disappears, if it possesses an obsessive character, or remains obstinately hidden when most wanted to appear, then it has the quality of a function rooted in the unconscious.

But such a function has still other noteworthy qualities ; there is something unindividual about it, that is, it contains elements which do not necessarily belong to it. Thus, for example, the unconscious feeling of the intellectual is peculiarly phantastic, often in grotesque contrast to an exaggerated, rationalistic intellectualism of the conscious. In contrast to the purposefulness and controlled character of conscious thinking, the feeling is impulsive, uncontrolled, moody, irrational, primitive, archaic indeed, like the feeling of a savage.

The same thing is true of every function that is repressed into the unconscious. It stays there undeveloped, fused with other elements not proper to it and remains in a certain primordial condition, for the unconscious is the psychical residue of undomesticated nature in us, just as it is also the matrix of our uncreated future. Thus the unevolved functions are always the fruitful ones, and so it is no wonder that in the course of life the necessity comes about for a completion and change of the conscious attitude.

Together with the above-mentioned qualities, the unevolved functions possess yet another peculiarity, that is, when the attitude of the conscious is introverted, they are extraverted in character, and *vice versa* ; in other words, together they compensate the conscious attitude. One could expect, therefore, to discover in an introverted intellectual extraverted feelings, and the idea was wittily expressed by such a type when he said : " Before dinner I am a Kantian, after dinner a Nietzscheian." In his habitual attitude that is, he is intellectual, but under the stimulus of a good meal a Dionysian wave breaks through his conscious attitude.

Just here we meet a great difficulty in the diagnosis of the types. The outside observer sees both the manifestations of the conscious attitude, as well as the autonomous phenomena of the unconscious, and he is embarrassed as to which to ascribe to the conscious and which to the unconscious. Under such circumstances the differential diagnosis can only be founded on a careful study of the material, that is to say, it must be discovered which phenomena proceed from consciously chosen motives and which are spontaneous ; and it must also be determined which manifestations possess an adapted and which an unadapted archaic character.

It is now quite clear that the qualities of the conscious dominant function, that is, the qualities of the general conscious attitude, stand in strict contrast to the qualities of the unconscious attitude. Expressed in other words, it can be said that between the conscious and the unconscious there is normally an opposition. This contrast is not noted as a conflict, however, as long as the conscious attitude is not too remote from the unconscious attitude. But if the latter is the case, then the Kantian is unpleasantly surprised by his Dionysianism because it begins to develop impulses that are far too unsuitable. The unconscious, in fact, if once brought into active opposition to the conscious, simply will not permit itself to be repressed. The conscious attitude then sees itself called upon to suppress the autonomous manifestations of the unconscious and thereby the conflict is staged. It is true that it is not particularly difficult to suppress those manifestations against which the conscious especially directs itself, but then the unconscious impulses simply seek other less easily recognisable exits.

Whenever such indirect safety valves are opened, the way of the neurosis has already been entered upon. By analysis one can indeed make each one of these false ways again accessible to the understanding, and so subject to conscious repression, but their determining power is not thereby extinguished ; it is merely pushed back further into a corner, unless, together with the understanding of the indirect way taken by the suppressions, there comes an equally clear realisation of the one-sidedness of the attitude. In other words, along with the understanding of the unconscious impulses there must come a change of the conscious attitude, because the activation of the unconscious opposition has grown out of this one-sidedness, and the recognition of the unconscious impulses is of use only when through it the one-sidedness of the conscious is effectually compensated.

But the changing of the conscious attitude is no small matter, for the sum-total of a general attitude is always more or less of a conscious ideal sanctified by custom and historical tradition ; solidly founded on the rock-bottom of innate temperament. The conscious attitude is always in the nature of a philosophy of life when it is not definitely a religion.   It is this fact which makes the problem of the types so important.   The opposition between the types is not only an external conflict between men, but also the source of endless inner conflicts ; not only the cause of external disagreements and antagonism, but also the inner instigation to nervous illness and psychic disorders.   It is this fact also that forces us as physicians to widen progressively what was originally our purely medico-psychological horizon, to include within its limits not only general psychological viewpoints, but also questions of a more general philosophical nature.

Within the necessary limits of a lecture, I am unable, of course, to present to you the extent of these problems in a thoroughly exhaustive way.   I must perforce content myself with sketching out for you in general terms the main facts merely, and the implications of the problems involved.   For all further particulars I must refer you to the detailed presentation in my book *Psychological Types*.

As a *résumé*, I would like to call to your notice the fact that each of the two attitudes of introversion and extraversion appears in the individual in accordance with the predominance, in a special way, of one of the four fundamental functions.   Strictly speaking, in reality there are no outright extraverts nor introverts, but extraverted and introverted function-types, such as thinking types, sensation types, etc.   Thus there arises a minimum of eight clearly distinguishable types.   Obviously, one may increase this number at will, if each of the function-types is split into three sub-groups, which, empirically speaking, would be far from impossible.   One could, for example, easily divide the intellect into its three well-known forms : first, the intuitive, speculative form ; second, the logical, mathematical form ; third, the empirical form, which rests chiefly on sense perception.   Similar divisions could be carried out with the other functions, as, for instance, in the case of intuition, which has an intellectual as well as a feeling side.   With such a splitting up into component parts, a large number of types could be established, each separate division being of increasing subtlety.

For the sake of completeness, I must also mention the fact that classification of types according to extraversion and introversion must by no means be looked upon as the only possible method. Any other psychological criterion could be equally well employed ; it only appears to me that no other possesses so great a practical significance.

SUGGESTION AND PERSONALITY

BY

WILLIAM BROWN, M.D., D.Sc., M.R.C.P.

Wilde Reader in Mental Philosophy in the University of Oxford; Honorary Consulting Psychologist and Lecturer on Medical Psychology, Bethlehem Royal Hospital, London; Lecturer on Psychotherapy, King's College Hospital

SUGGESTION AND PERSONALITY

BY

WILLIAM BROWN

HISTORICALLY, the problem of suggestion has been approached along two distinct paths. Up to quite recent times our knowledge of it has been a secondary result of the study of hypnosis : during the last few years the line of investigation has been that of mental analysis. There can be no doubt that the latter form of inquiry is likely to be the more fruitful of the two. In the work of Morton Prince we have both lines of investigation developed in a very successful way.

The problem of the relationship of suggestion to hypnosis is brought to a point in two distinct classical definitions that we have of the hypnotic state. According to the Salpêtrière School (Charcot, Janet, etc.), hypnosis is an artificial hysteria or mental dissociation. According to the Nancy School (Bernheim, Coué, Baudouin) hypnosis is a state of artificially-increased suggestibility. According to the former of these two definitions, we should expect suggestibility to be increased in hypnosis, because mental dissociation would tend to carry with it diminished self-knowledge and self-control, with the result that ideas elicited in the subject's mind would tend to realise themselves by their own momentum, as it were, unchecked by more far-reaching thoughts and higher forms of mental control. The difference between the two schools of thought would then seem to be this—that, whereas the Salpêtrière school puts mental dissociation as a cause of any increased suggestibility that may occur, the Nancy school makes no definite statement as to the cause of this increased suggestibility.

The problem of deciding between the merits of these two definitions can be dealt with by an appeal to experience. During the European War a great spontaneous natural experiment was carried out through the agency of the actual conditions of fighting. Soldiers suffered by the hundred from crude mental dissociation, showing itself by amnesia or loss of memory for definite terrifying events and experiences, together with loss of psycho-physical functions, such as the power of speaking, of hearing, of walking, the power of controlling tremors, etc.   Investigation of these patients immediately after their injury showed that they were readily hypnotisable. Moreover, that the ease with which they could be hypnotised was in direct proportion to the degree of their mental dissociation. In other words, one discovered a definite correlation between degree of dissociation and ease of hypnotisability.   Such a finding harmonises with the Salpêtrière definition of hypnosis, as an artificial dissociation.   On the other hand, in these cases it was found that the suggestibility, though certainly increased in milder degrees of dissociation, was often conspicuous by its absence in more pronounced degrees of dissociation

It is clear that we must here call to mind a fundamental distinction in the matter of suggestion.   If we define suggestion, as, *e.g.*, McDougall does, as the acceptance of an idea or proposition independently of logically adequate grounds for such acceptance, the further question arises—Whence comes this idea that is accepted ?   If it is elicited by the patient's outer environment, the people around him, the general physical and mental situation, the process may be called that of hetero-suggestion.   If, on the other hand, the idea arises spontaneously in the patient's own mind or is deliberately presented to him by himself, the process may be called that of auto-suggestion.   In cases of deep hypnosis, such as we have just referred to, where a patient's suggestibility seems sometimes to be diminished rather than increased, it may well be that it is merely a diminution of hetero-suggestibility—auto-suggestibility may be intensified.

Before passing on to a more detailed consideration of the nature of suggestibility, we must emphasise the fact that on the one hand crude mental dissociation facilitates hypnotism, and further, that this mental dissociation, although sometimes caused by mental conflict and repression, may often be caused by pronounced physical means, such as physical shock to the brain, and in a small proportion of individuals appears to be an inborn characteristic.   That is, in certain cases of physical shock to the nervous system, and in certain other cases, the state of hypnosis can be produced with exceptional ease, without any obvious psychological reasons.

If we remain in thought on the level of suggestion and suggestibility in our consideration of the causation and cure of psychoneurotic symptons, we have some such crude view as that of Babinski, who holds that hysterical symptons are produced by suggestion, and therefore are curable by persuasion.   In other words, the patient falls ill under the influence of pathogenic auto-suggestion, and recovers from his illness if these are neutralised by therapeutic suggestion, either given by a physician or others, *i.e.*, hetero-suggestion, or by himself, *i.e.*, auto-suggestion. So far as it goes, this explanation is not incorrect. In simple cases of hysteria, such as those seen almost in process of formation during the war, hysterical symptoms, such as loss of the power of walking, loss of voice, etc., were demonstrably the result of the patient's belief that he had become paralysed, or that he had lost his voice permanently, and the symptoms disappeared at once if the patient was informed that this was not the case, and was strongly assured that the power of walking, talking, etc., would forthwith return to him.

But even in so simple a case as this, the further question arises—"Why was the patient so susceptible to the pathogenic auto-suggestion, the suggestion of illness?" The answer can only be found in terms of desires in the patient's mind. Sometimes these desires are fully conscious, but, in the majority of cases, their true nature is not realised by the patient. In war neurosis, the desire for personal safety, to get away from the firing line, was a pronounced factor in the causation of these symptoms. The patient desired to get away at all costs from the firing line, and it was because he did not fully realise the nature and significance of this desire that he could become self-deceived and fall a victim to hysterical symptoms. He did, indeed, consciously desire to get away from the firing line, but with honour, without disgracing himself or betraying his comrades ; but at the back of his mind there was a more vigorous desire to get away *at all costs*. This desire welcomed the experience (say) of his being struck with fragments of earth thrown up by a bursting shell. The thought passed through his mind that he was paralysed, and this thought became a fixed idea because of the intense desire. It is sometimes said, as, *e.g.*, by Baudouin, that emotion is an auxiliary factor in suggestion ; in other words, that a patient succumbs more readily to suggestion when under the influence of some emotion or other. The truth is this : emotion is the subjective side of some instinctive tendency, such as the instinct to escape, the gregarious instinct, the sex instinct, etc., and these are not so much auxiliary factors in suggestion, as the essential factors. Suggestion only works in relation to the activity of some instinct or other. When in full consciousness, instinctive processes are controlled or directed by reference to the entire conscious self, and in such cases suggestion

X

has little or no scope. It is where, through conflict and repression, certain instinctive desires, associated often with definite sets of memories of the past, are dissociated from the main stream of consciousness that they can realise suggestions which would be unacceptable to the fully-conscious personality if their meanings were thoroughly understood.

One might provisionally harmonise the suggestion theory of causation and cure of symptoms and the analytic theory as follows : mental conflict and repression may produce hysterical symptoms as compromise formations which simultaneously satisfy repressed desires in the unconscious, and desires of another nature in the conscious mind, but the nature of the symptoms themselves is also partly determined by auto-suggestions arising as the result of diminished unity of the self—chance thoughts, they may be, which otherwise would have no influence over the patient's mental state, and to which he would not succumb. He is in a state of mind divided against itself: he is afraid for himself, afraid of ill-health, afraid that he may fall sick, and yet may desire sickness, for reasons that can be discovered by deeper analysis, (*e.g.*, as a self-punishment, or to tyrannise over relatives, etc.). So the idea gains a hold upon him. In this way the dissociation we have previously emphasised does favour the acceptance of auto-suggestion. On the other hand, what particular auto-suggestions, from among all the different possible suggestions, are accepted, is determined by the wishes, desires, etc., of the patient's mind. In order, therefore, to understand fully the realisation of suggestion, we must analyse the patient's mind and learn as much as we can about these mental factors.

One analytic view of the nature of suggestion and suggestibility is the well-known Freudian view that suggestion is a form of " transference " in which the patient reacts to the physician as he reacted in early life towards his own father, or towards others closely connected with him in childhood. In other words, the reaction is an erotic one, using the word " erotic " in the widest sense. The tie is an erotic tie. At first sight such a theory as this seems to be extremely improbable, since, besides the sex instinct, there are many other instincts which may be plausibly appealed to for an explanation of suggestibility in special cases. The instinct of escape, with its emotion of fear, the gregarious instinct with its own peculiar emotion, and the instinct of self-abasement, with its emotion of negative self-feeling, may be specially singled out in this connection. So much suggestibility seems, on the surface, to be the result either of fear, or of a standing desire to be in harmony with one's fellows. We must, however, remember that Freud has a definite theory of group psychology and of the gregarious instinct in terms of libidinal relationship of the individuals of a crowd or other group towards the leader of that group—the leader corresponding to the father of the horde in more primitive times. Such a theory brings the concept once more within the circle of Freudian doctrine, and recently Freudians have explained auto-suggestion in terms of narcissism. Indeed, Dr Ernest Jones explains all suggestion in terms of narcissism. He writes : " If the primary narcissism has been released and re-animated directly, by concentration upon the idea of self, the process may be termed ' auto-suggestion ' ; if it has been preceded by a stage in which the ego ideal is resolved into the earlier father ideal, the process may be termed ' hetero-suggestion '." ("The Nature of Auto-suggestion," *Brit. Jour. of Med. Psychology*, 1923, Vol. III, p. 209).

This is an original and important theory, and deserves careful testing by further psychoanalysis of patients, especially of patients who have previously practised auto-suggestion with success.

It is clear, then, that the problem of suggestion and suggestibility is far from being a question of the past, now superseded by analytical theory. It still remains one of the central problems of modern psychotherapy. Whether suggestion is always a libidinal relationship, is not entirely free from doubt. Instead of saying, with Freud, that all suggestion is transference, we are probably on safer ground in holding that the transference situation is, indeed, one of the conditions under which suggestion may occur, but that suggestion may also occur in psychological situations when there is no transference. But the question can only be finally decided by " deep " analysis.

In conclusion, a word may be said on the relation of suggestion and auto-suggestion to the will. It has been noted by many observers that over-anxiety counteracts the effects of therapeutic suggestion. If one feels anxious to get to sleep at night, one may become wider and wider awake. Similarly, in the attempt to recall a forgotten name, anxious effort to remember generally brings failure. Coué has summed up these and other similar observations in his so-called Law of Reversed Effort. " When the will and the imagination are in conflict, the imagination always wins." Such a formulation is only true of states of incomplete will, where fear of failure has prevented the full development of volition, and the word " will " should be replaced by " wish."

The completed state of will or volition is incompatible with any such fear or doubt. One of the best definitions of volition is that given by Professor G. F. Stout : " Volition is a desire qualified and defined by the judgment, that, so far as in us lies, we shall bring about the desired end because we desire it." The " judgment " in this definition comprises, of course, *belief*, and if completed, it is superior to " imagination " (suggestion) acting alone.

The advice given to patients, to avoid effort in the practice of suggestion, is a sound one, since effort tends to arouse the idea of possible failure and the fear of failure. If these do arise, they gain the mastery over the original suggestion. Most cases of successful auto-suggestion are characterised by avoidance of thoughts and fears of failure, and may, therefore, be considered as instances of supplementation and completion of the volitional process through adequate control of the imagination. To call the method one of auto-suggestion is really somewhat inappropriate and it might be more accurately described as a method of training the will. In practice the passivity of mere suggestion and auto-suggestion is quickly superseded by the activity of faith and calm determination to succeed.

What is acquired is a new mental attitude which protects the patient from suggestion of ill-health and incapacity. To make this protection complete, or as nearly complete as possible, the patient also requires a course of psychoanalysis or autognosis, to rid him of complexes and other dissociations and thus enable him to face the world with a unified personality.

THE UNCONSCIOUS IN PSYCHOANALYSIS

A CRITICISM

BY

HENRY HERBERT GODDARD, A.M., Ph.D.

Professor of Abnormal Psychology, Ohio State University ; formerly Director of Psychological Research, Vineland Training School

THE UNCONSCIOUS IN PSYCHOANALYSIS

A CRITICISM

BY

HENRY HERBERT GODDARD

It is fourteen years since Dr Prince published, in his *Journal of Abnormal Psychology*, the famous symposium on the Subconscious, and ten years since he wrote his illuminating book on the Unconscious, which, however, he says, is intended as an introduction to abnormal psychology. In the meantime, the literature of the subject has increased enormously, largely through the work of the psychoanalysts and the increasing interest in psycho-therapeutics.

The first plan of the present writer had been to summarise the various concepts of the unconscious, in the hope that out of the different views one could arrive at some sort of harmony by translating them all into a common terminology, which might be at least provisionally acceptable to each one, or which would not do violence to any one view.

This, however, has proved an impossible task. It is impossible from the standpoint of space, because each man's view is coloured by his whole philosophy to such an extent that it could not be expressed without giving something of the history of the concept in his own mind, as evidenced in his writings. And secondly, even when so reduced, the concepts are made up of such divergent elements that it seems impossible to bring them together into one general view. For example: we have the philosophical use of the term; we have a usage that is frankly mystical; we have discussions of the concept that, while ostensibly scientific, yet savour of mysticism to such a degree that they cannot by any means be considered exact and scientific. Then, we have a considerable number of writers who seem to use the term as a magic formula with which to explain natural phenomena (or imagined facts) that cannot be readily explained by known and accepted scientific concepts. The mere reference to Leibniz, Kant, Schelling, Herbart, Hartmann, Janet, Freud, Jung, Münsterberg, and

Jastrow, is enough to remind the reader of the truth of the foregoing statement. I have not included in this list the name of Dr Prince, because he, of all the writers, has come the nearest to a truly scientific treatment of the subject.

Under such conditions, the only procedure that seems likely to bring this article within reading distance of those who may be interested is to attempt to develop the concept of the unconscious in terms that will at least not be offensive to the scientific man, and will constantly reveal the intent and effort, on the part of the writer, to apply rigidly scientific criteria to the problem.

In order to achieve any satisfactory result, certain definite principles must be followed. First—there must be a body of accepted facts. Second—there must be theories or hypotheses put forward to explain the facts, which theories or hypotheses must not be contradicted by facts of other sciences, or be too much in conflict with other more fundamental and generally accepted theories. Third—due regard must be had to the meaning of terms already established in the language. Fourth—one must be constantly on his guard against the psychological tendency to make entities out of what in fact are pure negations of such entities. It seems to the writer that this last is the serious error of most of those who have discussed the unconscious. For example, Freud's fundamental concept is, that complexes have been forced " *into the unconscious*," " suppressed " or " repressed," and that they are kept in the unconscious by a " censor " who constantly guards the exit. The unconscious is thus a room, a safe, a prison, a place where ideas are kept when they are not wanted, a storehouse, a transfer file. Others assert that the unconscious is dynamic. It is a material or an immaterial *substance* which has stored up energy. Still others would give one the impression that the unconscious has *personality*, that it thinks, plans, contrives, struggles, and achieves. These concepts are, to say the least, hopelessly antagonistic, while to writers like Dunlap they are so ridiculous as to be almost nauseating. The only explanation the present writer can think of for such language is that it is " figurative." Even so it is unjustifiable because it leads to confusion rather than to clarity.

With these principles before us, let us proceed.

First, for the facts. We shall not, at this point, attempt to enumerate the facts. They will appear as we proceed. If anyone can satisfy himself that there are no facts of mental life except such as can be explained by the activity of consciousness, such a person is probably not reading this article, because he has no use whatever for the concept of the unconscious, and the very title of this article was enough to drive him on to the next articles to see if perchance he can find something there worth reading. We have already proceeded far enough to discover that we must define our terms. Etymology is always interesting, but not always a safe guide to an understanding of the concept connoted by the word used. In this case, however, the term ' *unconscious* ' can mean nothing but *not conscious*, without a distinct perversion of language. We come, then, to the question : " What is consciousness ? " Here we easily avoid the temptation to consider all, or any, of the philosophical discussions of what consciousness is. Everybody knows the state or condition of consciousness and, therefore, the state of *un*consciousness, whether it be absolute or relative. Granted that we cannot define or explain consciousness, we are no worse off than the physicist who cannot define or explain electricity. That does not prevent him from using the term intelligently, and calling certain phenomena electrical, without confusing the issue. The physicist can, however, tell us the conditions under which electricity is produced. Likewise, the psychologist knows the conditions under which consciousness arises, and some of the laws governing its appearance, activity, and disappearance. Psychology has been defined as the science of consciousness, which is equivalent to saying that we know enough about its manifestations to more or less satisfactorily systematise them and build up a body of classified knowledge. Now, the fundamental and indisputable fact about consciousness is, that it is connected invariably with a particular kind of action in a particular type of brain cell. Neither the psychologists nor the neurologists are entirely agreed as to either the exact kind of activity, or the exact type of brain cells, which give rise to consciousness. It is common to say that the seat of consciousness is in the cortical cells of the cerebrum. It is probably safer and more accurate to say that cortical brain cells must be included in any mechanism, the activity of which gives rise to consciousness. This distinction is like the distinction between the statement that " our food is our life " and the statement that " food is essential to life." It is not demonstrated that consciousness resides in the cortex, or is always produced when cortical cells are activated, but we may accept it as proved that no activity of nerve cells in the body results in consciousness unless some cortical brain cells are included in the mechanism. This, then, gives us our starting point for some definite understanding of consciousness and unconsciousness.

That there is brain and nerve activity without consciousness is an accepted fact which no one questions. The question whether such nerve action, which does not result in consciousness, has any influence either at the time or later upon that phase of existence which we usually designate as mental is the question which at once arises. Apparently some writers would not only maintain that it does have an influence, but even that it is of the most vital importance. When Freud, for example, maintains that the intra-uterine experiences of the unborn child may be the starting point for the neuroses of adult life, we seem to have an extreme example of such a concept. It may be maintained that we have no proof that such nerve activity is without the co-operation of the cortex, and therefore, of the type that we are discussing. However, in view of the known immaturity of the cortex, and the fact demonstrated by Flechsig, that even at birth, there are few, if any, medullated by neurones in the cortex, and that such medullation is necessary for consciousness, if not for any kind of function (in the case of cortical cells), we would seem to be driven to the conclusion that nerve activity under such conditions was for all practical purposes without cortical interference or connection.

For the sake of simplicity, let us take the simplest spinal cord reflex, and ask ourselves if there is any indication, or any possibility, that the nerve activity involved in such a reflex has any influence upon the mind. The importance of this question lies in the fact that, if our answer is negative, then a large part of what many writers include under the term " the unconscious " has nothing whatever to do with psychology, and no more to do with psychiatry than facts as to whether digestion is normal or abnormal. It is probably as hard to conceive that the nerve activity involved in the knee-jerk has any influence upon the mind, as it is to believe that it makes any difference to a man's future success in life, whether as a child he goes upstairs three steps at a time or two. But perhaps we are prejudicing the case by taking an illustration where the effect is so minute as to be impossible of appreciation. We have no better success, however, when we take large activities. We may even go into the vegetative system and consider those nerve activities which take care of digestion, respiration, and other processes, both those that make for health and those that are essential to life. And it is hard to discover that even the derangement of these conditions has any *permanent* effect upon the mind, unless they are of such a character that they overflow into the central system, reach the cortex, and produce more or less of consciousness. It would seem then, that the unconscious, in the sense of the *not conscious*, is of no more significance when we are speaking of unconscious nerve action than when we are speaking of any other tissue whose growth or activity is never thought of as having anything to do with mental processes. So far, then, we seem forced to conclude that the term "unconscious," in its literal sense, is simply the *not conscious*, and as such is of no further interest or significance.

If, now, we take into account the functioning cerebrum, we at once find ourselves facing a new set of facts. Here we find what Carpenter called years ago "Unconscious Cerebration," which expression, if it means anything, conveys the concept that there may be nerve action involving the cortex of the brain, which nevertheless does not produce consciousness. Here we have the group of phenomena which used to be called "Subliminal," and it was said that certain stimuli are too weak to produce nerve action that gets above the threshold of consciousness. There are sounds too faint to be heard ; there are colours not bright enough to be seen ; there are solutions too dilute to be. tasted, and so on. In these cases, however, it is possible to maintain that the phenomena are the result, not of *nerve action* that does not reach consciousness, but of a stimulus that does not overcome the inertia of the receiving organ, so that, as a matter of fact, no nerve action at all takes place.

But these are not the only phenomena that we have to deal with. Sounds that are loud enough to be heard are not heard, because, as we say, something else holds the field of consciousness. That there was *nerve action*, and that it was of a kind very akin to that which produces consciousness, is evident by the fact that it does influence our actions later on. As, for example, when we do not hear the clock strike, but later know the hour. This is typical of a large mass of experiences, which may properly be described as unconscious. These processes may be very elaborate, as is shown by what takes place in dreams and delirium, and still more striking, the solution of problems, the composing of poetry and prose in a state of sound sleep. It is conceivable that such phenomena are the result of the nerve energy finding its way among neurones that have been previously activated, but in a different arrangement, and which are now integrated into a more consistent system. It is further conceivable that such a neurone pattern, or neurogram, as Dr Prince has called it, having been worked out even without the accompanying consciousness, may retain its identity as a pattern, and if later aroused under conditions in which it gets into consciousness, it reproduces the state which would have been produced on the previous occasion, had not other neurones been more active. We need not dwell longer on these phenomena ; they are too well known to be denied or to need further elaboration for our present purpose.

We come now to another phase of unconsciousness. Consciousness has been defined as " mind now." According to this conception, mind yesterday, or even a moment ago, is *un*conscious, (or as some would prefer to say, " in the unconscious "). Apparently some people uncritically think of the ideas and feelings of the past as being *stored up* somewhere. Indeed, some writers use that very expression. They say, " the mind stores up ideas " as though ideas were commodities and the mind a storehouse. Here we seem to run into the question of what is mind, and what are ideas. And it would be easy to enter into a philosophical discussion of this perennial problem. But, for us, mind is a certain type of nerve activity, and an idea is a more or less complicated group of neurone activities. When those neurones cease to be active, the consciousness, or the idea which was that activity, ceases also. But the neurones are there, and if they can be set into activity in the same order as before, the same idea, or the bit of consciousness which we call an idea will reappear. As long as that particular group of neurones is inactive, so long are we unconscious of the idea which is the activity of those neurones. We have thus arrived at a point of view thoroughly consistent with our first definition, that *un*consciousness is the absence of consciousness, and that what we mean, when we say an idea has passed into the unconscious, is that the neurones have ceased to be active.

Illustration : The ideas of the preceding paragraph were expressed by the writer in audible words, and were spoken into a dictating machine. The sounds from that set of words have now ceased (gone into the unconscious), but there is on the wax cylinder a series of impressions. Those impressions are neither words nor thoughts. They are merely minute spacial variations in the surface of the cylinder. This cylinder may be laid aside and kept for a lifetime. Whenever the proper apparatus is applied, and the record set in motion, those words are again produced. In a similar manner an idea can be brought back into consciousness, because an impression has been made on a group of neurones, and their activity at any time will bring back the same consciousness as when they were first produced.

The experiences of life are constantly producing these neurone patterns in the cortex, which thus does indeed become a store-house, not of ideas, but of neurones whose structure has been modified by activity in such a way that a renewal of the activity gives life to the same consciousness that occurred with the first activity. And since consciousness *is* the activity of a group of neurones, there is, of course, no consciousness connected with those neurones that are inactive. If it is desirable, as it seems to be, to have a term to express the fact that there are these stored-up nerve impressions which have resulted from all one's past experiences, it may be proper to call them the unconscious mind, though, in so doing, we must cease to identify mind with consciousness. If there is objection to this, one might introduce the concept of potential mind ; the idea being that all these neurone patterns have the potentiality of becoming active and, therefore, producing consciousness. The objection to this might be that the term potential might equally well be applied to the unstimulated cortex, which, because of the nature of its neurones, has the potentiality of being stimulated and thus giving rise to consciousness. Thus the infant, whose brain has never been stimulated by many experiences, has a potential mind just as surely as the man of great experience, of most of which experiences he is now unconscious.

Up to this point, we have reached the conclusion that the term unconscious has no meaning and no use when applied to any activity of the nervous system, except such as involves cortical cells of the cerebrum and either actually produces a definite consciousness, or would have done so, had not the activity in the particular case been surpassed by the activity of other groups of cortical cells. These latter produced by their greater activity what we may call a stronger consciousness, with the result that we were not aware of the lesser activity.

The question may be raised : is there not nerve action that never has and never can involve the cortex and yet is of profound significance for the mental life of the individual, *e.g.*, the instincts ? Disregarding the possibility of success of those who would prove that there are no instincts, we surely recognise that there are inborn neurograms ready to be activated by the proper stimulus and produce specific action of great importance to the individual. But so are we born with blood of a definite composition, the circulation of which is of great importance. Is the one of any more significance for mind than the other ? The tendency of a muscle- or bone-cell to grow and divide is an unconscious activity of great significance and in the long run surely influences consciousness itself. But one would hardly include this in the concept of the unconscious.   Why then include nerve cells just because they are nerve cells, when they bear no relation to consciousness past, present or future ? May we not designate this cell activity—this activity of non-cortical neurones by some term which will not confuse it with consciousness in any way ?   To make the unconscious cover this seems to introduce troublesome confusion.

Our problem is thus enormously simplified, and a surer foundation is laid for an understanding of those facts which need to be explained.   The term "unconscious" may be accepted to express the fact that the great mass of nerve cells that were once active in consciousness are now inactive, but may at any time be reactivated, thus giving rise to the consciousness which belongs to them.   The use of the term "unconsciousness" in any other sense is not only unjustified by what we know of the functions of cortical and other cells but savours of the mystical and unscientific ; and, moreover, has proved decidedly misleading.   All usages of the term "unconscious" that imply that it is an entity, such as saying that ideas are *in the unconscious*, or that the unconscious is dynamic, show a thoughtless or uncritical attitude—or ignorance.   In any case it adds to confusion.

If our position is accepted it follows that all phenomena, especially those of so-called psycho-therapeutics, must either be explained in terms of cortical cell activity of a type that does or does not produce consciousness, or must be relegated to the limbo of imaginary science, along with magnetism, mesmerism, Perkin's tractors, drugs in hermetically sealed bottles, and the like.   To many, doubtless, the latter explanation will be the accepted one, and there is no need for further discussion.   To many others, however, among whom is the writer, this is not possible.   While the proverbial credulity of the untutored mind makes it possible for us to discard many of the reported instances, as not even warranting investigation, we have, on the other hand, too many instances, as well authenticated as any in medicine, to permit us to ignore them. Therefore, if they cannot be explained by reference to a reasonable hypothesis of nerve activity, conscious or unconscious, they must remain unexplained until such time as science shall have advanced far enough to enable us to formulate a new hypothesis.

The method and principles of psychoanalysis probably represent the best attempt at a scientific use and explanation of the concept of unconsciousness.   Psychoanalysis may, therefore, properly be taken as a source for facts to be explained, and as an illustration of the application of science to the problem of the unconscious, and also, unfortunately, of the careless use, as it seems to the writer, of unwarranted mystical concepts. The *argumentum ad hominem* is often fallacious, but, rightly used, has a certain value. The methods and principles of psychoanalysis are upheld and expounded, not by charlatans and ignoramuses—although the movement is not unmarred by the usual quota of these parasites—but, on the contrary, it is sponsored by some of the best minds of the age, men highly trained, of broad experience, conscientious and devoted to the welfare of humanity and the cause of science. It is neither just, scientific, nor wise to ignore the opinions of such men. Moreover, the principles and facts are recognised as true to life in too many cases to be ignored. Witness the *modified* disapproval of most of the opponents, or those who do not approve the movement. Moreover, the worst that the bitterest opponent can say of *some* of the principles, is that they are not new. It is true that many of them are not new, but it is equally true that the psychoanalysts have put many of the old familiar facts into a new and more useful light. It is the explanation and the terminology that jar us. For the most part, the facts are uncontroverted.

It is true that the analysts have given us very little, if any, evidence that their cures are radical and permanent, and it might be asserted with some show of plausibility that, since their field of operation is mainly the hysteric and the neurotic, the reported confirmations which the patients give them of their diagnoses are merely the accepted suggestions which the physicians themselves have implanted in the minds of these unstables, that the cures are temporary and the patients subject to relapse ; and thus the method has little or no advantage over the countless other methods that have had temporary results with this class of cases. It would be a satisfaction to many a questioner of the method to have presented a group of cases, each one of which showed the history and the results, more or less completely, to the effect that this individual has been hysteric or neurotic, useless to society and to herself for so many years, and, following the treatment by psychoanalysis, has been transformed into a useful and efficient member of society, which condition she has maintained uninterruptedly for a term of years. Bjerre gives us a history of a case in which he does just about that thing ; but we need a great many more. Furthermore, Bjerre's case is peculiar in that he says nothing about having used the technical methods of the psychoanalyst. There is no mention of dream analysis, and interpretation ; no mention of the association method ; no reference to the unconscious, in any other than the popular sense.   His whole procedure, while probably suggested to him by his psychoanalytic studies, nevertheless was a perfectly natural, simple, logical method.   It might have been used by anyone who understood the elementary principles of the human mind.

However, while we would like testimony of the kind suggested, we may nevertheless do what the analysts have evidently expected us to do, to accept their word for it, that great beneficial results have been obtained.   Indeed, as already stated, many points in the method are recognised as only a slight extension of principles that are well known.   For example : to start with the first case of Breuer and Freud, which gave rise to the term, " the talking cure," or to Freud's own term " the cathartic method."   This is only a somewhat new application of the well-known principle that it is a great relief to tell our troubles to some other person, or again, the proverbial phrase that " murder will out."   The murderer cannot keep his secret.   Or the still more universal experience of the difficulty that everybody has to keep a secret. Or, again, we say that suppressed grief is dangerous.   It is better for the individual to mourn and cry and otherwise give expression to the emotion.   All this is accepted even by the folk mind.   It is only when Freud tells us that the original experience was repressed, thrown into the unconscious, a censor placed at the door, and that this complex in the unconscious keeps struggling to rise to the surface, that we are compelled to say, the explanation is nonsense, and because the explanation is nonsense, we ourselves illustrate another Freudian concept, and transfer the nonsense from the explanation to the fact itself, and say the cure is ridiculous.

But if we cannot accept Freud's explanation, let us try, as we have already suggested, to explain the fact in terms of acceptable psychology and neurology.   In the first place, we have denied that there is any unconscious into which ideas are repressed. What then shall we substitute for this concept ?   Let us take a typical Freudian case, so that we may discuss the matter concretely.   A young girl (Freud says that unless the experience occurs before the eighth year of age it never leads to a neurosis), of good breeding and healthy-minded, allows herself or is forced to submit to some action of a sexual nature, which shocks her modesty and violates her ideals and her upbringing.   She cannot tell anybody and so has to keep her own secret, and in the Freudian terminology, represses it into the unconscious, where it continually struggles to rise into consciousness, being constantly opposed by the censor, until sometime in adult life she has a serious breakdown and becomes a neurotic or hysteric. She comes to a psychoanalyst for help. It should be remembered that not all the psychoanalysts agree with Freud in his explanation, and one might very well raise the question as to whether the inability to adjust the matter at the time was not itself a symptom of an abnormal mind, rather than the cause of the later abnormality. However, passing that, let us see what we have. As we have reiterated, there is no *unconscious* into which this memory is forced. If the child becomes unconscious of it, it is forgotten, and that is the end of it. There is no evidence that the neurone pattern, thus impressed upon her cortical neurones is in a state which can, by any stress of the imagination, be described as *struggling to get conscious*—struggling for activity, to use our own terminology. As we have said, if it is unconscious, it is forgotten. If it has made such a strong impression upon the nerve centres, or, as we more commonly express it, such an impression upon the mind that it cannot be forgotten, then it is not unconscious. It continually comes to mind, and, because it is unpleasant, the child tries to forget it. What is the process of trying to forget an unpleasant experience? There is no evidence that there is any other process, or any other method, than to " think of something else." Everyone has tried it, and has been more or less successful in forgetting unpleasant experiences. But, as long as we must keep trying to forget it, we are not unconscious of it. Whenever we succeed in turning our attention to something else, we are, for the time being, unconscious of the experience. If we finally get to the point, which usually happens in the course of time, that we seldom or never think of it, then we are totally unconscious of it. If this is what Freud means by its being in the unconscious, we say again, it is an unfortunate use of language. It is not *in the unconscious*; we are simply unconscious of the experience because the neurone pattern that underlies it is no longer easily activated. That such a conscious (not unconscious) struggle is unhealthy may readily be admitted and explained by reference to another system of the organism of which we know little, but of which what little we do know seems to warrant us in assuming that a satisfactory explanation may here be sought whenever our knowledge is adequate. I refer to the endocrine glands, and their relation to emotions on the one hand, and bodily welfare on the other. An unhappy experience constantly arising into consciousness may, through the unpleasant emotions

Y

attached to it, cause a derangement in the secretion of these glands that is in the long run quite serious, and possibly quite sufficient to produce all the symptoms of hysteria, or the neurotic constitution. The unconscious then, in this case, is nothing else than the more or less permanent forgetting. The repression is nothing else than the thinking of something else. And lastly, the censor is merely the idea already attained by the child, that her act was wicked, unbecoming, disgraceful, that people would not like her if they knew it, that she can never again be pure, etc.

There is another point that must be mentioned. We have said that if the child succeeds in forgetting the incident, she becomes unconscious of it and that is the end of it. The analyst tells us that is not the end of it, that his methods prove conclusively not only that the experience has been repressed into the unconsciousness, but that his methods of dream interpretation or association bring it into consciousness, and then, when the situation is gone over, and the individual goes through the same emotional experience as when the incident occurred, that this is the relief and the cure. But some of the analysts have themselves broken the chain. Even Freud admits that his patients frequently "*resist*" his efforts to get at the facts. They say they can't think of anything else, and he admits that that probably means that they don't want to think of it, and sometimes when they finally come out with it and he says "why didn't you tell me that before?" they say that they did not think it was important. Now, it seems not only probable on general principles, but the only explanation consistent with what we know of memory and other mental processes, and what we know of life and human ways, to conclude that the matter *was not unconscious at all*, and that the analyst's only task was to get the patient willing to give expression to what was already in mind.

There are several facts here that must be brought to our attention. In the first place, there are many people who can hardly bring themselves to speak to anyone of any of the bodily functions that are considered private. The reader who has been brought up in or who has acquired the habit of frankness in regard to such matters, will find it difficult to believe the following incidents. Nevertheless, they are not exceptional but rather common. A girl, sixteen years old, intelligent, and normal in every way, was ill and the physician was called. After he had gone she showed marked disturbance and excitement and finally explained to her girl friend that he had insulted her by asking her if she was constipated. A graduate student, some years ago, was making a study of the sex life of men, and sent a questionnaire to the graduate students of a distant university asking for data on certain facts of sex life. The answers were to be sent sealed, without name or other indication that might lead to identification. On some phases of this study the results were useless, because these men had refused to answer. The resistance of men and women to revealing such matters even to their physician, or to any one else, is not appreciated by very many people. Still more surprising would it be to many readers to know the extent to which patients refuse or think it unimportant to tell their physician their own symptoms, even those which do not relate to sex, and can have no mortifying association. Many a physician will testify, as many have done to the writer, that patients persistently " *lie* " about their symptoms even when their own health is at stake.

In view of the facts of which the foregoing items are mere illustrations, it would seem that the analyst is too easy when he assumes that, because his patient does not tell him these things, he has absolutely forgotten them. It is not necessary to assume that the patient wilfully lies about the matter. He always has a perfectly rational alibi that he " did not think that the repressed facts had anything to do with the case." To put the matter from the psychological standpoint, it is unthinkable that an experience of such a character as to have endured for years, and caused a serious mental disturbance, can yet be completely in that imaginary realm which Freud calls " the unconscious," and cannot by any possibility be voluntarily recalled. On the other hand, the reader will realise that this is not an argument against the method of psychoanalysis. The dream interpretation, the association of ideas, is all the more necessary in order to enable the patient, either to unintentionally give himself away, or to find an excuse for revealing, possibly in symbolical language, the facts that he does not want to speak of plainly. In other words, these methods are a somewhat refined kind of third degree, such as is practised by the police. Moreover, it should be remembered that in a certain type of cases the situation causing an emotional disturbance is forgotten while the emotion itself remains. The analytic method is useful to recall the original circumstance long since forgotten.

Perhaps no part of the Freudian theory has aroused so much opposition or had so much to do with preventing the general acceptance of Freud's views, as his theory of dream analysis, embodying, as it does, the symbolism. That, together with the fact that it all centres around sex, has caused many people to reject the whole system as utterly untenable, ridiculous, and all but disgraceful. It is no part of our purpose to defend the Freudian doctrine, although we could point out that, here also, Freud has at least called our attention to many very evident truths ; such as the fact that, for children, these dreams are frequently wish fulfilments and that, at least in many cases, the same is true of adults. But what we are particularly concerned with just now is the Freudian view that the dream is the expression of the complex that has been repressed into the unconscious, and because the censor watches so sharply the only way it can get into consciousness at all is by disguising itself by means of symbols and appearing in the dream. It would be unnecessary to emphasise that such a statement is as ridiculous to the neurologist and psychologist as it can possibly be to the most violent opponent of the Freudian theory, if it were not for the fact that there are many laymen with a tendency toward mysticism, and ignorance of neurological facts, who would see in this statement a wonderful mechanism for explaining a marvellous phenomenon. In place of this mystical theory, let us see if we can substitute one more in accordance with known facts of neurology.

It is supposed by neurologists that there are, in round numbers, approximately 10,000 million brain cells. Experiences of life are grouping these brain cells into what we have called neurone patterns or, as Dr Prince designates them, neurograms. When a neurogram is strongly activated, we have the consciousness that belongs to that particular grouping of neurones, while all those patterns that are inactive represent the ideas or experiences of which we are unconscious. In deep sleep all neurones are quiet. In a fully waking condition, every stimulus tends to arouse a pattern to activity and thus to produce consciousness. There is reason to believe that between these two extremes we have all gradations. From which it is easy to see that toward the sleep end of the scale we may conceive the brain as being in a condition that we, perhaps, for want of a better term, may call "dormant." Ordinary stimuli do not arouse any neurone patterns to activity. An excessive stimulus will arouse a small pattern which in turn may arouse a few cells that have been intimately connected with it, and these may arouse another group, and so on. The two situations may perhaps be likened to a surface covered with gun powder. When the powder is dry, a spark applied to any one grain explodes the whole mass. If, however, the powder has been wet, the spark will have no effect. But, if it has partly dried out and is drier in some spots than in others, there will be a slow burning, following irregular lines, the flame creeping along from particle to particle, until, perhaps, it reaches a little mass that is drier than the rest. There will be a flash, followed again by a slow creeping along of the combustion. This represents the dream. Now, our problem is, what determines the course of events. In our illustration, the determinant is the more or less completely dried-out part of areas or lines. In the dream, it is the groups of neurones scattered here and there through the cortex which, for some reason, are in a condition to be activated, either because the stimuli at these points are excessively strong, or because these patterns are all ready to explode, possibly because they have recently been active. The recency is shown in the accepted fact that a part of the dream at least relates to the events of the previous day, what Freud calls "the dream day," and it is quite possible that the dream in its entirety relates to the thought of the dream day—not necessarily the thoughts that have been at any time in the focus of consciousness, but perhaps largely thoughts that have been in the margin. And there may be neurone patterns whose activity did not even produce any awareness, because, as we have already explained, some other group of neurones was more violently active, and so monopolised the field of consciousness, so to speak. Moreover, it seems equally possible that the activity of cells that have been concerned with consciousness in the " dream day " may activate nerve patterns that have not been active for many days or perhaps for years. Thus we dream of things that we have not thought of for a long period, or that we cannot remember ever having thought of. These are the things that the analysts tell us are not what they pretend to be, but are symbols of other things. And thus we come face to face with the problem of symbolism.

For the psychologist, the fact that we dream in symbols can only mean one thing, and that is that we have some time *thought in symbols*. That we think in symbols, there can be no question. One has only to turn his attention to this aspect of our speech, or our thought, to realise that it is well nigh universal. Nor can it be denied, objectionable as it may be to us, that sex in some form or other constitutes a considerable portion of our thinking, and the more our conscience tells us that we should not think about such things, the more we tend to disguise it by symbolical language or thought. A perfect illustration of this is found in a recent volume

entitled *A Young Girl's Diary*, where a child confides to her
diary that she has discovered that certain words of common use
sometimes are used to symbolise various sexual functions, activities,
and organs.   She finally confesses that she is almost in a state where
she is afraid to talk at all, for fear her language will have some such
significance, and therefore would become a source of embarrass-
ment.   Not only do we thus have a symbol for everything of the
kind, but as fast as a symbol becomes accepted, well known and
understood, it so fully and completely stands for the thing it
symbolises, that it becomes just as objectionable as the thing itself.
Then we seek another symbol, and try to forget the plainer term.
The same thing is seen in the use of slang, or profanity.   The individual who feels that his social position, or his religious ideas, or
early training, or any influence whatever, makes it objectionable
for him to express himself in a slang phrase, or a profane word, will
invariably soften it to something simpler, which thus becomes a
symbol for the real term itself.   Such being the case, what is more
natural or to be expected than that in the dream the word, or the
idea, or the picture, will appear.   And whereas in our waking
moments, we have the thing symbolised more or less definitely
in the same field of consciousness, in the dream that may not
appear.   The symbol stands alone or perhaps associated with
something else which has been freely connected with it in waking
life, and so leads us away from the thing symbolised rather than
toward it.   For example, suppose I avoid the word " damn " by
using the term " darn," which in turn is generally (in all cases
except where one is expressing strong feeling) connected with the
idea of mending.   Thus the neurone pattern connected with consciousness of a hole in a garment which has been mended would
be quite as likely to become active as any other.   An illustration
or two from the writer's own observation may help to make this
clear.   On one occasion, the writer was introduced to a lady by
the name of Franklin, and shortly afterwards proceeded to introduce her to some one else as Mrs Marshall.   The mistake seemed
very strange until after some thought (analogous to the analyst's
free association method) he realised that *Franklin and Marshall
College* had been at one time much in his consciousness, that the
connection between the two names had become fixed.   A precisely similar experience was had, when a gentleman by the name
of " Morris " was referred to as " Mr Phillips," the explanation
being that some years previous a name constantly heard and
frequently spoken was " Morris Phillips."   Without going into this

matter, the reader may be reminded of the well-known principle of the conditioned reflex.

If we have succeeded in making our point, it will be clear that from this angle also, the analyst's notion of the unconscious, as used in dream analysis, is an appeal to mysticism, and as such is a dangerous concept for scientific psychology, the danger lying in the fact that it allows and even encourages us to accept the false with the true, and thus in the long run to confuse our problem instead of clarifying it.

Résumé.—In this paper we have tried to show that for the most part the unconscious, as conceived by the psychoanalyst, *does not exist*, and consequently cannot be used to explain in the naïve way, common to their discussion, the phenomena which they describe. Every experience that has at one time aroused the activity of cortical brain cells is recorded in those same cells, and the reactivating of these cells in whole or in part will at any time produce the same consciousness, either in whole or in part. Moreover, part of these neurone patterns may be recombined into new neurograms giving rise to thoughts or ideas, consciousness, which seem fully new to us because we have never made that combination before. Moreover, such new combinations may go on during sleep either in a fragmentary way, giving rise to the well-known incongruities and fragmentariness of the dream. On the other hand, parts may fit together more logically as when one solves in sleep a definite problem which he was unable to work out in his waking hours, because too many irrelevant ideas came into consciousness, through association with those elements of consciousness which were important for the problem. The term "unconscious" may have justification if it can be used in the right way. It may also be useful to designate that part of the so-called unconscious which is more easily recalled as the *fore-conscious* or *co-conscious*. When the psychoanalysts will thus translate their explanations into neural terms, or terms consistent with the known facts of brain physiology, much of the objection to it and many of the difficulties now encountered will disappear, and we will be on the road to a true science of psychoanalysis and the unconscious.

UNCONSCIOUS DYNAMICS AND HUMAN BEHAVIOUR: A GLIMPSE AT SOME INTER-RELATIONSHIPS OF STRUCTURE AND FUNCTION

BY

SMITH ELY JELLIFFE, M.D., Ph.D.

Managing Editor of the "Journal of Nervous and Mental Disease"; Co-editor of "The Psychoanalytic Review," and "Nervous and Mental Disease Monograph Series"

UNCONSCIOUS DYNAMICS AND HUMAN BEHAVIOUR: A GLIMPSE AT SOME INTER-RELATIONSHIPS OF STRUCTURE AND FUNCTION*

BY

SMITH ELY JELLIFFE

DR MORTON PRINCE has contributed so widely to our knowledge of mental mechanisms and their importance in behaviour, that I have thought it not without some interest to carry these ideas perhaps somewhat deeper and endeavour to show that even what may be called organic disease may essentially be concerned with what Prince would designate as co-conscious activities, but which the Freudian concepts deal with behind the hypothesis of the unconscious.

In contemporary pathology a great upheaval has taken place. Bacteriology came as a blessing and as a curse—the former in that it fastened very definitely some etiological factors beyond cavil, the latter because of a too facile displacement of its ideas to cover causality beyond its logical limits. The disposition or constitutional background which permitted infections to act or toxins to poison was forgotten and only in recent times has pathology resolutely turned its face back to dynamic ideas early taught by the Greeks.

Man is a social animal; he is one of a herd. He is not just a collection of organs. He is an entity, an evolutionary product with an enormous ancestry.

That ancestry began with cosmic physical and chemical forces. These still remain participants in aftercoming reactions : when life first insinuated itself into dead matter ; when crystalline laws were surpassed, because they were too rigid to allow for newer adaptations, a type of superchemistry arose, the behaviour of which

* See *New York Medical Journal*, April 5th, 1922, where some of these formulations were presented as a lecture given to post-graduate physicians, during the winter session of the New York Post-Graduate Medical School and Hospital, 1911–1912, and now revised.

science has symbolised under the term *vital* and which became condensed in structure. Vital structures in their turn threatened to limit the development of life's accumulations. The inexorable fact of duration (Bergson), that " piling up of the past upon the past," with its inevitable necessity for hanging on to the entire past, forced a supervitalism which finally in man was met by the masterly invention of the Symbol, by which this mighty Atlas of the past might be compressed, in tablet form as it were, to be used in the social machinery. Its most highly intellectualised form is language, although that is not by any means its only product, particularly for lower races and for earlier ontogenetic phases of the human animal.

Then, when as psychopathologists we speak of the psyche, we mean that *function* of man which operates by means of and through symbols. Psychical mechanisms are chiefly symbolic mechanisms. Their study is the study of symbology with its enormous phyletic past which is just being unravelled. By many who are mostly dealing with classroom problems, this study is more often called psychology. The average classroom psychology, however, only commences to fringe on the actualities of life. The psychology that is of any service is that which has this enormously rich past, of which the previously emphasised evolutionary hypothesis takes cognisance. It is the psychology which is tucked away, condensed, compacted in the symbol. It is best termed the psychology of the *unconscious*, or, as Bleuler (1) has termed it, deep psychology.

Through such a concept we can get into sympathetic touch with the past. Animal behaviour in its phyletic advancing stages becomes more and more comprehensible in that degree with which we discard categories and get in touch with the behaviour of things.

The *unconscious* contains all of the chemistry, the vitalism, and the symbolism. It has everything from the beginning. The psychology of the conscious is but a momentary flash of what the hundred million years of life have tucked away in the living human being. The conscious expresses the numerator of a fraction which represents life. The immensely more important part of life, which is hidden, is the denominator. Thus this idea may be put in the form of a proportion ; as the numerator, from minute to minute, is to the denominator, one hundred million years, so is our Conscious Knowledge of what is going on, to the Unconscious Dynamics which really makes it happen.

In his inimitable phrase Bergson has said, "What are we? What is our character if not the condensation of the history we have lived from our birth, nay even before our birth, since we bring with us prenatal dispositions? Doubtless we think with only a small part of our past, but it is with our entire past, including the original bent of our soul, that we desire, will, and act. Our past, then, as a whole, is made manifest to us in its impulse ; it is felt in the form of tendency, although a small part of it only is known in the form of idea."

It is, then, as readily may be seen, a long jump from the idea, the symbol, back to the beginning of that integration in man, the vegetative nervous system by which the physical and chemical forces were handled for the purposes of human behaviour.

This evolutionary attitude thus regards the vegetative or visceral (sympathetic) nervous system as regulating the metabolism of the human body; hence its function is related to the earliest part of the past in the unconscious denominator. The phyletically oldest part of the vegetative nervous system, and that part which still maintains structural relationships, the exact anatomical integers of which as yet are but imperfectly analysed (Küppers) is the endocrinous gland system. Some of these glands have manifest morphological resemblances to nervous structures, such as the pineal, the hypophysis, and the parasympathetic ganglia, while others, such as the prostate, pancreas, and thymus, have no obvious neurological structuralisations. A distinctly advancing series, however, may be hypotheticated in which the resemblances increase. Such a series, from the least to the most obvious nervous similarities, would be prostate, testicles, ovary, thymus, pancreas, suprarenals, thyroid, parathyroid, choroid plexus, neuroglia, sympathetic paraganglia, pineal, and hypophysis.

It has been assumed by many physiologists that each of these structures elaborates some specific substance to which the name *hormone* (energy carrier) has been applied. Although only one of these hormones has thus far been definitely isolated, epinephrine (adrenaline), yet it seems fairly well demonstrated that substances, specific in some sense at least, exist within each of the structures mentioned. Kendall's thyroxin is possibly another and insulin a possible third.

Intracellular metabolism in simple cellular organisms is a physico-chemical affair. The colloidal state of the protoplasm permits this. But with succeeding complexities, channelings and bindings became essential ; these, foreshadowed in the fibrovascular bundles of the plant, slowly progressed into the vascular, muscular, neuromuscular, and nervous structures of the vertebrate animal.

In these higher animals the chief hormones are now carried through the body chiefly by means of the blood current, and there occurs an amazingly complex interplay between the vascularly brought hormone supply and the behaviourist craving, in which the receptor end of the nervous arc touches the hormone stimulus and the effector end, after connector integrations, brings about the appropriate and adequate response in trophic, secretory or motor action which equilibrates the craving and adjusts the behaviour.

It is not too extreme a hypothesis that designates carbon dioxide as the original and phyletically the oldest of the hormones, parhormones (Gley). The phylogenesis of its successors has not yet been traced. Physiology is looking for a Mendelieff to trace out the hormone evolutionary products. A better knowledge of the chemical evolution of our present hormones is still lacking. No reference can be quoted on this subject, but such must exist.

Nevertheless, while dealing with carbon dioxide, let us stop a moment here and point out a relationship between it and respiration and the further function which man has developed as an accessory to his carbon dioxide hormone need, namely, aspiration, which has developed into that chief distinguishing attribute of human animals, speech.

Lung function is closely related to the psychical function of social integration through symbolic language. I hope to raise several concepts for consideration relative to the psyche and to the vegetative nervous integration of the lung structures, which are, I believe, very pertinent in human pathology (Guth, E.). For, just as man cannot live simply to eat, so the man who utilises his lungs only to breathe will surely suffer some form of the *lex talionis* (retributive justice). He must do something more with them. They form a part of the mechanism for the delivery of his creative energy, and through the expression of new ideas he alone lives. In terms of the Parable of the Talents, if he simply wraps up his respiratory gifts in a napkin and does not put them out to usury, *i.e.*, to create and exchange ideas with his fellow man, *i.e.*, sublimates his respiratory libido (Stärcke) he will be in the position of the one who "hath not and shall have taken away from him even that which he hath." I beg of my readers not to get ultra-scientific—criticism not infrequently being thought of as pseudoscience by many—and remind me that deaf-mutes can live healthy useful lives (see Menninger).

Should the expression of a conviction be hazarded that the problem of the conquest of the chief enemy of the respiratory organs, the tubercle bacillus, is taking place through a better and better distribution of respiratory psychical energy—libido—I trust it may be taken as something to think about and study in your individual cases along lines which it is the general purpose of this lecture to outline. If one were able to trace, step by step, the psychology of the unconscious so far as respiratory needs were concerned, the pathology of tuberculosis and of many respiratory affections would be seen with an enlarged vision. The old truths are still true, but inadequate. This has been done for certain asthmas, for enough is known of these cases to be able to show some of the unconscious mechanisms which probably interfere with harmonious (hormone ; suprarenal) activity, and thus bring on the asthmatic spasms.

An extremely important topic for human pathology is here broached. It has been approached through a respiratory pathway, but it could have been approached by a number of different avenues, that is, similar questions can be brought for many other diseased organ patterns. Shall we say, as I have preferred to phrase it, that unconscious mental mechanisms induced a modification of the suprarenal glands or other hormone-producing bodies, which in their turn so changed the vegetative nervous system control of the respiratory organs—unstriped musculature, as to induce an asthmatic attack, or shall it be phrased, as it most frequently is in present-day orthodox pathology, that a disorder of the suprarenal gland alone or with other related endocrinous glands has brought about the altered action of the vegetative nervous system, and thus caused the asthmatic attacks, leaving the psychical situation out entirely ?

Here the importance of the title to this paper may be emphasised. In the first place, there is not the slightest doubt that there are asthmatic attacks in which neither the psychical system nor the hormone systems are involved. Such attacks are due to direct involvement of the sensori-motor structures themselves, from tumours, caseous nodules, or syphilitic processes within the posterior mediastinum pressing upon the main nerve trunks. Then again there are other endocrinous neurological disturbances, asthma being only one in which the involvement is primarily of endocrinous origin. These are due to acute inflammations or other direct somatic implication of an endocrinous gland. But, and here is the chief point in our discussion, there are also certain other affections of the vegetative nervous system which are pre-eminently or even solely psychogenic in their origin. Surgery or pharmacotherapy is essential for the first group and other therapies are illusory. Psychotherapy is hocus-pocus for the second group and opotherapy or X-ray therapy is indicated, while for the last group psychotherapy is alone rational and other therapies are usually " hokum."

To which group, or rather to what preponderance of action, a given disturbance belongs can be determined only after a most painstaking neurological analysis, with special methods devised to determine the specific vegetative nervous system anomalies, as well as a thorough acquaintance with the conscious and unconscious life of the patient. It is of no avail to speak of neurasthenia, or psychasthenia, or hysteria, or dementia præcox, or autointoxication ; these are not terms which explain anything. They may make interesting discussions relative to etymologies—Galen said this *apropos* of hysteria—but of the " behaviour of things " such word designations lead to sterility. Above all, let us not be thrown off the track by the cheap trick of the superficial dogmatist, for there are medical demagogic slogans as well as political ones, that pooh-pooh that which makes man what he is, his psychical as well as his metaphysical subtleties.

In the past ten years certain methods of investigating the vegetative nervous system have come into use which promise great assistance in sizing up a large group of patients who have been much neglected because of the inconstancy and bizarreness of their symptoms. Few will be in doubt concerning a diagnosis of cretinism or myxœdema, of exophthalmic goitre, Addison's disease, diabetes, acromegaly, dwarfism, achondroplasia, Raynaud's disease, scleroderma, or psoriasis. Yet it must be emphasised that for every single evident and well-marked vegetative disturbance there are one hundred atypical, irregular, incomplete or mixed cases.

It may be said that approximately fifty per cent. of the cases which now are frequently looked upon as abortive or mild cases of hypothyroidism or hyperthyroidism, ten years ago were diagnosed by the self-same physicians as neurasthenia. I have done so myself in many instances, and with each periodical revision of my histories, following out the later histories, I find many important things which were entirely overlooked. Ten or twenty years in the future there will be a different way of grouping the accumulated facts, each new generalisation, symbolised by a diagnosis, helping " more of the patients more of the time " than the preceding ones.

In order that our considerations may not be too diffuse, a clinical case is offered as a contribution to this discussion. It is to be thought of, not as an isolated situation, but as a paradigm, *i.e.*, a general example of scores of related occurrences. These are to be found in all branches of medicine. Here is taken up an endocrinopathy, but related reflections refer to some diseases of the skin, of the bones, of joints, of the blood-making organs, of diabetes, of tuberculosis, of the cardiorenal system and of others.

Case History*

Case.—A woman, thirty-five years of age, of Scandinavian parentage. She had been married about fourteen years and had one child, a girl four years of age. Her husband had a good retail business, was moderately prosperous, a hard worker, and because of his greater interest in money-getting than in making a " home " for himself and his wife and child neglected her and made her shift for herself for her own development. About five years ago she had her first upset, which came to the surface in the form of a mild exophthalmic goitre. This quieted down because she had a humane and good common-sense doctor, an obstetrician, by the by, who did not insist on " operation." During the whole time she was nervous, easily fatigued, and during the time she was under treatment, a period of three or four months, she showed—retrospectively interpreted—a typical vagotonic reaction. She had a slight

---

* This case history has had to be somewhat distorted, *i.e.*, disguised, a familiar device well known in Russian literature (see Stragnell, *Psychoanalytic Review*). Since the days of Hippocrates, medical ethics has wisely (?) insisted upon the " medical secret." If doctors (or priests) told the truth (from the housetops) which dramatists since the days of Æschylus have done and are doing—symbolically—(and are paid for it), they would be " burned at the stake." In 1923-1924, see on the New York stage : *1 he Spook Sonata*, by Strindberg ; *Rain*, by Somerset Maugham ; *Roseanne*, by B. Stevins ; *Outward Bound*, by Sutton Vane ; *Spring Cleaning*, by Frederick Lonsdale ; and *Tarnish*, by Gilbert Emery, and others, all satirising the hypocrisies of wickedness in high places. Socrates was one of the earlier victims of this mass psychological response to unwelcome knowledge of what man fears and hates concerning the devil within himself. This fact renders it very easy to use demagogic slogans, political, medical, economic or ecclesiastical. (See Walsh, J., in his recent humorously-deceptive propaganda, *Cures*, Appleton and Co.) Also consult Martin, E. D., " Some Mechanisms which distinguish the Crowd from other forms of Social Behaviour," *Journal of Abnormal Psychology*, 18, 1923, 187-203, which shows how " *prejudice* " as a form of repressed self knowledge may be used to defeat honourable public servants and elect " tools " of dishonest politicians.

z

struma, somewhat larger on the right side, which became worse, following an attack of tonsillitis, to which disorder, she stated, she had not been subject.

She was slightly agitated, had a very fine tremor, her face was slightly flushed, and there were reddish patches on the skin. The eyes were not markedly protruding, the palpebral fissures were slightly unequal, the left somewhat larger than the right, the pupils were unequal, and her eyes glistened. As she looked down, the eyelids followed slowly. There was no tachycardia. She said she had some respiratory hunger and felt oppressed at times. There was a sense of globus hystericus, and the history (kindly furnished by the said obstetrician) showed some visceroptosis (X-rays). She had lost fifteen or twenty pounds in weight and had attacks of looseness of the bowels without diarrhœa. Her blood pressure was fairly high. She was vivacious in her manner, lively, and inclined to laugh and be happy. She said she slept poorly and dreamed little. Internists, called in consultation, had told her she was suffering from autointoxication. Eosinophilia was five per cent., but gastrointestinal therapy had been inefficacious. Rest in bed had not been of particular service.

Attention might be directed to the fact that she had an increased suprarenal reaction, a mild hyperadrenalemia, also a mild hyperthyroidism. If statistics were being collected from the adrenal point of view, she would be the former ; if from the thyroid, the latter. If one had just been reading Cannon's work on the reciprocal relation between the adrenals and the thyroid, it might be assumed that these glands were overfunctioning. From the knowledge that the patient had had tonsillitis which was followed by an exacerbation of her symptoms, one might assume the presence of an infectious thyroiditis of a mild grade. Any and all of these points of view would be perfectly valid. At all events, her tonsils should be cleared up and possibly X-ray applications might help a possible infection. The patient might be given a rest cure or a surgical operation, but I hazard the opinion that, if one went no further, the woman would not be helped very materially. She would probably move into another hospital or go to another doctor.

If, as was learned after many hours of careful investigation, her psychical situation was known, she was in a sorry mess which on no logical ground could be excluded in the chain of causality. If this were neglected, one would really know nothing essential about the dynamics involved in this endocrine behaviour.

Our patient married, not for love, as she expressed it, but because her family thought it was a good match. She was almost shoved into it. She " carried on," however. The sexual adaptation was only so-so. She was excitable and her husband precipitate, and always too busy to be with her much. She was mostly unsatisfied. " He did not marry her for *that*," he would say as an unconscious defence against his relative impotency (money preoccupation). She managed to get along, however, presenting only mild anxiety neurosis symptoms for which she was " bromided " for about ten years by numerous physicians, who called her hysterical. She remained sterile throughout this period, at no time taking any precautions or preventives. Much could be said about her creative wishes—unconscious—all this time. Of course, there were curet-tages. As if the uterus did not know its job better, after millions of years of experience, than we medical blunderers ! The only really interesting thing was that for a time she menstruated every fourteen days. This I correlate, with apologies to my gynecological confrères, with the conflict between an organic uterine craving for doing its work, and the unconscious component that knew that this was *no love* situation (Ego Ideal, Freud).

After all these years of frustration she found someone who, she thought, really was interested in *her*, and letting down the conventional barriers, under most conflicting and stirring situations, that month became pregnant. She had had intercourse with her semi-impotent husband and her lover the same week. It was then she commenced to worry as to whose child it was. Which parent would it resemble when it grew up ? What would her husband think ? Would he throw her out ? And a host of other extremely disturbing doubts and inquiries. It was just then that the first attack of hyperthyroidism (and tonsillitis) came on. She was in an extremely agitated state for some time.

Whether it was the thyroid that produced the agitation or the agitation that produced the hyperthyroid activity, I leave the reader to decide, according to his prejudices and his honesty.

She was perturbed for some time during the pregnancy. Luckily all of the triangle were blue-eyed and light-haired, and as our patient was not disturbed by any knowledge of Mendelian recessive factors, she finally came to a moderate state of adjustment. The hyperthyroidism slowly disappeared and she " carried on." For a time, during the nursing, she was better. Her husband was much more attentive and, although he was still far from being satisfied, she managed to get along, presenting only some anxiety neurosis symptoms. Later, however, the husband became very busy. He had to get up very early in the morning ;· he had to go to bed early in the afternoon or evening. Little by little he left her more and more alone. He was exhausted from his day's work and would go months without intercourse, and when he did attempt it, it was finished in a second. She either masturbated or anxiety symptoms came on and she developed a rich phantasy· life.

Some years later (and, now for the first time, the present writer enters directly into the situation) we faced a new and severe flare-up. Just what determined this flare-up, I do not think the ordinary methods of inquiry would give us any dynamic clue. The Goetsch test might be interesting, study of her basal metabolism might tell something, but we suspect these are has-beens rather than causes. The reader may be assured that these and similar " tests " were not thrown out of court on *a priori* prejudices. That such " tests," used in all situations of pathological inquiry are not depreciated, must be emphasised, but far and above these statistical after-resultants, we would here emphasise the more dynamic situation : What is the patient striving to accomplish ? What are her cravings ? What is the Freudian wish ? (Holt). Here we stand firmly on an empirical basis of actual findings and turn to the " royal road " into the unconscious and ask what does the dream life contribute to our understanding of this behaviour ?

This is the formulation : The individual *as a whole* is the subject of our inquiry at this or any particular time ; we are not interested in any of its *parts*, save indirectly. *As a whole*, the human being functions in his *wish capacity* ; he is constantly forming plans to carry out desires and cravings. In a specific way this formulation states there are two chief modes of expression for these human instinctive cravings. They follow two broad roads, as it were, which run parallel toward a goal which, for lack of a better term, let us call happiness. One might change the metaphor and say that this stream of wishes could be compared to a twisted strand of rope made up of innumerable intertwined smaller strands in which two larger groups of strands could be distinguished. These roads, these strands, following the German poet Schiller's example, we roughly call *hunger* and *love*. They constitute the great wish forces of life. *Self-preservation* and *race-propagation* are their ancestral and present-day patterns. Do we eat to live, or do we live to eat ? An answer to this question tells us that whereas life's energy flows more strongly now through one, now through the other, yet, if one could put a pressure gauge upon these two forces, the highest pressure would be found on the *race-propagation* side, and the old dictum that self-preservation is the first law of Nature will be found to be false. It is but a weak-kneed concession to what human beings have attempted to repress since Adam and Eve ate of the tree of knowledge. The phylum, the race, is more important than the individual. In the swing of Nature's pendulum which oscillates alternately but never just equally—for Nature does not relish being caught on a dead centre—the push is greater on the race-propagation side. The fly-wheel of the race-propagation side is loaded. Creative evolution is thus made possible and the game goes on. It has come from protozoon to man, a lively contest of new models for anywhere from one hundred to a thousand million years. During all this slow ascent organic memory (the Mneme of Semon) has been laying down useful bits of biological structure, building them finally into a fabric which we call man. These old bits of structuralised function—for this is what the organs of the body can advantageously be conceived of as being—contain much that is not available to conscious control. They function automatically, yet are not out of actual contact with the rest of the body.

The body *as a whole* is an organisation of all of these, a synthesis made possible by the nervous system. Not at the receptor surfaces, not in the spinal cord, not in the midbrain, not in the motor or sensory cortical projection fields, but only finally in the frontal cortex is this ultimate synthesis made effective. Here intuition or instinct meets with intelligence. Control of the bodily movements to satisfy its cravings has an arbiter. This control factor, however, has been building itself up just as long as any organisation was found to be an advantageous scheme of things. When there were no conflicts, intuitive action went straight to its goal and satisfaction was implicit. When obstacles arose, however, then a new scheme of things arose. We call it *consciousness*. It was a *by-product* of faulty intuitive action. It was only needed because intuition became clouded. The *unconscious*—for such can be named this vast series of intuitive, instinctive syntheses—tended to be blocked by as yet ill-assimilated conscious contacts. The *Individual* and the *Crowd* are in conflict. Man's intelligence and his instinctive reactions are in conflict, and his vaunted intelligence is wrong. When we say that " *conscience doth make cowards of us all*," are we not only saying that the unconscious is wiser really than our intelligence ? (See Samuel Butler.)

" Beyond Good and Evil " is the title of a study by Nietzsche.

He has seen that force, neither good nor evil, is present within our unconscious. How shall we utilise that force? For good or for evil? That determines health or illness! Then our unconscious is very badly maligned. Yes, it is. It is the source of both good and evil, yet is it neither.

What then is good or evil? Everyone has asked the question. So long as mankind dealt with conscious psychology, anybody could make his own definitions, and everybody did. " What is one man's meat is another's poison," and we have every possible brand of good and evil, according to climate, to race, to custom, and to fashion. From this point of view my " doxy " is orthodoxy and your " doxy " is heterodoxy. Everybody who thinks differently from me will be damned. So has mankind come up, getting freer and freer from certain dogmas, and yet chaining himself tighter and tighter to other dogmas.

In the unconscious, however, will be found truth in simple form. Here we can see what we are after without all the currents and counter-currents of camouflage and hypocrisy. The dream is the royal road to the unconscious. Such is Freud's well-known and well-tried-out suggestion. We shall, therefore, look to the dream.

The first day I saw the patient I obtained a full history of her family, her father, mother, brothers and sisters. Her mother had always kept an eye on her. As to her dreams she told me she rarely dreamed. A great many people say the same, but everybody dreams just as everybody breathes, secretes bile or urine, but not all people remember their dreams. As to nightmares, she said she had had one recently. It was as follows :

She was going to a party. She had a lovely time. She was glad to see a stranger. (She awoke with palpitation.)

I did not attempt an analysis of this nightmare and shall not now, only remarking that the word " party " may have a double significance, a " double entendre," as our Latin races express it. She saw a stranger and woke up. Waking up = conflict. Whether the wish was to have a *party* with a *stranger* and that gave her nightmare—for it will be recalled how a similar " *party* " gave her a " *baby* "—will be left for the moment and the next dream will be considered ; for we must be interested in the specific rather than the general problem.

At the next visit she recalled with some difficulty the rambling dream she had had the night before. She dreamed as follows :

I met a man on an elevated station. It was at .... Street, where there was a shuttle train (going backward and forward). He did not recognise me. Then there was a lady there whom he seemed to know. I was with someone then, and as I watched them I said to this someone (a woman), " Oh, if Mrs P. (the wife of the man) should know this." I decided it was the best policy to say nothing about it. (She had anxiety and some palpitations when she awoke.)

Notes on the Dream

Question : " Mr P. ? "—" Oh, he was her husband. He spoke several languages. He had kept a hotel. He ran around with many women. His hotel was foreclosed. She was a hard-working woman. She had had some business with Mrs X.'s (the patient's) husband. Her husband, Mr X., was greatly worried about business. He might be foreclosed. He was thinking of moving or changing his business somewhat, had thought of supplying (things) to hotels."

Question : " What comes to your mind about shuttle ? "—"He got out at .... Street. I was going to take the downtown train."

Question : " The woman Mr P. seemed to know ? "—" Oh, she seemed to be someone I knew. A fast woman. She was a fly person. She laughed and giggled. She was short and stout." (Patient was tall and thin—disguise of censor—fair—patient was fair.)

Question : " What comes to your mind ? "—" I've lots of friends, I know lots of people. I know no friends like her. Mrs D. V., she's a little suspicious. But I'm broadminded, I don't believe in being narrow-minded. Of course, people like that, they must live —what sort of a life ? How much nicer and how much worse it must be. She is beautiful (patient was a handsome blonde). People have different ways of living, after all. Terrible, in a way, but then they can love one another. A mistress, sometimes, may be possible. Companions, they can get away from each other when they get on each other's nerves. Still a married woman is the best. It is safer."

This then leads to a long discussion as to her young womanhood and her girl friends, and the " fellows " that called. She liked life and wanted a good time, but with X., " he was all for business." " He never liked to be gay." " He was tired all the time." She wanted to go out, play cards, dance, see the shows. But my mother, she had her heart set on my marrying a steady fellow. I respected him highly. He was always very serious. He never flirted at all. He is very kind, but is not my real mate. At first everything was terribly painful (dyspareunia). After a few months it was all right, but he never seemed to care much for " that." " Had not married me for *that*." Practically always unsatisfied.

The chief features in the dream have been presented and some of the free associations of the dream are recorded. As this material is reviewed, it will be quite clear that the patient was seriously disturbed over the temptation of being some man's mistress. She was resisting it, as the free associations tended to show—" A married woman is safer," etc. I did not disturb the patient too unduly, and I did not attempt to bring into consciousness whose mistress she wanted to be, but let her tell all about her troubles with her mother, about her husband and the hard work she had to go through on account of the baby, the difficulty with maids, with the cook, her husband's irritability, etc.

For a few days she had no dreams. Then a few about the child. In one dream, *her girl had peculiar white and green stools which worried her.* These were also left only partly analysed. Speaking from the standpoint of psychoanalysis it may be of very little service in a beginning of an analysis to try to bring into the consciousness of a woman that her child, especially a girl child, may be a nuisance to her, from certain aspects of her personality. Such truths can only be discussed rationally when a patient knows much more about the selfishness of her *ego* and its conflict with her better self, *i.e.*, her love for her child.

Then she had a dream of " *having triplets, two blondes and one with black hair and brown eyes.*" This brought out a great deal about whether the child she had had was her husband's child or the lover's child. If her lover had brown eyes and black hair, what would have happened ? There was much material, but I waited, feeling certain that I would soon find the " man with the brown eyes and the black hair." For two weeks the resistances prevented any advance.

One of the dreams in the interim contained material which dealt with a doctor who curetted her and who had been very friendly. Her transference to him was very strong and the dream discussed whether I should be entitled to as close a place in her confidence as Dr Z. Two or three neurologists who had been consulted also appeared in the dreams. (Who they were, and what they did and said, contains much material why jealousies exist between members of the profession.)

In about six weeks after I had begun to see her she presented the specific situation. She dreamed :

There were two gray automobiles standing in *……… *Street* (the *street where she lived), between* ……… *and* ……… (*parallel streets i.e., parallel wishes*). *One was adorned with draperies, with bright colours on the body. There were red bandannas in it.* " *I don't like this car. Like a fortune-teller's wagon.*" *Out of each one came a Mr L. with a woman. She was a fast woman. There was another woman and another man I knew. Both go to Mr L.'s house. Then I say, "if Mrs L. were alive, what would she say ?"* *Then in another dream the same night : I visited Mrs L. She was alive and the place was very upset.* " *It looks as if you were going to move,*" *and she picks up some artificial hair, puts it on her head. It was black in colour, and she said : " Is it not awful the way my husband abuses me ? "*

At this point it seemed not injudicious to bring the issue up on this situation, and from the dream associations it soon developed that Mr L. was the " dark-haired, brown-eyed man " who was trying to persuade her to be his mistress. He was a widower, a lawyer, wealthy. (He told her so, but she had her suspicions. He was not so generous.) There was some doubt about his generosity, as a previous dream about rings and jewellery had partially revealed ; he was rather stingy with his money (took a street-car and not a taxi), and also, possibly, as a lawyer, he would get out of the divorce possibility with her husband, and leave her " stranded " after all.

It would be nice to exchange *her situation* (comparative poverty) with an *automobile situation* (wealth and comfort) but (red bandannas) was he only a slick fortune-teller, after all, and where would she land in the interchange when she went to Mr L.'s house as mistress (urged) or as wife of wealthy man (promised), and concerning which the office, his clothes, his niggardly attitudes, etc., made her doubtful ?

Of course, for ordinary mortals without such temptations (for, remember she had a husband who neglected her) there is little need to be agitated and disturbed, but for her, as she used to go to the lawyer's office to " discuss the possibilities of divorce," and he would make passionate love to her " on his very ample sofa," it does not take a wizard (fortune-teller, *myself*) to see her dilemma.

---

* Omitted, because of the " medical secret " situation already alluded to, as being a matter of discretion.

This complicated story could be elaborated into a three volume novel, and novelists deal with just such realistic (human) material, and we sit up into the small hours of the morning reading them. Why? Because, as novelists, they put it all into intelligible (and fantasy) terms, while we, doctors, as scientists, deal with the impulses that need all this long-drawn-out terminology to render them intelligible to mankind. As a *scientist*, one deals chiefly with the bare framework of the forces which are pulling this woman. Her cravings and her fears, money, comfort, automobiles, sexual satisfaction on the one hand ; a secure home, her daughter, her marriage security, meaning social support, on the other.

Why should the hyperthryoid activities be considered as a mediating mechanism? I do not altogether know. If I did know, possibly I would know as much as God knows, and, with all my pretensions to knowledge, I have not yet gone so far as to approach the Omnipotent. As physicians, all that can be said is that there is a definite series of wish components on the one hand, and an equally definite series of bodily reactions on the other. If Pavlov's dogs show gastric juice reactions to conditioned stimuli, and Cannon's cats show physical reactions to other types of stimuli, can it not be said that the " prostitution-mistress-money-comfort " stimuli have something to do with the hyperthyroid physical reactions? I seriously ask you to consider the possibilities, yes, the probabilities of this connection. It is a specific stage of the parental complex. The future may help us as scientists to build up the relations between structure and function.*

And here we must leave it, but before I leave it I cannot refrain from alluding to an important reflection. The situation, on the outside, and partly from the inside, is very widespread. Many human beings are caught in just this kind of a dilemma, yet hyperthyroid reactions do not develop in all. I can only say : So be it. I agree with you absolutely in all your doubts and conservatisms. There must be a definite chain of events which lead to a definite outcome.

Is this hyperthyroidism (or other organic situation) alone conditioned by the factors which I have all too hurriedly sketched? I do not think so. There are complex constitutional factors which are a part of the structure. These are to be resolved as well.

* Since this initial presentation, in 1911, these anatomical structural correlations have advanced very materially. But this is a subject of another presentation. See References.

In the meantime, while we are busy with the biochemical and hereditary and hidden structural parts of this integration, we are faced with the present real situation. The patient *wants*, and yet *does not want*, to run away with the dark-haired, brown-eyed man, sacrifice the husband and the daughter, and get even with the mother who had always bossed her, and who had thrust this worthy husband upon her. Can she stand it? She cannot! Her physical disease is her reaction to the conflict. It is a compromise between her conscience (God's Law, Ego Ideal) and her craving (Individual wish). It is the symbol of her sacrifice.

We, as physicians, must first straighten out her ethical conflict. Removing her thyroid does not do this, even if we admit that she has gotten her body into such a mess that she would rather die than renounce the wish. For this happens, and only surgery may prevent the unconsciously arrived at physical suicide.

What happens afterward, even if the thyroid be removed? Will it be morphine, alcohol? Will it be " bridge " and a round of hideous attempts at forgetting? Will she go to the devil or will she be an exile, shut up in her apartment, devoted to the only resource left, to see that the daughter does not get into the mess that she got into? Will she sacrifice the daughter, as many do, or will she triumph and come through? *Quien sabe:* Who knows?

REFERENCES

Küppers (E.), " Der Grundplan des Nervensystems und die Lokalisation des Psychischen," *Zeitschr. f. d. g. Neur. u. P.*, 75, 1922, 1–46.

Küppers (E.), " Weiteres zur Lokalisation des Psychischen," *Ibid.*, 83, 1923, 247–76.

Küppers (E.), " Ueber den Sitz der Grundstörung bei der Schizophrenie," *Ibid.*, 78, 1922, 546–52.

Guth (E.), " Lungentuberkulose und vegetatives Nervensystem." I, II, III, IV : *Beiträge zur Klinik der Tuberkulose*, Vols. 53, 54, 55, 1922–3.

Mühl (A. M.), " Tuberculosis," *Psychoanalytic Review*, 1923.

Stärcke, " The Apnœic Phase of the Pregenital Libido Pattern," *The International Journal of Psychoanalysis*, 1923.

Menninger (K. M.), " Deafness and the Psyche," *Kansas Medical Journal*, 1923.

Laignel-Lavastine, *Pathology of the Vegetative Nervous System*. (Here the chief results of the past ten years are collected). Paris, 1923.

SMITH ELY JELLIFFE

Kappers (Ariëns), *Comparative Anatomy of the Nervous System of Vertebrates*, 1920.

Winkler, *Anatomy of the Nervous Ssytem*, 1919, 1920.

Jelliffe (S. E.), " Paleopsychology," *Psychoanalytic Review*, April, 1923.

Jelliffe (S. E.) and White (W. A.), *Diseases of the Nervous System*, 4th Edition, 1923.

Jelliffe (S. E.), " Psychopathology and Organic Disease," *Am. Archives of Neurol. and Psych.*, December, 1922.

THE METAMORPHOSIS OF DREAMS

BY

JOHN T. MacCURDY, M.D., M.A.

Lecturer in Psychopathology, Cambridge University

THE METAMORPHOSIS OF DREAMS*

BY

JOHN T. MacCURDY

I<small>T</small> is a scientific misfortune that so much psychoanalytic work is therapeutic in its aim rather than primarily investigative. This is, of course, inevitable : few people can be found ready to sacrifice time, money and personal comfort in the interest of psychology. Naturally, then, the vast bulk of dream analysis is carried on with the definite object of unearthing the hidden tendencies, which are causing the patient's symptoms, not with the hope of discovering laws concerning the structure of dreams. Every analyst has daily opportunity to verify the fundamental claims of Freud as to dream mechanisms—the " dream work " ; but he is forced by consideration of the patient's need to forgo the pleasure of reconstructing the dream after it has been analysed, since this is largely of academic interest. Again, we have all of us the constant experience of confining ourselves to one chapter, one act of the dream, or one dream of a number presented in one night. If we should attempt to run to earth every detail in a long panoramic dream, we would find ourselves spending days, even weeks, with the productions of one night, and taking little account of the progress of the patient's nocturnal autistic life.

We feel comfortable enough in directing our attention mainly to the latent content of a dream because we know that this is of more importance to the patient than any prolonged consideration of the manifest content, or any discussion of the nature of the symbols employed to express the underlying thought. We are confident that some opponents of psychoanalysis have made a great mistake in seeking to explain the dream in its obvious form as a distorted echo of the experience of the previous day. A repetition of events of the " dream day " in a dream is to us an indication of a hidden significance in those experiences. Perhaps it is a fear of this meticulous superficiality which has kept psychoanalysis from

* This paper was read at the Sixth Annual Meeting of the American Psychoanalytic Association in Washington, May, 1916.

any serious study of the dream as it is actually remembered. An example may make this plainer. The patient may dream of a Cathedral spire, a maypole, a sword or a snake. The opponent finds a recent experience to determine each picture and is satisfied with that. The psychoanalyst applies his technique, finds a phallic significance in each and says that all are the same, regarding the manifest difference as largely or entirely accidental.

Now in the investigations which Dr Hoch and I have made of the manic-depressive psychoses we have come to have some respect for the manifest content. We find the same latent content with almost dreary iteration, no matter what the clinical picture may be. There is in this, then, ample evidence that the same dynamic factor is responsible for all these dissimilar states. When we come to examine what is constant in any one type of disorder, however, we discover that the mood corresponds to the form in which the underlying thought reaches conscious expression. In other words, the patient is anxious, guilty, elated or depressed in consequence of unconscious tendencies coming to expression in rather specific form. Another phenomenon is of no less interest : the idea may be in consciousness but for a fleeting moment, while the abnormal mood may persist apparently independent of it.

When one considers how closely analogous dreams are to delusions or hallucinations it is natural to ask how far these principles may apply to dreams. I may say that the application of these psychiatric laws to dreams has enabled me with few exceptions to predict the emotional state of the patient during the day following a dream when once that dream has been revealed. It is, therefore, immediately evident that the manifest content of the dream has a profound significance for the patient. In fact, one might even claim that it determines his waking health and happiness.

There is another problem bound up with this. As has been stated, much attention has been given to the waking thoughts that determine the content of a subsequent dream, but little has been written about the fate of these fantastic ideas. Not a few neurotic symptoms have been traced to dreams, it is true, and Jones has given us an example of " The Influence of Dreams on Waking Life," but no attempt has been made, as far as I know, to trace the mechanism by which our dream thoughts pass over into our waking activities. It is the object of this paper to present a few suggestions on this topic.

It is necessarily a rather speculative subject of discussion for reasons which will be immediately obvious. We have to rely almost entirely on subjective, introspective data, and it is a peculiarity of such material that it is almost necessarily incomplete. We dream, of course, infinitely more than we remember ; the censorship sees to it that we forget our nocturnal adventures with all possible speed ; in fact, the instantaneousness with which an elaborate memory of dream experiences can be wiped out of consciousness is one of the most astounding phenomena in all psychology. As a rule our attention is fixed with sufficient intensity to register in waking consciousness only one or a small group of many dreams which we have had. This applies to true dreams. There is also a drowsy state of half sleep when dreams seem partly true and the real environment is also grasped in part. For this period we also tend to be amnesic. If we attend to this, then the previous incidents—the real dreams—are lost to consciousness. Now, for our present problem we need to have succinct memories not only of our dreams proper, of our thoughts in the twilight state, but also of what we think and do when fully awake. Naturally, we cannot hope to obtain this full sequence frequently. More often we can get fragments that enable us to reconstruct the gradual transition from sleeping to waking thoughts which our amnesia has made to seem abrupt.

It has long been a commonplace of psychoanalysis that the same theme tends to run through all the dreams of any given night. Sometimes a careful noting of all details immediately on waking may enable one to demonstrate the latent content in such a sequence by the mere principle of equivalents. That is, details may vary so little from one act to another of the drama that the patient can see for himself the meaning of the symbols. A condensed example may make this plainer. A young woman has three dreams, of which these are the central incidents : First, she sees a bull and a cow mating in a barn yard—she is disgusted but morbidly attracted to the spectacle ; second, she spies on a boy and girl cousin who are flirting ; third, she watches her father with much interest pouring gasoline into a motor. In all three curiosity is expressed. The transition from the crude to the innocent sexuality and from that to the pure symbol is evident. This much the patient can see for herself. The analysis showed by definite associations a specific curiosity which was the common latent content of all three dreams. The important point for us to note here is that the manifest content is changing as she comes nearer to waking so that the reaction to it is more comfortable. In the first dream she is highly uncomfortable ; in the second (she

AA

complained) she felt *de trop* ; in the third she is comfortably interested. It could never disturb her peace of mind to see her father put gasoline in a car in waking life. This familiar type of sequence is still in the pure dream stage.

The next example gives us the birth of the dream into waking thoughts and actions. The patient is a physician whose father died of a lingering illness while the patient was still a young boy. He has specialised in the treatment of tuberculosis and is head of a hospital where many incipient cases are successfully treated. He appeared for analysis one day very depressed, apparently as a result of a dream where the latent content of eliminating his father from the family was not sufficiently distorted to be comfortable. (This is typical of the depressive idea or dream. An anti-social tendency comes to consciousness in a form which represents something repugnant to the patient's normal standards of conduct.) The analysis obliterated the depression. The next day he appeared elated and reported an extremely active, successful day's work. His first thought on waking was the problem of telling an older married man that he had a serious tubercular infection. Next he recalled that he had to examine several cases which were suspected of early tuberculosis. He looked forward to this and when the time came made extraordinarily good examinations and was able to satisfy himself that his suspicions were correct. This buoyant efficiency lasted through the day. When asked for his dream, however, he had to make a confession. On rising, he had jotted down a few headings, but on looking at them later in the day they were meaningless to him. The dream was gone. Fortunately a few associations from his notes led to the recovery of it. His room mate at college had died from tuberculosis after some years of unhygienic life during which he had been in ignorance of his disease. The patient had felt that if only a diagnosis had been made earlier he would never have succumbed. The dream fulfilled this wish. In it he was back at a house party where they had been fellow guests some years before (at the time when the friend's symptoms first developed, only to be disregarded). The patient examined his chest, discovered the lesion and turned him over to the head nurse of his hospital for treatment. A brief analysis made the whole sequence transparent. His father dying of a wasting disease had created the patient's interest in tuberculosis. It was a sublimation of the idea of death in connection with his father. His friend and the old married man who was doomed were father-surrogates. What had been the night before a depressing theme was changed to a sublimation—it gave an outlet in the underlying wish in a form that met the approval of the patient's every standard.

The fact that this dream was forgotten deserves some comment. It was not of an unpleasant nature; in fact, it passed the censor long enough to allow the patient to make notes of it. Moreover, it returned to consciousness after a short analysis. For this amnesia one probably does not need to presume such a desire to forget as is necessary in most cases. Entirely apart from dynamic reasons we tend to remember best what is connected with our daily life, simply because it is more in our waking consciousness—more associated to our waking activities. This probably is one factor accounting for the topical memory of stages leading from pure dream thoughts to pure waking ones. One object of the process is to give a form to the latent thought that is adaptive to our waking needs. Each one is a substitute for the last and so there is always a tendency to remember only the last. This accounts merely for such amnesia as is here described ; the effectual hysterical type of amnesia is obviously not adaptive and can be explained only on dynamic grounds.

The next example from the same patient shows a less extended sequence, but again illustrates the transition from dream to waking life. He was a man of 36 years, superficially normal, but suffering from enough inhibition to have adopted the belief that he was not " a marrying sort." He had resigned himself comfortably to the idea of celibacy until suddenly an ejaculation while examining a boy patient startled and depressed him. He recognised at once a homosexual tendency previously totally unconscious. The resulting depression impaired his efficiency seriously and finally he applied for psychoanalytic treatment. The results were rapid and before long hopes of marriage filled his mind. There were two not unimportant difficulties in the way : there was no one in whom he felt sufficient interest to begin a courtship and his income was hardly large enough to support a family in the same comfort that he enjoyed as a bachelor. In a more or less conscious effort to surmount the first obstacle he began to indulge much more in social activities than had been his wont, which caused considerable comment among gossips. It was at this period that he awoke one morning with the thought which he could not identify with certainty as either a dream or an actual experience at a dance the previous night. It was this : He was watching one of his patients dancing with his fiancée and wondering how they could get married,

as the man had little money. This was all he could recall till on
his way to the analysis, when he remembered a real dream : " I
was in a doorway of the ballroom. Toward me came a patient who
has owed me money for some years. He and his wife began talking
to me about this bill, which embarrassed me very much, as all the
other guests were looking at us. He shouted at me that he would
pay it soon—next month." In his associations, the embarrass-
ment led to his sensitiveness to the gossip about him, as it was said
he was looking for a wife. The public promise to pay led to the
idea of his demanding the money, which he needed for
marriage. This shows at once the significance of his drowsy
thought.   The problem was transferred from his own to
another's shoulders ; it was then a real situation, not a dream
imagination, and moreover its contemplation gave him no
discomfort.

Part of the following dream sequence was reported by me two
years ago* to exemplify the mechanism by which a day-dream
experience precipitates a dream. At that time I spoke of the waking distortion as an example of what Freud has termed " secondary
elaboration," but on more mature consideration I feel that Freud
does not intend to include such complete metamorphoses under
that term. The following account is quoted, in part, from this
previous article.

This dream was produced on the seventh day of the analysis
of a woman suffering from morbid anxiety. From the very
beginning a strong " transference " to the physician was evident
from her dreams, which had been readily understood by her as an
expression of confidence, reliance and gratitude. Then came, as
soon as the analysis began to touch her vitally, the opposite feelings
of hate and distrust, coming to consciousness during associations
as an expression of the fear that the analyser would abuse his
privilege as a physician, a feeling that he was exposing her life
history for his own gratification, that he was " outraging her
innocence." These ideas came relentlessly to expression, and for
several days were regularly accompanied by harrowing attacks of
anxiety that interfered temporarily with the analysis. The underlying wish for erotic satisfaction—an idea repugnant and foreign
to her conscious personality—remained unconscious, however, till
she read in the newspaper about some deal that J. P. Morgan had
put through by unfair means, she thought. The following night

* " A Psychological Feature of the Precipitating Causes in the Psychoses,
etc.," *Journal of Abnormal Psychology*, 1914, Vol. ix.

she had this dream, which I quote from her written record of it:

" This dream is really too vague to tell. *I feel it has changed its form at least three times before I finally got it into my mind.* This is it: There was a financial deal to be put through. Several people were going to do it, but at the last they were afraid, and Morgan went in alone and managed the thing. An element of indignation and scorn on Morgan's part. *Before the dream changed to Morgan, it was something about the wheat pit, with a feeling that I was connected with it. Before that it was something about myself.* [My italics.]

" I awoke with the impression that someone was knocking at my door. Somehow a vague thought in my mind of something— the word ' modesty.' There was no connection between the knocking and the thought in my mind. I seemed to pick up this vague thought when I realised that no one was knocking."

Associations showed, with multiple overdetermination, that Morgan represented the physician, who scorned her " virtue," and who would abuse his medical privilege to seduce her. The scorn was, of course, in turn a projection of her hatred of the analysis, consciously, and unconsciously, her opposition to seduction.

Now, how did this dream come into being? Reading of the financial operations of Morgan, who " betrayed a confidence," touched off the unconscious wish to be betrayed. She said that, while waking, she had the feeling that she must record the dream, and knew that it concerned herself; but, while thinking of it, it turned, like the Old Man of the Sea, into the dream of the wheat pit, with which she was somehow identified. To the wheat pit she associated directly the " lambs " who are ruined, and her own innocence. Already there is here the staging of the financial world, but the wish was not sufficiently distorted to be acceptable to the waking consciousness, so it again underwent a complete metamorphosis and became the final Morgan dream. The loathsome caterpillar had changed into the butterfly and she was witness of the change.

The same latent idea is carried over into the semi-waking stage of consciousness with the hallucination of someone knocking on her door (attempting entrance to her bedroom) and the apparently irrelevant word " modesty." The truly unusual feature of the sequence is, of course, that the patient was herself conscious that the three dream formulations were somehow all one.

I have recently had an opportunity to confirm this theory experimentally. The patient is an unusually competent nurse whose psychosis has been as puzzling clinically as it has been baffling therapeutically. Anything like an adequate description of the case would require a fair-sized volume, but the features essential for our present purpose may be given briefly. She is now 36. In her late teens she began having attacks of depression, a number of which were severe enough to demand confinement in institutions for the insane. The attacks increased in frequency, so that for the past few years she has never had more than a month or six weeks of continuous mental comfort. What the earlier attacks were like, it is impossible to state, but all the later ones have been characterised by a gradual onset with irritability towards women in her environment followed by compulsive thoughts that she must kill or otherwise injure different people, often her fellow nurses, often a child or all the children where she had been working in a children's hospital. With these compulsive ideas there begins a certain amount of clouding of consciousness. As this last increases, the compulsive ideas become delusions—she has killed these people, is the wickedest criminal living, and so on. Sooner or later there is an insistent demand to go away or to kill herself. If she can't do one of these things, she will lose all control of herself. In this state she usually packs a bag and leaves her hospital or her case, is absent for a week or several weeks and finally returns, much better, but able to give only a meagre account of where she has been. Ordinary psychoanalytic methods have failed for this reason : She has had a rich dream life to report, and these dreams have led to the recovery of many important childish memories plainly related to her symptoms, but, unfortunately, significant associations have always been produced in a sort of twilight state for which she is largely amnesic afterwards. As a result she has never been able to bring her unconscious ideas into the limelight of her fully waking and critical consciousness. Nevertheless, much has been accomplished in aborting attacks, although no permanent health has yet been obtained.

A few months ago, however, when in an attack, she was trying to recall some ideas at my request, and became dizzy and nauseated. Persisting in her effort, she suddenly went fast asleep, " as though I had fainted," she said later. This sleep was evidently a deep somnambulic condition, for she answered all questions put to her in a dreamy, almost emotionless, far-away voice. Since then the same state has been produced artificially by suggestion, with ease when she has been partially clouded already, and only with great difficulty when her mind has been clear. Her productions in these somnambulisms are unique. It is apparently a condition where all resistance is removed and the unconscious speaks unimpeded. She has given with ease detailed memories of significant events ; and her thoughts at the age of two and three, with as much directness, explain the meaning of contemporary symptoms in unconscious terms. In these séances she has explained that her father found her little brother (two years younger than herself) in a hollow tree and brought him home to her mother. He should have given him to her, however ; her brother is really the child of her father and herself, as she often insists, " He is *my* baby ! " Both her parents died when she was three years old, but she speaks of them in the present tense when questions are asked referring to the period in her life when they were alive.

In a recent attack she had come to the point where she felt an ungovernable impulse to go away. Before doing so she came to see me. She was too upset for ordinary advice to affect her, so an attempt was made to hypnotise her. This produced only a mildly dreamy state where she told of a dream the night before of going with somebody who had a baby carriage ; that she had had compulsions to steal children on the street ; that she had been thinking of asking her brother (who is now married) to give her one of his children. Finally she said : " If I could only find a baby of my own ! " At this point she was told she would go to sleep if she continued to think of the baby. A minute later she was asked : " What else about the baby? " Immediately came the reply, in her typical somnambulic voice : " The baby ! My father gave me my own baby ! " She then gave explanations of her symptoms. She had wanted to go away to find this baby. It must be lost. She must have her own child, she did not want to nurse some other mother's child. After more questions, not relevant to our present purpose, she was asked to say what she was dreaming. Her reply was :

" Crossing Queensborough bridge—sky and clouds—cherubs ; there are children in the clouds, playing. I cross the bridge and I look at the children in this cloud. Beautiful day. I look in the shops and buy presents for my brother's baby." (" Is that all ? ") " Going to the home in the hospital—babies ; their mothers have gone away and left them. They are my children ! The king comes to see the children." (" Is that all ? ") " Yes."

She was next asked if she would not be able to wait till next summer, when she could take a position as head nurse in a hospital for children, where she had previously been ; if that would not be better than going away now. She agreed to this. Then she was awakened by counting five. I asked her at once what she had been dreaming. Her reply was :

" Queensborough bridge—blue and white clouds—walking home on Queensborough bridge—something about a hospital or home— about children—some little boys and girls—nice place—belonged to somebody—somebody had charge of it. Seemed like they said it was the king—but we don't have a king. A nice man—he came to see it—he stays there most of the time—he had charge of it." (" Was he the superintendent ? ")　" Yes, I think so." (" What had you to do ? ")　" I had charge of it—took care of the children —part of it. Had nice things for the children." (" Presents ? ") " They had toys—they belonged to the place." (" You gave them any ? ")　" Yes, I bought them, but not with my money, but with the money of the place ; it was a nice place. They had lots of money and took good care of the children. I took care of it and looked after them."

On waking, her symptoms had totally disappeared.

We have, then, this sequence : A dream of going with somebody who has a baby carriage. The next day compulsion to go away and to steal children ; in a somnambulic state these are both explained as the unconscious desires to gain possession of her brother as her child. Still in this sleep she has a dream representing proprietorship of children. On waking she recalls the essence of this dream with elaboration and distortion, both of which adapt it to reality, making a sublimation of this wish her professional activity and, with this, her symptoms disappear.

With this evidence before us it is plain that the normal sequence of dream thoughts is their gradual metamorphosis into a setting which is adapted to reality and to the patient's adult ambitions rather than his infantile cravings. A failure of this process can be remedied only by complete amnesia for the dream or analysis of it. If neither occurs, there is an abnormal mood during the following day, usually elation or depression. It seems to be a peculiarity of depression that it coincides with the presence of an idea, ethically unwelcome, on the fringe of consciousness. That is, depression corresponds to an unsuccessful effort at repression. The repressing forces having failed specifically seem to become diffuse and inhibit all interest, making the patient inert and all activity unattractive. Forel seems to have glimpsed the gaseous tail of this idea in his book on *Hypnotism and Psychotherapy*, where he speaks of curing depressions by suggestions of amnesia for unpleasant dreams.

These principles are well shown in the following dream. It may be well to remind you that a frequent idea of the anxious depressions in the puerperal psychosis is that of the death or injury of the child. This is a particularly painful idea because it is the last thing the mother consciously wishes. The determination of the unconscious wish to destroy the child need not be discussed here ; it is necessary, however, to mention that this unconscious wish is responsible for many symptoms of pregnancy with which there is a ready *somatisches Entgegenkommen.* The patient in this case was a young married woman, six months pregnant. She came to see me late one afternoon, complaining of considerable depression, which she felt was somehow connected with a dream of the night before. She confessed that, although she suspected the association of her mood and the dream, she had not been able to bring herself to think of it. The dream was—omitting unessential details— that there was some trouble on the inside of her left thigh that demanded surgical attention. When asked what the trouble was, she first claimed it was a sore, but then remembered it was a tumor. Associations to " tumor " led almost immediately to the idea of pregnancy—another form of " new growth." When asked for a further description of the tumor, she said there was a pain in it and that the pain was like that she felt in an old appendix scar consequent on the abdominal distention of her pregnancy. When she had said this, the depression instantaneously disappeared and she remarked : " If I had only thought of that pain I would have seen the meaning of the dream immediately ! " It was obviously a thinly disguised wish for an abortion—a wish that had been neither recognised nor completely repressed.

Another example of a depression dream may be cited which is also interesting as a part of a cycle of settings for the same basic idea. The patient is a Swede, aged 39, who had suffered much from an unconscious antagonism to his father, which led to unnecessary rebellion against authority and friction with superiors. It is also necessary to state that he has a fierce antagonism to the paternalistic institutions of the *Vaterland* where he spent a number of years studying, and then practising, engineering. He appeared one day depressed and stated that the one bright spot of the day had been when he had heard one Italian labourer address his companion as " Pig of a German." The dream of the previous night was this : He was in a boat sailing out of the harbour of Stockholm for Finland with three companions of his rather riotous youth. The captain and owner of the boat had been left behind, and some discussion took place as to whether they should proceed or put back for him. The dreamer urged that they keep on their course, and his argument prevailed. In this dream a crime—stealing the boat—is all but directly expressed, and the patient is the chief of the thieves. Analysis revealed that the captain stood for his father, the dream, as a whole, representing his leaving home and using his father's money in activities, largely sexual, of which his father disapproved. The next day he was distinctly elated. He awoke amnesic for his dream, but with a picture in his mind of a painting of a Swedish artist representing two eagles sweeping regally over the surface of the sea. A few associations brought his dream to consciousness. He had been flying the night before in an aeroplane over the Western Front, dropping steel bolts on the German lines. Analysis was not necessary. He recognised at once a sublimation of the wish to destroy his father, now represented by the " Fatherland." The flying of the dream had been transformed into something real on awakening, but the elation of the sublimation had persisted.

So much for case material. One cannot resist the temptation of a little theorising, which, though admittedly speculative, is still perhaps justified by the material.

The sequences described above are not to be observed every day, but this does not mean that they are not regular phenomena. As has been pointed out, we remember the barest fraction of our total dream productions and the tendency to find a setting for the underlying theme which is adaptive to reality is a tentative one which seems to eliminate the unfit settings. This means, of course, an amnesia that follows close upon the constructive process, wiping from memory each stage, each formulation, as it is given up. Not unnaturally, a prime characteristic of this embryology is that it is unknown to introspection.

If we assume, however, that this is a normal and constant process, a number of interesting conclusions may be reached. The first of these is that there is no sharp line dividing sleeping from waking thought. One type is nearer the unconscious, less adaptive to reality, that is all. It is because the dream thought is cruder and more primitive that we choose it for analysis. There is no theoretic reason why we should not analyse waking thoughts instead of dreams. In fact, we are sometimes forced to. I have had two patients who produced almost always nothing but dreams which seemed to be excerpts from their daily lives. They were naturally difficult of analysis, as the distortion and elaboration from the primitive initial thought was so extreme. In fact, the telling analyses were almost entirely those made of occasional nightmares or other unpleasant dreams. If our hypothesis be correct, we have no reason to suppose that there is any conscious thought which has not its root in the unconscious. When this statement is put in another way it may appear less startling. It is undoubtedly true that we can have no thought, no interest, which has not a history back of it. My simplest action is a product of the development of my total personality. If this history be traced back far enough it leads to the period of primitive tendencies where the roots of what are later sex impulses are inextricably intertwined with the roots of other impulses whose conscious fruition is far from sexual. To claim, then, that every dream has a sex basis is equivalent to claiming that every waking thought is similarly determined. This is ridiculous, if by that we mean that there are no other factors ; but, taken in a more liberal sense, that the analysis may demonstrate factors potentially sexual and therefore subjected to the same developmental influences as are plainly sex impulses, in this sense it is reasonable. An example may make this clearer. A chemist may dream of, or actually make researches with, some chemical compound. The analysis of this leads back to the development of his interest in chemistry, which is shown historically to have grown out of a curiosity as to the construction of things, with which is mingled a sex curiosity whose repression resulted, as compromise or compensation, in a stimulus to all other curiosity. The superficial psychologists who reconstruct a dream out of recent experiences are not wrong ; they simply say the house is made of bricks and eliminate the architect and contractor. The question for them to answer is, " Why the interest in these experiences ? "

The next point is : May this hypothesis explain the problem of the mechanism by which a person reaches a solution of some difficulty by sleeping over it ? As we have seen, there is good reason to believe that every conscious thought has unconscious roots; in fact, it is likely that the ideas present in consciousness represent only a few of the many concepts which tend to come up from the limbo of the unconscious—only those which are adaptive to reality in the broadest sense of that term. Now, if such be the case, a man confronted with a problem is, presumably, offered many solutions by his unconscious. Many of these are fantastic and so imaginative that he represses them. In this repression he inhibits himself from imaginative thinking, and so no solution of his difficulty " comes into his mind." Now, if this man goes to sleep, however, his inhibitions are lifted, the unconscious roots of the problem bear fruit in numerous dreams, fantastic, perhaps, and crude, but still good building blocks for practical thoughts. The new idea is warped gradually into a form compatible with reality, and in the morning he wakes with the desired solution in his mind, amnesic probably for any dream.

In this connection there are some phenomena worth mentioning. It is a commonplace that when we first begin to wake we exhibit some symptoms of typical depression—lethargy, lack of initiative and retardation. The reason for this is now clear. At this time we are repressing our crude dreams and elaborating (unconsciously) the themes of these dreams into settings adaptive to reality. When this process is complete we are " awake." This phase in the dream metamorphosis is also responsible for the phenomenon so many of us exhibit, that, unless we get our half hour from 7.30 to 8 (or whatever it may be), we are tired all day. We seem more dependent on being allowed to have even fifteen minutes to wake up in than we do on being given a definite total number of hours of sleep. We must be allowed time to change our dream thoughts to waking thoughts. The first sign of a developing neurosis or psychosis is not infrequently an extension of this period. As we all know, a certain type of invalid makes this waking state last all day. I have had one patient who complained that in the prodromal periods of his mental attacks he would be depressed till noon, unable to apply himself to any work and never sure whether the environment or his dreams were real.

My next claim, is, perhaps, a little more speculative. Dreams are, as we all know, more allied symptomatically to the psychoses than the neuroses. They consist of hallucinations, delusions and abnormal mood reactions. In both unconscious tendencies are the dynamic factors. May there be a clinical parallel? We know that in dementia præcox we get open expression of infantile sex wishes ; in the benign manic-depressive group these tendencies are in evidence, but never with the same directness; here they are " adultified." As in real life the infantile object is represented by a substitute, or, if it be present as such, the outlet does not appear in its crude form. On the other hand, in epilepsy we have a condition that leads to a state where there is no content at all, apparently a regression to a period before ideas of any sort are well developed.

It may be possible that in sleep we reproduce each night these different types of insanity. The depression and elation dreams I have cited are certainly closely analogous to the content of the manic-depressive psychoses. But we know that people do have cruder dreams than these. As far back as Sophocles, there are reports of actual incest dreams. May not these correspond to a dementia præcox level in sleep ? I have had one patient who could distinguish in a vague way different " levels " in his dreams. One which he said was very " deep " was of his mother coming into his bed. Other dreams of the same night which had not this " deep " feeling were adultified versions of the same theme. If we go still deeper, we would come to a level corresponding to epilepsy, where the content is extremely vague and impalpable or where there is no content at all, as in physiological unconsciousness, which may perhaps exist in deepest sleep.* Dreams of this level would be formless, consisting of vague feeling, hard to put into words. A typical example is the dream with which De Quincy closes his *Confessions.* It consists almost entirely of metaphors, word pictures, not real incidents. Its content (if we judge by the metaphor and the free associations which follow) is a birth experience. From this standpoint, we could describe the metamorphosis of the mentation in sleep as proceeding from waking thoughts, to fantasy allied to reality, to a manic-depressive phase, then a dementia præcox level and finally an epileptic stage. On waking the reverse process would take place. It is possible that the physiological repair goes on only in the epileptic period, although great mental relief may be obtained from a brief flight into fantasy such as takes place in a light nap. This, however, pending rigorous investigation, is mere conjecture.

From all that has been said, it is obvious that mental health is secured by a completion of this development before waking. To employ the obstetric parallel, the fœtus must come to full term. Our final problem is, what may produce an abortion ? A complete answer would, of course, be equivalent to a final settlement of all psychopathological problems, which is an absurd demand. Never-

* The mere fact that experiments of waking people at different times have always revealed a dream is no proof of dreams being constantly present. That a dream can be manufactured instantaneously is notorious. (I have known one case where a man fell asleep between two words in a sentence and had a long dream, although his hearer noted no pause.) Now, if a person comes to life out of a deep sleep, that waking process involves some time, long enough for some dream thoughts to be elaborated. In fact, it is hard to imagine an absolutely instantaneous orientation, and, if we admit any delay in these perceptions, we have admitted the conditions necessary for the fabrication of a dream.

theless, a formulation may be given which relates this problem to others.   All psychotic and psychoneurotic conditions are dependent on a lack of balance between the regressive and progressive forces.   The same cause which forces regression would undoubtedly prevent elaboration of a dream thought from a crude to an adaptive setting.   But there are in this case specific disturbing influences as well.   I refer to waking stimuli.   These have received large attention from non-psychoanalytic investigators, but have been deemed less important by psychoanalysts with good reason. Jones has given the excellent formulation that, when a dream bears an obvious relationship to the waking stimulus, the latter operates as does the day-dream experience in providing a setting for a latent theme.   With this I agree heartily.   In the light of " dream metamorphosis," however, one may see a wider importance to this factor than has been granted it.   If waking is accomplished before the development of the idea is complete, the subject faces the world with non-adaptive thoughts—which always cause trouble. Moreover, as the setting of the dream corresponds to the stimulus, development is apt to proceed to that point and no further.   For example, a painful stimulus may inhibit development further than a painful setting for the dream thought.   The ethical censorship may be satisfied, but a comfortable, " normal " setting has not yet been reached.   It may be this mechanism which accounts for a great difference between the dreams of men and women. The former frequently remember frank unvarnished sex experiences in their sleep, the latter rarely do.   In the light of this theory, a satisfactory explanation can be given.   The male genitalia react to sex thoughts by erections and emissions which cause much more physical disturbance than do any analogous reactions of the female.   In other words, the erection or emission of the male wakes him up while the dream thoughts are still at a crude sex level of development.   It is astonishing to find how " præcox " so many emission dreams are, when note is taken of them ; they are not merely sexual, but infantile sexual.   In quite a similar way we can explain the nightmare after the proverbial Welsh rarebit. The gastric distress wakes the subject and provides a painful setting for an imperfectly elaborated dream thought.

To sum up : There is evidence to show that our dream life shows not only regression but progression.   That there is a tendency for crude ideas to be completely metamorphosed—as far as the manifest content is concerned—until a point is reached where a thought is present in the subject's consciousness that is fully adaptive to his diurnal life.   At this point the individual is awake.   The sequence of settings for expression of the latent content is analogous to the types of ideas seen in different types of psychoses.   Mental health is dependent on the continuity and completeness of this process. If, to use the obstetric parallel, the thought is born before coming to full term, the abortion disturbs the subject and produces an abnormal mood during the day, at least until it can be repressed and a new formulation found.   In this way the waking period is the crux of the whole day ; if it be disturbed, the psychic processes proper to that time are carried on through the day with disastrous results.   In our sleep the strain of adaptation is relieved and we regress to the primitive type and content of infantile thinking, but if we are to be normal and efficient this process must be reversed, we must have developed an adult type and content of thought before fully waking to face the world.

CONFLICT AND ADJUSTMENT IN ART

BY

HERBERT SIDNEY LANGFELD, Ph.D.

*Professor of Psychology and Director of the Psychological
Laboratory, Princeton University*

CONFLICT AND ADJUSTMENT IN ART

BY

HERBERT SIDNEY LANGFELD

ALTHOUGH there is much divergence of opinion and confusion about the nature and purpose of art, æstheticians have always agreed that art is sought for its own sake. This opinion is so universally held that it has become a platitude. We find it appearing in various forms, such as " Art is self-contained." " It is without any purpose beyond itself." " It is detached from the practical world of affairs and holds a uniquely isolated position." " The artist works without any idea of use or gain and we behold the results in a state of entire disinterestedness." One or more of these phrases may be found in almost any treatise on beauty. At first glance their truth seems obvious and yet they contain a paradox which demands a solution.

It is beyond dispute that art is considered to be one of the most valuable of human possessions. It has been desired and fostered in one or more of its forms by races in almost every stage of cultural development. No matter how indifferent a nation may be to ethical values, it will cherish its art treasures. They are a possession of rich and poor alike ; even a criminal will pause to listen to a song. A drive as universal and persistent as that which induces artistic production and appreciation leads us to conclude not only that it is a fundamental factor of human behaviour, but that it plays an important rôle in the struggle of the organism to overcome the difficulties with which it is constantly confronted by the ever-changing conditions of its environment. Art then, although in a narrow and specific sense falling under the category of the non-practical, becomes through a wider and more generalised view of its functions intrinsically practical. The purpose of artistic activity extends beyond the creation of beauty merely for its own sake, even though we may admit and perhaps demand that the artist, *qua* artist, should be unconscious of this wider purpose. In like manner we must interpret the terms " disinterestedness " and " detachment," which only vaguely describe an attitude intrinsic to the appreciation of art.

It is my aim in this paper, therefore, to seek the ultimate function of art. I shall attempt to describe the nature of the drive which results in art and to show that artistic activity both in the sense of creation and appreciation plays a fundamental and, therefore, invaluable part in the adequate adjustment of the human organism. I am aware that there are many persons who think of the purpose of art in terms of the ideals and sentiments which objects of beauty inspire and of the so-called spiritual harmony which results from æsthetic contemplation. No one can well deny the value of such an approach, but ideals and sentiments must lead to action, and spiritual harmony, if it means more than a mere emotional state, must indicate a unification of impulses. We thus come in the last analysis to human behaviour and it is on this level that we must conduct the inquiry in order to discover the fundamental facts.

If we start with the phylogenetic origin of the art impulse, we find many theories at hand. They embrace sex attraction with the related impulse of self-display, self-exhibition and the desire to attract by pleasing, imitation, play, self-defence, utility, and the like. These theories are too well known to require further description. Undoubtedly there is some truth in all of them, in that they enumerate factors or describe situations which contribute to the development of art in general or one or more of its forms in particular.

A treatise which deals more specifically with the development of the form in art, especially that of the drama, than with the origin of the impulse, but which contains implicitly a hint of the nature of the latter, is the exposition by J. E. Harrison in *Ancient Art and Ritual*. She shows that the origin of primitive ritual is to be found in the seasonal rites connected with the harvest and she, therefore, correctly concludes that the drive underlying this more or less formal activity is hunger or at least the desire for food. The ritual always had a practical end. It was an integral part of the life of the people, and even when it developed by gradual stages into the Greek drama or appeared in static form in sculpture, it still reflected the original human motive that gave it birth. Whether ritual is the only source of art is difficult to decide. Harrison herself avoids a dogmatic assertion ; " . . . ritual is, we believe, a *frequent* and *perhaps* universal transition stage between actual life and that peculiar contemplation of or emotion toward life which we call art."* What seems to me to be one of the most important contributions to this theory is the emphasis upon

* Jane E. Harrison, *Ancient Art and Ritual*, p. 205. (Italics are mine.)

human longings and needs. As Miss Harrison has expressed it, " All our long examination of beast-dances, May-day festivals, and even of Greek drama has had just this for its object—to make clear that art, save perhaps in a few especially gifted natures, did not arise straight out of life, but out of that collective emphasis of the needs and desires of life which we have agreed to call *ritual*.* That these needs and desires are related primarily to food-getting makes the theory none the less plausible.   In fact, it is very refreshing, for there has been so much importance given to the sex drive during the last decade that it has become for some psychologists the only source of action.   One sees, of course, how the Freudians can reduce in some fantastic manner the food-drive ultimately to sex as they have every other action, but such simplification by the breaking down of essential differences obscures rather than clarifies the issue.†   No one would deny that the various drives, as we find them in actual experience, differ in essential qualities and that they must all be taken into account in explaining the details of the structure of mankind.   Whether any one drive is fundamental to the rest, and which it is, seems irrelevant to our present problem.

It is the longing, the vaguely defined seeking and restlessness common to all drives that is the starting point of our discussion. Such inner states are indicative of a wish or desire which is unsatisfied because of an inner conflict that must be resolved, or, as in the case of food, an external deficiency that must be overcome by new adjustments.   They are accompanied by the feeling of unpleasantness or pain, which persists until satisfaction is obtained. It is this restless, unsatisfied state of the organism which forms the basis of action and the drive towards increasing synthesis of impulses and therefore of progress.   As has been frequently pointed out by psychologists, the condition of the organism which is accompanied by pleasure is one of tranquillity.   Only restlessness with its uncomfortable feeling tone produces change.   Nor is it the idea of future pain any more than future happiness that is the driving and guiding force of our actions,‡ but the present discomfort which we may speak of as a state of dissatisfaction.   An illustration of the frequent mistake of confusing cause and effect may be taken

* Jane E. Harrison, *Ancient Art and Ritual*, pp. 205–6.
† It is interesting to note in this connection that in one of the most recent and authoritative entomological studies it has been shown how the hunger drive is the determining factor in the social organisation of insects.   *Social Life among the Insects*, by W. M. Wheeler.
‡ See W. McDougall, *Outline of Psychology*, p. 188.

from Gregor Paulsson's otherwise admirable treatise on " The Creative Elements in Art." " Joy," he writes, " is the origin of play," and he further explains that " the aim of joy is simply to preserve an unchanged relation to an object,"* and when the child experiences an opposite emotion he ceases to play. I would say rather that when the child finds the play adequate for a synthesis of his present impulses he will continue to play and that he will cease as soon as a change occurs that is in conflict with his determining set. The joy which he will probably feel during the play period is a conscious indication of successful adjustment. When this adjustment alters, he will experience discomfort or some other unpleasant emotion such as anger or fear, and on account of the maladjustment, and not because of the unpleasantness, he will either turn from play to some other situation to which he will be better able to adjust himself, or he will alter the form of the play to suit the present requirements of his organism.

We have in this revised interpretation, it seems to me, a description of the essential mechanism of behaviour, which always begins with the random restless movements of the infant resulting in better co-ordination and which continues through the long series of habits forming the more or less successful development of the individual. The environment presents an infinite number of situations to which the individual may become adjusted. The difficulty of the adjustment obviously depends both upon the degree of integration which the individual organism possesses at the time and upon the complexity of the situation. Any new situation to which the individual is not yet adjusted will cause a conflict of impulses which will be experienced as more or less unpleasant. These new situations have a tendency to be avoided by many individuals and thus arises that conservatism which is a barrier to progress. There are persons—one suspects that they form a large part of the world's population—who are satisfied with the minimum amount of co-ordination necessary to live contentedly in the small bit of the environment in which at an early age they have found themselves. Their action patterns are soon fixed and they become almost as stereotyped as a series of phonograph records. Either they remain safely in their circumscribed world or, if they choose rather to wander afield, they frequently meet with disaster, in which case they are apt to refer to their " bad luck." Persons with a greater amount of nervous energy are constantly seeking new situations to which their impulses must

* *Scandinavian Scientific Review*, 1923, Vol. II, p. 19.

conform.   They are the type of the scientist, the discoverer of new relations.   I use the term " scientist " here in the broad sense of having the characteristic dispositional pattern, although the persons so described may never figure as scientific to their companions, inasmuch as they may seldom put their experiences into communicable form.   They are well organised to respond to the complex situation of reality and their emotional life finds an easy outlet in conventional behaviour.   The conflict of their ideas is resolved in either chance experience or systematic observation and experimentation, and their imagination is accompanied by the constant hope of eventual verifications.   Finally there is the individual who finds reality as he experiences it inadequate.   His conflicts seldom find complete relief in ordinary experiences and his imagination, therefore, shapes life not always perhaps as he would wish it, but at least as he finds it must be shaped if it is to offer a satisfactory means for his own inner adjustment.*

This last type is that of the artist.   It is also the same type that we recognise in the young child at play.   Whether, however, the play attitude is the origin of the art impulse seems to me a purely academic question.   The form of play may surely be viewed at times as one views a work of art, and wherever we draw the line between art and play the decision remains an arbitrary one. Both attitudes, that of the artist and of the child, have essential points in common—a conflict and a resolution in a situation of their own making.   All children, we may well say, are artists. The demands of the world, however, will not allow them all to remain artists.

We may see the close relation of play to art in Paulsson's description of experiments which he made upon the progress of drawing in young children.†   He has shown how the child's earliest scribbling in the form of random movements, which one might be inclined to call play, soon goes over into a form so definite that the child will repeat it and seem to take refuge in it as an agreeable co-ordination at intervals in its random scribbling. The result is an embryonic bit of art, indicative of a well-organised series of movements which, through lack of strength and experience, the child probably could not have attained in the manipula-

* The above types are, of course, abstractions.   The scientist can be and often is an artist, and as to the first type even the most satisfied and least imaginative individual has some small trace of the artist in him.   Nor do I intend the description to cover all existing types.   There are obviously many transitional stages.

† *Scandinavian Scientific Review*, pp. 36 ff.

tion of more cumbersome material. It might be asked why the child could not as well have swung its pencil or merely moved its hand about in some co-ordinated way. In the first place the random scratches on the paper were helpful visual clues for the formation of the unified figure and, secondly, the completed form was on record, so that the child's interest was more likely to be revived than it would have been if the child had merely waved its pencil in the air. Permanency, while theoretically perhaps not an essential characteristic of art, has been as practical a necessity for its development as language has been for thought.

The attribute of permanency is also essential for that social quality which so many writers on æsthetics have rightly insisted belongs to art and which most likely distinguishes it from play. As Hirn has stated : "The work of art presents itself as the most effective means by which the individual is enabled to convey to wider and wider circles of sympathisers an emotional state similar to that by which he is himself dominated."* The point that I desire to make clear, however, is that the communication of emotional states as such is not the important function of art any more than is the communication of ideas. It is not the social quality that has made the function of art one of the most valuable assets of the race, but rather the characteristic of unification which indicates that the artist through the medium of his art has been able at least in part to integrate his own impulses into an effective form of behaviour. It has not only been possible for him " to express his inner life in outer form," but also to give balance and proportion to his ideas and emotions and thus to overcome his inhibitions to a degree which he has probably found impossible in the practical situations of his life. As the form is permanent, he has the opportunity of returning to his former experience at will. He thereby also offers to his fellow-men a means by which they, too, may find relief in conflicting motives and forms of action and in addition may learn more varied and more highly organised habits of response. It is in this aspect of art that we find its social rôle. To the extent to which the artist has been successful in his own integration will his works be considered beautiful ; to that extent also will he give pleasure and satisfaction to others. And the more the conflicts of the artist resemble those which are common to the race, the greater will be the influence of his works and the wider will be their appeal. Individualism in art is necessary in so far as the artist must express the answer to his own inner problems.

* *The Origins of Art*, p. 85.

The roots of his motives must be in his own personality and not in the convention of a " school," but these motives must have a functional meaning beyond himself if his art is to live.

In order to explain the relation of art to action patterns of the nervous system and more especially the function of art to the organisation of these patterns one must assume the theory of dynamogenesis, which in its most general form may be said to imply that all afferent nerve impulses and, therefore, all ideas eventually find an outlet through the efferent system to striped and smooth muscles. The action may either be overt or implicit. In either case every new sensory pattern is the cause of a new synthesis of motor paths. What particular motor paths are stimulated depends upon the state of the organism at the time. There is not necessarily any one-to-one correspondence between stimulus and response. The visual perception of a wavy line, for example, need not be followed by eye-movements and if it is, these movements cannot possibly be identical in form with that of a wavy line, for it is well known that the eye can only move in the form of jerks.* It may quite well be that the visual perception will go over into weak efferent impulses toward the limbs or some other part of the body. It is also possible that there will be an effect on glandular secretions, which in turn will intensify the response of striped muscles.†

When the motion, either implicit or explicit, becomes identified with the objects of perception and imagination, we are accustomed to speak of empathy. I realise that this is a revision of the theory as formulated by Lipps, inasmuch as he denied motor response and remained in his description on a purely " mental " level, but I believe it is the form in which the theory is at the present time generally understood, if it is accepted at all. This projection of our own experience forms the basis of our apprehension and appreciation of beauty. Empathy, however, is not a *sine qua non* of our adaptive processes. When the sculptor, for example, is in the act

* Bullough is one of the latest writers to use this ancient argument in regard to the restricted movements of the eyes in order to discredit a " functional theory " of art. He makes the assertion that " the same fate [definite disposition of the eye-movement theory] may be anticipated for various other theories which make the easy functioning of muscular or organic action in the apprehension of beautiful objects the basis of æsthetic values." (" Recent Work in Experimental Æsthetics," *British Journal of Psychology*, 1921, Vol. XII, p. 91.) It is evident that this is a personally biased prophecy as yet unwarranted by the facts.

† With the *Gestalt* theory as represented principally by Koehler, Koffka and Wertheimer in mind, it should further be stated that the integrated impulses are in themselves a form of structure at what Koehler would name the psychophysiological level.

of modelling, there may be no projection of his impulses into the object, nor can we rightly speak of projection and, therefore, of empathy when the painter is conscious of the brush stroke. In other words, when we are conscious of our movements as such there is no empathy. Further, when I stated that empathy is the basis of the apprehension of beauty I did not mean to imply that it is a factor of the æsthetic appreciation which distinguishes that appreciation from our other activities, since it is obvious that empathy occurs in many situations that could in no way be termed æsthetic.*

I have given this brief sketch of the nature of responses as an explanation of the possible mechanism by which the inner conflicts of the individual find expression, although I am aware that those persons who consistently avoid behaviouristic terms will prefer to remain on the mental level of ideas and motives and of meaning as a content of consciousness. Irrespective, however, of the terminology in which it may be expressed, most persons will probably accept the theory of conflict and release through art, which is generally traced to Aristotle's doctrine of *katharsis*. The interpretation of this famous theory has been a subject of historic discussion and the meaning of the original statement is prone to be coloured by the psychological knowledge of the interpreter, so that to-day one usually understands it to imply a freeing or purging of the individual from unpleasant emotions through his reaction to tragedy. The question naturally arises whether the mere expression of emotions will purge the individual of them, unless the underlying cause is removed ; that is to say, whether the expression of emotion for emotion's sake, as we find it, for example, among the frequenters of motion-picture performances, is of any particular benefit ; whether, in fact, such expression is not rather more harmful than beneficial, even when it is aroused by the unreal situations of a tragedy. Certainly we get no intimation from Aristotle that

---

* I have attempted to explain in *The Æsthetic Attitude* what I believe to be the distinguishing feature of our reaction towards objects which we call beautiful and ugly. As it is the purpose of this paper to describe the function of art and not the nature of beauty, I may refer the reader to Chap. III, especially pp. 59 *ff.* of that book. In Chap. V, I have tried to define the term " empathy " as it seemed to me it should be employed, since there is an unfortunate tendency to use the term to denote any situation which has the characteristic of inner mimicry, irrespective of whether there is present the element of projection or identification of the subjective state with the external object. For instance, Southard's " empathic index " is frequently taken to mean that mechanism by which we judge another person on the basis of an imitation of his behaviour. Our own state will under such circumstances be one of introjection rather than projection and it is therefore hardly correct—in fact, it is misleading—to call it empathic.

internal conflicts are reconciled by means of the technique of tragedy, nor is there any hint as to their rôles in art production.

Freud and his followers have most clearly emphasised the fundamental importance of conflict in the genesis of art, although they have not given much attention to the technique and practice of art itself in its relation to the resolution of the conflict.   One may not always desire to follow them in their insistent search for a sex motive—we have previously referred to the fact that there are other fundamental drives such as the food drive—yet one can agree with them that art, which is not merely the imitation of an established form, does not spring " from a tranquil soul." The lives of the great artists have given us sufficient examples of a nature at war with itself to make the theory an almost obvious fact.

A number of analyses of artistic production which have been made by Freud, Jones, Abraham and others, although not always convincing in all their details, are extremely suggestive in that they indicate the intrinsic function of conflict in the construction of well-known works of art.   The article by Ernest Jones on Andrea del Sarto is particularly illuminating in that it shows that Andrea's art never reached the highest perfection, because circumstances prevented his expressing his innermost conflicts in his work.   As Jones has stated it, " How could Andrea sink himself into his art (flight into work) when there was Lucrezia in the body with him at every moment ? " and further on " .   .   .   she forced the internal battle, which is necessary for all artistic creation, to be fought out in the current details of everyday life,* and so allowed him no opportunity to gather strength and inspiration that could be applied to higher aims."†   With sufficient freedom from his wife's influence he would have gained complete freedom for himself in his art and the world might have had greater masterpieces from his brush.

Where I should disagree with the Freudians is in their belief that conflicts must always have their origin in unconscious repressions and that the artist is unaware of their real nature.   Not that inspiration does not spring from the unconscious.   Such a state-

* But was never completely resolved in his everyday life any more than in his art.

† " The Influence of Andrea del Sarto's Wife on his Art," *Essays in Applied Psychoanalysis,* p. 242.   The following is a characteristic reference to conflict in its relation to art, such as one finds in the Freudian literature : " It is also possible, at any rate in many cases, to show how these images [in poetry] are symbolic expressions of some conflict which is raging in the mind of the poet."—*Conflict and Dream,* by W. H. R. Rivers, p. 148.

ment would contradict the obviously intuitive nature of that state,
nor can it be denied that the artist is frequently a dual personality.
His characters often seem to play their parts in what Morton Prince
terms the co-conscious, in seeming independence of the control of
foveal consciousness, as the statements of such writers as Steven-
son, Hearn, and Barrie bear witness, but the meaning of the
artist's restlessness and urge towards expression may at times be
completely known to himself.   We have a typical instance of this
self-knowledge in the life of St. John Ervine : " The starting-
point for *The Magnanimous Lover* was the abrupt souring of his
own narrow and bigoted Protestantism within him.   The fierce
intolerance of his native city, Belfast, against Roman Catholics
infected him as a child.   One day he awoke and shook off the
incubus of Presbyterian self-righteousness.   A sudden revulsion
of feeling ensued.   Repressive hatred cried out for some adequate
redress or conversion into expansive liberation from prejudice.
The shock of self-recognition, as is customary in such cases, fought
for an outlet and in Ervine's experience it took the form of a one-
act play whose sole object, in his own words, was ' to hit that
prejudice and hit it hard.' "*   There seems no necessity in this
instance to seek further by means of the psychoanalytical method
for any deeper motives.

As has been previously stated, man is not freed from his conflicting impulses, whether conscious or unconscious, merely by giving
them voice. This is only the first step to which must be added
some form of reconciliation and resolution.   Generally he is able
to make an adjustment to life directly either through his own
efforts or those of a physician.   If his impulses are too much at
variance with life as he finds it, he resorts to the intermediate stage
of fantasy, which may at times have the strength of hallucination,
but as such imagery is of a transitory nature and not necessarily
well integrated, it may not be permanently satisfying.   If the
individual has artistic talent, he has the means at hand of adjusting
his conflicts in the permanent form of his art.   He finds a certain
peace in the balance of lines, colours and tones and in the resolution of opposing motives.   This balance is the essence of beauty.
And, further, by giving to the world the solution of his problems he
presents a situation in which his fellow-men may find a similar
adjustment and become more capable because of the better integration of their own actions.

* " St John Ervine's Method," by Pierre Loving, *The Drama*, January,
1921.

The objection may be made that, if the function of art is to offer a way for adjustment which cannot otherwise be made, why is it that artists are so often unhappy and discontented? In the first place it must be remembered that an artist is a man of unusually intense and conflicting motives. His art is, therefore, at times inadequate for the relief of all of his inhibitory tendencies. He is not maladjusted or abnormal as some would say, because he is an artist, but he is an artist because of his maladjustments. The fact that he is " awkward " and " out of place " in real life, is the reason for his living as much as possible in a world of his own creation. That this world is not always large enough for him is due either to his own limitations of creativeness or to objective circumstances as in the case of Andrea del Sarto. Secondly, a work of art may not always be a permanent release even for those conflicts which were the cause of its inception. And, finally, art cannot be, except in very rare natures, a complete substitute for life. The function of art is not to displace life, but to supplement it. Art can only have a meaning beyond itself if we return from our excursion into the realm of fantasy better equipped to meet the prosaic currents of existence.

PRINCE'S "NEUROGRAM" CONCEPT
ITS HISTORICAL POSITION

BY

LYDIARD H. HORTON

PRINCE'S "NEUROGRAM" CONCEPT*
ITS HISTORICAL POSITION

BY

LYDIARD H. HORTON

SOME YEARS before the publication of "The Unconscious" (1914) by Morton Prince, I had occasion to attend, very sedulously, a certain seminar at one of our large universities, at the conference table of which Memory and the Association of Ideas was the topic of study. We gave due credit to Ebbinghaus and ran the gamut of his nonsense syllables and paid our respects to all the great authors who have dealt with the subject of How We Think, albeit most of them have agitated it at a distance, as it were, with a ten-foot pole.

Toward the end of the sessions, the professor in charge of the seminar made a summing up. With his usual detachment and perspicacity and clarity, he reviewed all that had impressed us as outstanding conceptions of the mental associating machine. In deliberate fashion, and fumbling somewhat for the right words, he averred that a great deal of work remained to be done; that it was not altogether clear how far the conceptions he had reviewed were really final or could be regarded as representing the essence of the thinking process. He weaved back and forth a good deal in an endeavor not to underestimate the contributions of the various schools we had discussed.

Finally, realizing his scientific humility and his fear of approach-

*"Whatever may be the exact nature of the theoretical alterations left in the brain by life's experiences they have received various generic terms; more commonly 'brain residua,' and 'brain dispositions.' I have been in the habit of using the term *neurograms* to characterize these brain records. Just as telegram, Marconigram, and phonogram precisely characterize the form in which the physical phenomena which correspond to our (verbally or scripturally expressed) thoughts, are recorded and conserved, so neurogram precisely characterizes my conception of the form in which a system of brain processes corresponding to thoughts and other mental experiences is recorded and conserved." ("The Unconscious" page 131.)

CC

ing anything like scientific arrogance, I ventured to risk, on my own account, a distinct violation of the scientific amenities:

"Professor," I said, "is it not a fair statement, seeing all that we have been through together at this table, to say that, to all intents and purposes, the knowledge of the mechanism of Memory amounts practically to nothing at the present time—that we really have not got anywhere?"

This remark did not shock him as I had feared; it seemed to fit into the current of his thoughts, for it hardly disturbed the semi-revery into which his effort to take a wide view of our subject had plunged him.

"Well—yes," he began, as if with reluctance, but then with apparent relief, he went on meditatively to agree that the statement was, on the whole, a fair one.

Naturally, in this seminar, there was no question of emphasizing the three-sided aspect of Memory as *registration, conservation*, and *reproduction* of experiential records. For this would have been adopting *de parti pris* the angles of approach that are characteristic of the Principian psychology, with its trenchant subordination of *recognition* as only a more perfect kind of reproduction with consciousness. Yet it was not long before the professor in charge became attracted to the theory of neurographic records by the publication of Prince's lecture-course on "The Unconscious."* But this did not stimulate the professor to revise his mode of presenting "association" to his classes; rather, it aroused in him an unexpected interest in the formulation of the Coconscious. Because this feature of the book became a sort of entering wedge in a mind thoroughly versed in all the other kinds of discussions relating to the association of ideas, it is worth while here to quote some relevant passages.

Concerning the Conservation of Memories

Although not touching the essential feature of the neurographic theory, the following shows Prince's mode of approach toward the general problem of memory.

"It is hypothetically possible that our thoughts and other mental experiences after they have passed out of mind, out of our awareness of the moment, may continue their psychological existence as such although we are not aware of them. Such an hypothesis derives support from the fact that researches of recent years in abnormal psychology

---

* These were delivered 1908–10, one of the earliest courses in Abnormal Psychology. Published by MacMillan, 1914; enlarged edition 1923.

have given convincing evidence that an idea, under certain conditions, after it has passed out of our awareness, may still from time to time take on another sort of existence, one in which it still remains an idea, although our personal consciousness of the moment is not aware of it. *A coconscious idea, it may be called."* (*"Conservation considered as psychological residua," "The Unconscious," page 110.*)

However interesting the developing of the Coconscious may be, and whatever may be the acceptance that it is finding, it is important here only as leading up to the conception of the nature of the conservation of ideas. It brings into view that parting of the ways between the extreme behaviorist who takes the somato-centric view that modifiability of thought and action are *merely reflex* and the other extremist, who falls in with the psycho-centric doctrine of the Subliminal Mind of F. W. H. Myers. The distinction is important; it is relevant to the fact that Prince affirms an intermediate position He says:

"So far then as coconscious ideas can be discovered by our methods of investigation, they are inadequate to account for the whole of the conservation of Life's experiences." (*The Unconscious," page 112.*)

In other words, we have to pass on to the physiological forms of "conservation." Prince regards as unthinkable the hypothesis (implied by Myers) that *"The great mass of mental experiences of our lives which we have at our command . . . from which we consciously borrow from time to time, would still have persisting conscious existence in their* original concrete psychological form."

"Such an hypothesis, to my mind, is hardly thinkable . . . " (*"The Unconscious," page 114.*)

In this way, Prince indicates his independence of those theories of the subconscious mind which teach the doctrine that our personal consciousness is but a small portion of the sum total of our actual consciousness; and that personal consciousness is but a *"sort of uprushes from this great sum of conscious states which have been called the subliminal mind, the subliminal self, the subconscious self."* (*"The Unconscious," page 115.*)

Here, at once, we have the Principian independence and divergence from certain prevalent views that lean toward what I may call the grab-bag theory of memory and recall. Prince says:

"The facts to be explained do not require such a metaphysical hypothesis. All that is required is that our continuously occurring experiences should be conserved in a form, and by an arrangement, which will allow the concrete ideas belonging to them to reappear in consciousness whenever the conserved arrangement is again stimulated."

This requirement, Prince points out, is fully met by the theory of "conservation" (of physiological dispositions) which harmonizes particularly with psycho-physiological studies. ("The Unconscious," page 115).

"We have . . . in the concept of brain residual neurograms the fundamental meaning of the Unconscious *. . . the great storehouse of neurograms which are the physiological records of our mental lives. ("The Unconscious," page 149.)*

Neurographic Records as Archives of Consciousness

Prince develops the concept of the neurogram as contrasting with alleged *psychological*—i. e., non-physical—dispositions. Here we reach a field of vagueness in which, ostensibly, Freud and Jung have made their habitat, assuming on their part a standpoint which fits with what I have called the grab-bag theory of Mind; in this view almost any sort of mental mechanism may be looked for without much reference to any concrete physiological form of conservation. Prince, accordingly, would like to know whether Freud or Jung view the unconscious as psychological or as physiological.

Prince's position in the matter is much clearer, although he avoids exaggerated definiteness, in view of our lack of knowledge, as shown below:

"In other words, without binding ourselves down to absolute precision of language, it is sufficiently accurate to say that every mental experience leaves behind a residue, or a trace, of the physical brain process in the chain of brain neurons. This residue is the physical register *of the mental experience.* This physical register may be conserved or not. *If it is conserved, we have the requisite condition of memory; the* form *in which our mental experiences are conserved. But it is not until these physical registers are stimulated and the original brain experience is reproduced that we have memory. If this occurs, the reproduction of the brain experience reproduces the conscious experience,—i. e., conscious memory (according to whatever theory of parallelism is maintained). Thus in all ideation, in every process of thought, the record of the conscious stream may be registered and conserved in the correlated neural process. Consequently, the neurons in retaining residua of the original process become, to a greater or less degree,* organized into a functioning system *corresponding to the system of ideas of the original mental process and capable of reproducing it. When we reproduce the original ideas in the*

*form of memories it is because there is a reproduction of the physio-
logical neural process."* (*"The Unconscious,"* page *120.*)

In contrast to the trend of Behaviorism, it is characteristic of
Prince's development of the neurographic concept that it does not
militate against his interest in such features of Memory as
may be ascribed to "psychic stuff." That is, I see in Prince's
message no warrant for the view that his insistence upon the
definiteness of neurograms is, in any way, of the old style icono-
clastic and materialistic type which aims at excluding the concept
of "psychic stuff" or at bolstering such pleas as "thought is a secretion of the brain!" In last analysis, he says, everything can be
reduced to psychic forces as the actuality of the physical forces.

Futility of Psychology without Neurology

Prince's unfolding of the neurographic picture expresses his own
intensive clinical familiarity with the detailed and copious manner
in which specific memories are conserved. His application of the
neurogram concept permits him to move at ease through a gamut
of mental phenomena that is scarcely touched in the laboratory-
man's approach to the problem of Memory. At the same time, he
makes us comprehend the immensity of physical detail involved in
the conservation of any single experience. For both range and detail
have to be dealt with in any effective study of human personality.
Therefore, he conceives something very much more definitely
brain-traced than the alleged "faculties" of the soul, or than anything else contemplated by the ordinary workers in the field of
Association. For, until recently, psychologists were mainly concerned with refining their observations within the limited range of
mental phenomena originally made noteworthy by Aristotle, but
coupled by him with suggestions leading away from physical
correlations. To be sure, we may honor Aristotle, the reputed
father of Association, as having been a great thinker of antiquity
and a contributor to psychology, but we should not forget his
inevitable ignorance of the natural history of the organism — only
lately revealed by modern biology. Accordingly, it is a fact that the
Aristotelian tradition has been, and still is in many quarters, a
wet-blanket on practical studies of the mental life, in spite of
Cardinal Mercier's attempt to liberalize it.[1]

"In most universities today," exclaims Prince, *"Psychology is
classed as a department of Philosophy! How long is this attitude to
be continued?"* (*Footnote, "The Unconscious,"* page *530.*)

[1]Mercier, "Les Origines de la Psychologie Contemporaine."

In many seminars, problems of body and mind are being discussed seriously and earnestly with entire forgetfulness of the fact that thinking is in a large part of its course an operation of nerve filaments acting as specifically in their way as telephone wires, instrumenting or mediating long-distance telephone conversations, but much more intricately. We owe a debt to Morton Prince as a writer on extensive problems of psycho-pathology in that he has never lost sight of these mechanistic bases of memory and that he has always written into his papers safe reservations against the day when the neuro-mechanism of thought should become experimentally more manifest. May we not dismiss the semblance of a materialistic trend arising from some of his work, and think of him as exclaiming with Emerson:

"I believe in the material world as the expression of the Spiritual or the Real; and in the impenetrable mystery which hides the mental nature (and hides through absolute transparency), I await the insight which our advancing knowledge of material laws shall furnish." (From *Natural History of Intellect*.)

The knowledge of material laws necessary to comprehend the mental machine was scarcely dawning when Emerson wrote. But the progress of the last hundred years has opened our eyes to the ethereal structure of matter, thus cutting the ground from under the feet of Nineteenth Century materialism.

It is not, however, my intention to suggest that writers like Aristotle, DesCartes and Hobbes, did not, considering their times, take a remarkably vivid interest in reaching precision about the material side of the mind's working. What concerns us is the fact that most of them did not get far with it and that, until very recently, philosophers and psychologists were content to follow rather unclear scholastic and *a priori* reasoning on mental association.

Crude Mechanistic Views of Earlier Ages

Take Hobbes, for instance; he veered strongly to the calculating machine view. Association was nothing but a system of accounts:

"When a man 'reasoneth,' he does nothing else but conceive a sum total, from 'addition' of parcels; or conceive a remainder from 'subtraction' of one sum from another; which, if it be done by words, is conceiving of the consequence of the names of all the parts, to the name of the whole; or from the names of the whole and one part, to the name of the other part. And though in some things, as in numbers, besides adding and subtracting, men name other operations, as 'multiplying' and 'dividing,' yet they are the same; for multiplication is but adding together of things equal; and division but subtracting of one thing, as often as we can. These operations are not incident to numbers only, but to all manner of things that can be added together, and taken one out of another."

This is interesting even if hopelessly schematic; it was useful because it was a scientifically-minded effort to take the mystery out of the working of the machinery of the mind.

While we are dwelling on the history of the topic, it would be unfair not to note how early the striving for mechanism made itself felt. Aristotle is strikingly mechanistic in certain passages of *De Motu Animalium:* —

"When beings endeavor to do something. . . . The case is exactly like that of automata, which are started by the slightest movement as soon as the springs are let go, because the springs can proceed to act the one upon the other; for example, the little chariot which moves by itself. At first you push it in a straight line; thereupon its movement becomes circular, because of its wheels being unequal, and that the smaller wheel on one side acts as a pivot, as we see in cylinders. It is absolutely thus that animals do move. The instruments of this motion are, both the apparatus of the *neurons* [muscles and tendons] and that of the bones. The bones are in some way the timber and the iron of the automata; the *neurons* are like the springs which, once released, stretch themselves and move the machine.

"At the same time, in the automata and in these little chariots, there is no internal modification. . . . In the animal, on the contrary, the form can change, when the different parts expand under the influence of heat or shrink later under the influence of cold; and also, when they suffer from internal alteration. These alterations can be caused by the imagination, by sensation and by thought. That is, the sensations are indeed a sort of alteration that one experiences directly. As to imagination and active thought, they have the same power that objects possess. For example, the *species*—the idea—of heat and of cold, of pleasure or of pain which is formed in thought, is approximately what is each of these things. It is enough to think of certain things to be chilled or to tremble with fear."[2]

This hodge-podge of mechanism, idealism and physiology may sound very much out-of-date, but on the whole it represents the

[2] Translated from Barthélemy St. Hilaire's version of "Des Mouvements des Animaux."

sort of interpretations that were still running as an undercurrent in psychology when Prince began to write. They aimed at a premature simplification of the facts of organic life and disregarded what I may call the bee-hive or ant-hill feature of the brain, which operates busily through a hierarchy of coöperating systems. A similar insufficiency of thought still prevails wherever psychology follows the old Aristotelian tradition and where philosophizing is an intellectual sport pursued for its own sake. Indeed, as Bacon says: "Knowledge derived from Aristotle can rise no higher than Aristotle."

While Aristotle made a very important distinction between Memory and Reminiscence, he was too deeply occupied with the empirical and terminal stage of memory, as recall, to give due attention to all the phases of the process as a whole. The registration and the conservation of memory in the nerve mass, which occupy Prince and a few of his contemporaries, were subjects too big and too infinitely perplexing for a man who, however precocious as an historical figure, did not know the difference between a nerve and a tendon. And, following Aristotle, nerves were long overlooked as merely a kind of tendon. Let us not forget that this sort of confusion is at the bottom of much of the mystic philosophy that Prince has so long protested against for being an interference with psychological progress, and for delaying the recognition of the detailed functioning of the neurone web as the substrate of memory.

Vicissitudes of Locke's Famous Essay

As a sidelight on the curiously inconsistent way in which the psychology of thought-linkages has developed, we learn that "John Locke had, meanwhile (that is, before Hume raised express questions as to what are the distinct principles of association) introduced the phrase: 'Association of Ideas' as a title of a supplementary chapter incorporated with the fourth edition of his Essay meaning it, however, only as the name of a principle accounting for the mental peculiarities of individuals, with little or no suggestion of its general psychological import."[3]

Anyone reading this chapter, after digesting the Essay, must recognize that Locke's remarks were a sort of an unwitting "crawl" back into the fold of the Cartesian School from which he had early severed himself by denouncing their theory of unconscious mental activity. What Prince properly called, in 1891, "Association

[3] Encyclopaedia Britannica, Article on "Association."

neuroses," and explained in terms of the Unconscious, are precisely the phenomena of semi-automatism that Locke sought to understand. This is pathological association, and therefore Locke was studying what has since been called "the morbid laws of the association of ideas" rather than the normal ones.

This departure of the meaning of "Association of Ideas" from the original morbid implication intended by its author, is only one of several historic blunderings that Morton Prince has had to reckon with in his attempts to gain medical recognition for psychology. For Locke's thesis, with all its hints to education and psychotherapy was lost sight of in the vaguer use of his term.

It is still germane to note that Locke made an egregious error when he attempted to refute the Unconscious as conceived by the Cartesian School. Sarcastically he says: "This is something beyond Philosophy; and it cannot be less than Revelation, that discovers to another, Thoughts in my Mind, when I can find none there myself."[4]

Locke's animus in this controversial writing touching the Cartesians was such that he could not recognize the thread of identity that stretched from the Cartesian Automatism to his own theory of habitual "Connexions of Ideas." Even after he has propounded as puzzling those unreasonable "antipathies" that are not natural but acquired, he fails to see that his explanation that they are "Trains of Motion in the Animal Spirits" should imply not only, on the one hand, *reflex action* but on the other should open the possibility of trains of thought *below the threshold of awareness.* Yet the chapter "Of the Association of Ideas" contains in germ all the questions that the concept of the neurogram tends to answer. Not until the Nineteenth Century do we see a glimmer of light upon Locke's puzzle. Sir William Hamilton's "latent thought" and Dr. Carpenter's "unconscious cerebration" are phrases heralding the slow recovery from the psychological confusion left in legacy by Locke.

Later Conceptions of Automatism and Subconsciousness

When Huxley revived Cartesian Automatism (1874) it was without any specific reference to "the unconscious," which notion was still a matter of philosophical conjecture.

"The epoch-making researches of Janet on hysterics and almost coincidently with him of Edmund Gurney on hypnotics very clearly

[4] The Essay, Book II, Chap. I, §19.

established the fact that these phenomena are the manifestations of dissociated *processes outside of and independent of the personal consciousness. Among the phenomena, for example, are motor activities of various kinds such as ordinarily are or may be induced by conscious intelligence. As the individual, owing to anesthesia, may be entirely unaware even that he has performed any such act, the process that performed it must be one that is subconscious."* ("*The Unconscious," page 157.*)

"*The phenomenon of subconscious perception of sensory* stimulations applied to anesthetic areas *tactile, visual, etc., in hysterics, first demonstrated by Janet, is of the same order, but has been so often described that only a reference to it is necessary. I mention examples here merely that the different kinds of phenomena that may be brought within the sphere of memory shall be mentioned."* ("*The Unconscious," page 56.*)

We shall find in the work of Morton Prince, as early as 1885, a constant drive to correlate conscious and unconscious mentation with the principle of reflex action. Among writers on psychopathology, he was to be one of the first to make the *reflex arc* a common denominator in terms of which all levels of mental functioning might be expressed, compared and accounted for. In the meantime, Charcot's studies in hysteria had lifted hypnotic experiments out of the muck of mere charlatanism; and Janet, by his clinical demonstrations, had liberated the notion of sub-consciousness from the domain of speculation.[5] The neurogram concept was not to be developed till later. In Prince's hands it turns out to be a sort of algebraic equivalent for the underlying nerve-process, that furnishes a convenient formulation for mapping specific complexes of mental functions, normal and abnormal, in the play of temperament, in the growth of experience, in recovery from split personality and in such usually untouched things as sudden religious conversions. He has also extended the neurogram concept to the subconscious fabrication of dreams, both natural and induced.

Prince's View of Subconscious Fabrication

"*Residual processes underlying dreams—When citing the evidence of dreams for the conservation of forgotten experiences I spoke of one type of dream as a symbolical memory. I may now add it is more than this; it is a fabrication. The original experience or thought*

[5]Pierre Janet: "L'automatisme psychologique," Paris, 1889, and numerous other works.

may appear in the dream after being worked over into a fantasy, allegory, symbolism, or other product of imagination. Such a dream is not a recurrent phase of consciousness, but a newly fabricated phase. *Further, analytical and experimental researches go to show that the fabrication is performed by the original phase without the latter recurring in the content of the personal consciousness. The original phase must therefore have been conserved in some form capable of such independent and specific functioning, i.e., fabrication below the threshold of consciousness."* ("*The Unconscious,*" page *98*.)

Much yet remains to be garnered concerning that mysterious weaving which can only be called now by the name of subconscious fabrication or subconscious maturing of thought (Jastrow[6]). It is the fullness and the facility of such processes, as revealed in the experimental reactors of Gurney and Janet and Prince and others, that has required a sharper defining of the subliminal mind. It is no wonder that Prince, in the present almost hopeless confusion of the '*sciousness* family of words, has essayed tabulating coconscious and unconscious mentation as divisions of subconscious phenomena; and we must not forget to credit him with having done so in the hope of paving the way for a clearer description in neurographic terms. Now so well authenticated, this re-arranging of the neurographic web by an invisible spider transports our scientific imagination far beyond the formal categories imposed by certain writers who, since Locke, found the denial of unconscious cerebration a dogma too formidable to upset offhand. For, as regular philosophers, they could not afford the amateurish daring of an Emerson calling for "bold experiments with the mind." The Concord Sage, little impressed by Phrenology as he was, appears to have been still less awed by alleged principles of association: "There is no book like the memory, none with such a good index, and that of every kind, alphabetic, systematic, arranged by names of persons, by colors, tastes, smells, shapes, likeness, unlikeness, by all sorts of mysterious hooks and eyes to catch and hold, and contrivances for giving a hint."[7]

Inadequacy of Cut-and-Dried Principles

To finish with classical psychology, we need not re-echo the encyclopedia by discussing Hume's Principles of Association, as resemblance, contiguity in time and place, cause and effect; nor

[6] Jastrow, Joseph; Chapter VIII of "The Subconscious," Houghton, Mifflin & Co., 1906.
[7] Emerson, R. W. Works, Vol. XII., p. 66. "Memory."

Dugald Stewart's resemblance, contrariety and vicinity in time and place; nor the somewhat sophomoric views of Reid. They fall under the reproach of attempting to logicalize the mental processes on the Aristotelian model, in a rigid way that William James effectively set aside by his discussion of Redintegration.[8]

Now, out of all these attempts to reduce the mental process to the formulas of logic or to the principles of a calculating or logical machine or to a group of "faculties" and association types, very little has eventuated except the spurious method of approach and the habit of trying to win the attention of the reader by professing to exhaust the mystery of thought linkages.

In the last two decades of the Nineteenth Century, much had happened in the field of the Association of Ideas that would seem to penetrate that mystery. It has been approached from the standpoint of Galton's "psychometric experiments," and we have a right to be much impressed by the knowledge won in the field of *learning technique*, not to mention in detail the enlargement of the field by Cattell, Yerkes, Thorndike and others, through mental tests and animal experiments. Yet any candid student of the history of Association Psychology cannot but see that, a decade or so back at least, even the most advanced students were taking a very naïve view of the mechanism of thought. It would seem that their situation was that of being willing to tolerate a considerable amount of mystery, which, until recent years, fully obscured such subjects as Sleep, Dreams and the Mechanism of Thinking. For this, as Morton Prince has very definitely indicated, the philosophic attitude of a traditional type is largely to blame. It is precisely because Morton Prince has had no feeling of indulgency towards this situation that it seems important not to overlook the historical development since 1885 of his neurographic theory, the theory that treats of the registration, conservation and reproduction of experiences. Itself, this tripartite division, with its significant omission of recognition or recollection as a separate rubric, indicates the freshness of his view of the mental mechanism.

Pragmatic Treatment of Recall

Intent upon an inclusive theory that will help the psychology of association to find its feet on a basis different from the old philosophical psychology, Morton Prince has not concerned himself very much with "recall" through such alleged "fundamental"

<hr>

[8] James, William, "Principles of Psychology," pp. 579-581.

principles as contiguity, similarity and contrast, which, as Sir William Hamilton has shown, were pretty clearly anticipated by Aristotle. It is well to note that in his lack of preoccupation over these categories of association, and by his placing his emphasis elsewhere, Morton Prince is doing for psychology what logicians like Alfred Sidgwick are doing for dialectics by showing up the needlessness of cut-and-dried principles, and, like William James by indicating that the old principles of distinction are not fundamental but merely schematic. For instance, the formal aspect of logic is being set aside in favor of a pragmatic study of what underlies logical thought.[9] We are being waked up to the idea that logic is a sort of device for winning an argument, instead of constituting a law of nature!

Similarly, Prince does not stress classifying the *content* of recall, but rather his first care is to dispose the mind of his pupils and readers to study the natural history of the subject. His own tendency is to trace the dynamic motives underlying the registration, conservation and reproduction of experiences and thus to reach a *biological* conception. Prince seems to have guessed that Association is a trick of the individual to make his nerve-records help him along the way to a goal. He detects the influence of enduring, though secret, thoughts and motives even in disordered mentalities, in a manner that makes him join with Cannon and McDougall in their findings of physiological purposiveness and of social "drives."

"*In the survey of life's experiences which we have studied we have, for the most part, considered those which have had objective relation and have been subject to confirmation by collateral testimony. But we should not overlook the fact that among mental experiences are those of the inner as well as outer life. To the former belong the hopes and aspirations, the regrets, the fears, the doubts, the self-communings and wrestlings with self, the wishes, the loves, the hates, all that we are not willing to give out to the world, and all that we would forget and would strive not to admit to ourselves. All this inner life belongs to our experience and is subject to the same law of conservation.*" (*Page 85, "The Unconscious."*)

Value of the Cell Theory

On the objective aspect of conservation there is a peculiar message of Biology to Psychology that Prince is passing along through his neurographic concept.

---

[9] Alfred Sidgwick: "The Application of Logic," MacMillan, London, 1910.

Modern biological research, casting its net into the ocean of possibilities, announces that it has dragged to the surface a great simplifying fact in the study of all life. It is that, in any living body, the function and the structure alike reflect definitely and necessarily the life-activities or behavior of its individual cells, which make of the animal a composite of cell colonies. The nervous system is made up of billions of "elongated amoebas" with pseudopodia ranging from a fraction of an inch to a yard in length. They are the threads which, being tied together in the throes of growth by experience, make up a neurogram.

Prince finds it conceivable that we may some day understand how groups of these filaments become chemically sensitized so that they conserve the power to combine again and again into a characteristic pattern, bearing the stamp of some particular life experience. For this we are prepared by the knowledge of sensitization in other cells and in their surrounding fluids.

As biologists have advanced in the study of the various cells, and in the examination of their nucleus, they have brought us to the threshold of a new world, almost transcending the material. As seen in the discovery of immunity and of anaphylaxis, cell life is complicated by the "humours" of the blood:—"humoural memory" for particular poisons seems to rival or surpass that memory which we ascribe to the colony of filamentous cells called the nervous system. It is too early to say what lies behind such recent discoveries, fraught as they are with intimations of colloid mechanisms as complex as any astronomical system. Perhaps, as Prince would appear to believe, the substrate of both mind and matter is coming within scientific ken.

The kind of memory that is taken to be mediated by the nervous system alone is a very old problem, and has long been pressing for solution. If the solution has been delayed, it is due to the habits of authors in clinging to Locke's type of thought, when studying memory, without taking into account what I have called, for picturesqueness, the beehive or ant-hill nature of the nerve mass and the phenomena resulting therefrom. These require open-minded attention to the vast hinterland of automatic mentation that lies outside of consciousness. Unquestionably, the *a priori* attitude tends to shut out the kind of subject-matter that Prince has majored in. In psychology, Prince's neurographic theory is an eye-opener comparable to colloid study in chemo-physics—not because he is unique in averring a belief in definite traces or graphs in the lattice-work of nerves, but essentially because he performs the rare service of carrying the neurogram theory into his practice.

There has been a failure to form a picture of personality based upon a due recognition of the immense number of permutations and combinations of connections among those cell-filaments which compose the nervous system, as a substrate for experiential registration, conservation and reproduction. Thus, few people have conceived the variegated organization of neurographic complexes. And it would seem that Morton Prince has served quietly but insistently a good turn to philosophy and psychology and psychopathology (not to mention the psychiatry which is so *démodé*) by warning visitors to the mental realm that they should not go on counting without their host, the nervous system. From the beginning, he has held to the *reflex* picture, as shown by the following passage from "The Nature of Mind," published in 1885:

"I think it is possible to show, by reference to the facts of physiology and pathology, that from the simplest muscular act, such as the winking of the eyelid, to the most complex muscular actions and trains of thought, there is never a difference in kind, only one of degree, that we can pass from one to the other by a series of gradations, step by step, and find them all of the same nature, reflex in character." (*Page 96*.)

Yet the fact that he never fully accepted the seductive teaching of Huxley along this same line witnesses the independent spirit in which Prince has held himself free from entanglement with more recent doctrines. He rejects "epiphenomenalism," the idea that makes consciousness a mere steam-whistle in the mental power-plant.

Consciousness as Interacting with Reflexes

Further, in his "Nature of Mind," by his striking analysis of Dr. Mesnet's case of human automatism (cited so forcefully by Huxley) and by his remarkable plea for *consciousness as a link* in that very chain of automatic behavior, Prince proves himself restless to unify Body and Mind. He synthesizes into one picture the nature of mind-beyond-matter with that which is reducible to neurone patterns,— these being viewed as a hierarchy of physiological dispositions. Scarcely a writer on practical neurology in recent times, unless actually inspired by Prince, has had such a determination to bring the sphere of consciousness and the sphere of automatism into a synthetic view, and that without slighting the one for the other, as most authors are wont to do.

It is this fact, working its way into his writings and reflecting itself in the practical examples he adduces, that gives a peculiar tang to his neurographic formulas, and invites delicate appreciation.

II

IT IS NOT customary, in estimating scientific progress, to judge an author's contribution from the standpoint of taste, unless it be merely literary taste as an ornament of scientific writing. Yet, in judging of any work that goes beyond scientific routine into the subtler things of the mind, one may perhaps make free to ask oneself whether good taste may not have played a deciding part at many junctures. That the reflection is not utterly senseless may be suggested by the experience of Charles Darwin who, in the later years of his life, found reason to bewail his voluntary misfortune in having excluded himself from the domain of taste in Art and Literature by having dwelt too exclusively on dry details. Such exclusiveness forms no part of Prince's fate; and there is every reason to speak of a certain "guardianship of taste" that has presided over his scientific work as a factor in his avoidance of ugly pitfalls. Now, taste involves implicit aversions as well as positive selections. And, among the things that Prince has almost intuitively (by that I mean *implicitly*) avoided, are those overloaded and encumbered concepts that still block the way to psychological discussion. In particular, I will take, for example, his view of the still undefined term "intelligence," as characterizing his striving to avoid obscurantist views.

"*I cannot help thinking that 'intelligence' is a pragmatic question, not a biological or psychological one. It would be much more conducive to a clear understanding of biological problems to use intelligence only as a convenient and useful expression, like sanity or insanity, to designate certain behavior which conforms to a type which, without strictly defining its limits, popular language has defined as intelligent. Sanity and insanity have ceased to be terms of scientific value because they cannot be defined in terms of specific mental conditions and much less in terms of mental processes. So intelligence cannot be defined in terms of conscious and unconscious processes. Any attempt to do so meets with insuperable difficulties and becomes 'confusion worse confounded.'*" ("*The Unconscious,*" *page 240.*)

This instances the rejection of an outworn tool of thought in the form of a term—"intelligence"—which has been overloaded with denotations and connotations until it ceases to make any sharp effect upon discussion. Recent debates among psychologists indicate that Prince's distaste for the abuse of the term has been fully validated. Other examples here and there show the up-to-dateness of his anticipations of the trend of modern psychological discoveries; but it would be tedious to cite instances at length. One has only to note the significant omissions in his work to realize that he is not wandering in a maze of by-paths and blind alleys, and that the neurographic conception leads into a region free from pitfalls and opening a visualization of mental phenomena of which psychologists have not yet taken sufficient advantage.

Doctrinal Confusion Regarding Mind

To appreciate the historical position of Prince's neurographic concept is to come nearer to appreciating the struggles of those who have wrestled with the problem of human personality. It should be remembered that Prince is distinctive among modern or recent writers in regard to the kind of a hold that he has taken on the problem as a means of grasping its fundamentals and preventing the subtleties from slipping out of ken. This is another way of saying that Prince's uniqueness is marked by the *level of explanation* which he has adopted as a basis for thinking about the mechanism of so-called Mind. This basis has long been so distinctive that his outlook on the subject has tended to make the word "Mind" itself appear curiously meaningless.[10] To my notion, Prince's discovery that this term is almost hopelessly overloaded with denotations and connotations, and thus not scientifically useful, points to the fact that he has sought and found, at least, a refreshing viewpoint. It is one that cannot commend itself immediately to the popular demand nor to the ultra-simple outlook that students are required to assume in experimental psychology. As time goes on, it will be seen that the visualization presented in Prince's theory is related to a more helpful level of explanation than the ones commonly resorted to.

For, among contemporary writers on Personality, there are few who maintain their standpoint and who do not confuse their levels of explanation and present us, as it were, with mixed metaphors drawn from different levels. There are at least three distinct levels. Today, we see the behaviorists descending austerely to the reflex and reflex-conditioning level; and again, we discern an important

[10] "Nature of Mind," page 148. Pub. by J. B. Lippincott, Philadelphia, 1885.
DD

contingent of workers who are making themselves at home on a high plateau where a vast horizon is filled in with instincts and instinctive dispositions in a varied panorama. Again, there are those who dwell, by preference, on the mountain tops where behavior appears as emerging peaks jutting from a sea of clouds that hide the illimitable possibilities of the subliminal mind. Prince's neurographic conception is not out of keeping with the phenomena contemplated by any of the theorists on these various levels, which range all the way from extreme materialism to extreme idealism. Prince can fit these explanations into his formulation, exactly as a food expert can take into one consistent picture the views of the chemist, physiologist and culinary artist.

Pan-Psychism Admits of Neurone Organization

If Prince has ever seemed to be losing himself either in materialism or in idealism, his book "Nature of Mind and Human Automatism," of 1885, should set us right as to the path he has followed. The essence of this exploration has not been omitted from "The Unconscious" where neural dispositions are spread so large upon the page:

"In the last analysis, matter and mind probably are to be identified as different manifestations of one and the same principle—the doctrine of monism—call it psychical, spiritual, or material, or energy, as you like, according to your fondness for names. For our purpose it is not necessary to touch this philosophical problem as we are dealing only with specific biological experiences." (Footnote, page 148.)

With this warning that there is something ultimate in reserve, Prince, the neurologist, makes the most of his observations of human personality in explaining memory in its proximate sense, as based upon the physiological residua of past experiences, and still without excluding the participation of inherited dispositions. It is as if he intended to make us understand that when dealing with neurograms, he is after all dealing with proximate units and not ultimate psychical elements. Is he not somewhat in the position of the food expert, maintaining a well-poised interest as between the two main aspects of food, which are the *proximate* food elements such as protein and carbohydrates and the *ultimate* chemical elements? As a consequence of this position, conditioned reflexes and instincts (even sentiments) are regarded by Prince as so many "complexes" in the broad medical and architectonic sense in which he employed the word currently many years ago. (*N. of M., p. 138.*)

In explaining these complexes in "The Unconscious," Prince has not attempted the definiteness of H. R. Marshall, with his patient and ingenious parallel between neururgic and noetic emphases.[11] Nor has he occasion to develop the neurographic conception, like Max Meyer [12] to the point of diagramming an apparatus for what I may call the machine-switching of nerve impulses. Such pictures are merely complementary to Prince's exposition. He does not elaborate upon them beyond the scope of his own purpose, which is to call attention to the signs of *organized* working of neurographic records in their every-day manifestations.

Neurographic Combinations as a Key

Prince has a restless drive to find a better hierarchy of the sentiments. I shall not forget sitting on the porch at Nahant and watching Dr. Prince and Professor McDougall marking a piece of bright yellow paper with such apparently light-hearted legends as "I love Nellie." "Here," said Dr. Prince, "is a sentiment. Nellie is the object; love is the emotion with its instinctive dispositions; where shall we place the 'settings'?" Then he went on to discuss the alternative ways in which the union might be conceived of those different dispositions of experience and of instinct that go to make the unity of a sentiment which contains within itself a striving for its own ends. To be sure, in all this, Prince gives much credit to McDougall and Shand; but the "drive" to go ahead straight on the road to explaining personal experience in terms of interconnected and elaborately organized dispositions (regardless of the exaggerated simplicity of behaviorism and regardless of the mythological entities of psychoanalysis) is distinctly the Principian trend. He stresses the fact of organization as such rather than the details of the neurographic substrate.

Is not this entirely in keeping with the latest disclosures of physiology and psychology? Does not Sir Charles Sherrington allow that recent work shows an unexpected simplicity underlying the process of mental activity, in other words, that nerve centers may not possess their own special kinds of mechanisms, but may have simply the properties of nerve impulses in combination?[13] The combination is the thing. Does not this justify Prince's algebraic method in working up the concept of neurograms without

[11] "Consciousness," MacMillan Company, New York, 1909, Chap. II & III.
[12] "The Fundamental Laws of Human Behavior," R. G. Badger, Boston, 1911.
[13] Sherrington, C. S., Presidential Address, British Association for Advancement of Science, Sept. 22, 1922. Reprinted in "Mental Hygiene," quarterly, 1923.

undue attention to the specific neural picture? The way experiences are stitched together is what counts. Carrying this idea in the back of our minds when reading Prince's formulation of neurographic mechanisms, we shall not encounter in it anything inconsistent with the recent progress of physiologists toward Sherringtonian insight into "nerve impulses in combination." Perhaps this is the long-sought formula which has hidden the mental nature by its "absolute transparency"—to echo Emerson.

Adherence to the Canalization Concept

Surely modern neurology has been ready for this simplification for some time, witness the prevalence among neurologists and physiological psychologists of the teaching that, potentially, every neurone has access to every other neurone. It is just as well that Prince should not have obscured this potentiality by any too ambitious scheme for neuro-canalizations, considering the use that he makes of the concept. Let us be thankful he has found it unnecessary to deny "the stuff the soul is made of" in order to make room for neurograms, and that he has refused to populate the brain regions with a "censor" or other entity of the psychoanalytic type, in order to hold the fort for consciousness. Nor has he in any other way planned a premature simplification of the field of investigation; but he did accept in advance "nerve impulses in combination" as the unit of investigation. Both his cautious restraint and his insight were fed and sustained by his having saturated himself with observations of conduct and of character-phenomena on every plane of mental life, even at a long distance from the laboratory and the clinic. The result was that the peculiarities of his neurographic substrate, hypothetical though it might seem, were impressed upon him with the definiteness with which the housewife comes to know and count on the action of yeast in bread-making, even though she may not form a definite cell picture of the yeast enzyme. Under the circumstances, the neurographic conception could be safely carried only far enough for Prince to steer clear of the formalized thinking into which his predecessors had fallen. He kept to the path of realism.

May I, in this connection, submit it as my personal opinion that if Freud, Jung and Stekel had been thinking along these lines since young manhood, as Prince's record shows he did, they would have been better prepared to interpret their own rich and even unprecedented collections of material of the psychic life, without succumbing to that fever of extreme theorizing from which they are but slowly recovering as yet.

To make a long story short, Prince has not stumbled into the pitfalls set for unwary theorizers. Specifically, after 1909, he was one of the few who did not go to extremes of denunciation of or adherence to the newly circulated views of psychoanalysts concerning the Unconscious. The result is that his neurographic conception has steadily developed and stands today in perfect harmony with what we may call the canalization concept of neuro-action.

Inconclusive Views of Various Schools

A practical contribution to the immediate situation in the psychology of Personality has been that he filled the office of a snowplow: keeping the channels of intellectual progress open to all sorts of traffic of opinion and never allowing the school of Freud or of Jung or of Behaviorism, or any other school, to snow under any avenue of discussion. Indeed, he was cricitized by some for opening his Journal of Abnormal Psychology so widely to the most divergent opinions. Its pages, be it said, are the proof of the variety and confusion among levels of explanation while, at the same time, they exhibit Prince's personal striving for a simplified and unified level to which all honest thinkers might repair.

With the advent of the Gestalt theory in America, we sense the upsetting of the preconceived notions of Learning and Association, against which I have inveighed in the first part of this paper. I regret, however, that Prince's modest way of writing makes it hard to show in his actual language how long he has felt that the old Associationism was dead anyway. In their attack on Associationism, the Gestalt School will be killing a moribund idea, not to say a dead dog. They have, however, the signal advantage of introducing a captivatingly clever formulation into the field of Memory at a time when this is still beset by obscurantism and hopelessly conflicting viewpoints.[14]

Increasingly in recent years, Prince has striven to remove anything like obscurantism from his formulations. Difficulties of language and of physiological statement are enough to explain

[14] Koehler.,W."ZurPsychologiederSchimpansen,"Psychologische Forshung, 1921. Kafka, G., "Tierpsychologie," Leipzig, 1914. See McDougall's comment on Formreizen, page 69 of the "Outline of Psychology," 1922.
Koffka, K., "Grundlagen der Psychischen Entwicklung," 1921.
See translations in International Library of Psychology: Kegan Paul, Trench, Trubner & Co.. London; Harcourt, Brace & Co., New York, 1924.

whatever remains of unclearness in the neurographic conception. Still there are those who say Prince has not yet "put over" his theory. Such critics now greet the recent onrush of the Gestalt School. These exponents of "configurational dispositions" seem to have located a weak spot somewhere between the animal psychology of Thorndike and the behaviorism of Watson.

As it happens, the milk in the coconut of the Gestalt theory, is a juice that has been running in other fruits of research. For Yerkes long ago had made it clear that trial and error was in a sense suspended as a principle of learning-behavior in certain chimpanzees. He still speaks of *ideation* in chimpanzees. What Koehler and Koffka see at work in "configurational dispositions" and maturation" are processes that often trespass upon what Prince and Jastrow call subconscious fabrication and subconscious maturing. Also, not new is the hint that some of the configurational dispositions of the chimpanzee may be associated with a reflective consciousness similar to our own.

To take the liberty of citing my own papers, I have intimated as clearly as I could what was suggested by my own studies of natural dreams:—that subconscious trials and errors fill in the gaps that are observed in problem-solution whenever it reaches resolution without externalized trial and error. The abrogation of external trial and error does not imply the non-continuance of the process neurographically:—i. e. in conscious or subconscious procedures.[15]

Can the configurational dispositions of the Gestalt School bring more clarity to the things of the Mind than Prince's neurographic dispositions? To answer this point one does not need to detract from the excellence and suggestiveness of the Gestalt School's experimentally simplified observations upon quasi-human chimpanzees. Like our American comparative psychologists, they find it an excellent thing for one's study of behavior and learning technique to train one's observational powers by keeping chimpanzee pets under vivarium conditions. Already, Professor Yerkes tells us that the protocols of his actual experiments can hardly give an adequate idea of how much more the observer sees in the behavior of the chimpanzee than can ever be set down. The sense of the *familiar* touching observed animal behavior and *the accompanying emotion of conviction* are thus coming into the field of

---

[15] See *Resolution of the Unadjusted* in paper by L. H. Horton: "Scientific Method in the Interpretation of Dreams," p. 388, Journ. of Abn. Psychology, Feb.-March, 1916,

scientific statement, whereas, a few years ago, it was not correct experimental form to advert to such elusive things! Yet, during many years, Prince and a few others were studying human beings under conditions of virtual vivarium existence which (considering that humans were studied, and not chimpanzees) could properly be regarded as "experimental"—because sufficiently controlled to ward off error and to carry conviction. Nevertheless, it is a fact that Prince's conception of Association Neuroses was not given full credit by his contemporaries. He spoke with "the voice of one crying in the wilderness." Today, after the exuberant agitation of the psycho-analytic movement and after the shock of experience with war neuroses, the pendulum of medical belief has finally swung in Prince's direction; and the idea is now seriously entertained by advanced diagnosticians that neurographic idiosyncrasies may be functioning to produce this or that symptom formerly attributed without question to purely bodily causes.

Possible Fallacy in Comparison of Man and Chimpanzee

Undoubtedly the psychology of learning will greatly profit by the simplified studies of chimpanzee life. They may clear the ground of old lumber. But the results cannot illuminate such human behavior as flows from social sentiments and *savoir faire* nor from other higher mental processes. Therefore, the experimental queries put to the chimpanzee should not be overestimated like the famous quest for the philosopher's stone, nor yet as a hopeful hunt for the pot of gold at the end of the psychic rainbow. When all is said and done, we shall only have reached the end of a chimpanzee's rainbow of intellectual promise. As we come nearer to human goals in the problems of comparative psychology, we experience a paradoxical slowing-up in the yield of information from animal experiments. To paraphrase Bacon, we may say that knowledge derived from chimpanzees can rise no higher than chimpanzees. The proper unit of investigation of humanity is man! Chimpanzee study will bring mostly knowledge of chimpanzees and not insight—as hoped for—into some new open-sesame to unlock the secret of mentality. For, to re-echo the Sherringtonian formula, the behavior of the nerve-mass (including, I think, the higher learning process of the chimpanzee) should still be reducible to the strategy of *nerve impulses in combination*. We are not, I say, to expect the discovery of nerve centers possessing particular kinds of intelligence of their own, or differing radically from reflex action. That such breaks in the chain are absent, is quite consistent with what Prince has assumed right along in his neurographic formulation. When the experiments with chimpanzees are as finished as a squeezed orange, there will still be left out of account the especially *human potentialities* of nerve impulses in combination. For human mind will not have been disclosed to be a mere multiple of chimpanzee mind-units, however alike may be the behavior of child and chimpanzee, and however similar may appear certain brain zones possessed by man and chimpanzee—in common, as it were. The hierarchic and architectonic features of the human integrations of purpose, of learning and of sentiment will still require the system of accurate notation afforded only by a truly neurographic formulation.

III

IT IS NOT very long since science first took up the Trial-Error-Success formulation of animal behavior. Its mainstay has been the observation of some imprisoned animal trying to get out of a "trick" cage, and its extension has been contrived with more or less fruitful results, by studying animals running in a maze.[16]

As a result, we have a wilderness of single instances which has grown up around the experimental psychologists, who are now trying to find their own way out so that they may not "fail to see the forest for the trees." I submit that what they need is a visualization conforming to the neurographic concept, in order to coördinate the observations upon animal behavior—indeed, upon all behavior.

Trial-and-Error in Visualization

Jacques Loeb, in the *Yale Review* of July 1915, has argued more brilliantly than I can for the sort of visualization here alluded to. According to his notion, the value of visualization can sometimes transcend that of experiment itself. But, curiously enough, Loeb begs one of the questions at issue by setting the goal of biological research in the direction of pure mechanism, as if it were something necessarily apart from trial and error. He even cites the automaton or selenium-eyed "dog" of John Hays Hammond, Jr., as behaving in a manner that does "not support the theory of 'trial and error.'" Loeb's pre-conceived idea of mechanism, far from

[16] A piquant departure has been Professor McDougall's discovery at Harvard of the advantages of the water maze for studying the behavior of rats in learning to swim their way to food at the end of the maze.

weakening my appreciation of his argument in favor of visualization, tends, on the contrary, to strengthen it. For Jacques Loeb would not be regarded today as having overshot the mark and become ultra-mechanistic if he had himself practised what he preached and had relied more on visualization and less upon jumping at conclusions from too narrow experiments. In failing to make sufficient use of visualization, he was, as it turns out from a study of his biography, stringently limited by an ingrained prejudice against the abuse of religious conceptions and all allied obscurantist notions, to which he likened the Trial and Error Theory. Had he known what was going on in his own mind, from the neurographic standpoint of Prince, he would have corrected his own bias, and his own process of "trial and error" would probably have reached "success" in explaining human behavior!

At this stage, I may as well admit that I am intent on spanning the alleged gap that exists between the concept of mechanism and the concept of trial and error. My proposition is that we need to visualize the nerve system as a biological mechanism contrived to afford a facility for "learning" by trial and error and success. This brings me back to defining Prince's neurographic concept as useful to that end. In this sense, I shall review the registration, conservation, and reproduction of experiences in order to make clearer how much Prince's formulation already affords to the would-be visualizer. In preamble, however, I should again recall the fact mentioned earlier in this paper, that mechanistic visualizations of memory processes have played a prominent part since the earliest days of ancient psychology.

On Visualizing the Neurographic Mechanism

The idea of some pattern impressed upon the memory is not a modern idea. Plato had his conception of wax tablets as receiving the impress of experiential stimuli, like the cachet of a signet ring. (This is a registration analogy.) Aristotle paid attention to traces left in the memory, in the form of ruts along definite retraceable paths. (This is a conservation analogy.) And, more recently, Thomas Hobbes sought to express the *train of ideas* by the simile of drops of water following the finger on the window pane. (This is a reproduction analogy.) DesCartes, who was the first to schematize a consistent picture of registration, conservation and reproduction, came nearest to modern knowledge by his "waterworks" supposition, to wit: that the nerves were little canals which, irrigated by the first effect of experience, would retain a disposition to conduct the "animal spirits" more easily a second time. It was admitted by Huxley that very little improvement over this canalization theory of DesCartes had ever been developed.[17]

The difficulty seems to have been that no one could carry in his mind the picture of the conservation of canalization-forms. And even Prince has felt somewhat the effect of this discouraged attitude on the part of thinkers. For, to the average student, the jungle of nerve connections is an inextricable mass and there are very few who have carried out, in one personal experience, what Wm. McDougall has advocated, namely: an intensive analysis of nerve processes and of mental processes in parallel. Thus, few thinkers can "get it into their head." Yet practical neurology, especially in brain localization and in the kinetics of nerves, is sufficiently advanced today to meet halfway the students who would undertake such analyses of mental function. It is really an Emersonian "chalk line of imbecility" that keeps the neural and the psychological conceptions so far apart. To be sure, the *rapprochement* had been made, as far as possible at the time, by William McDougall in his highly valued "Physiological Psychology" (London, 1905). But the lesson has not been generally assimilated, as a context for psychological thought, to the degree that Prince's work demands.

Those who are technically equipped to understand psychological language should read between the lines of Prince's message and not be lazily expecting the nature of mind to be formulated for them with the simplicity of street cries—"Behaviorism!" "Libido!" "Reflex-action!" "Gestalt!"

I trust it may not seem presumptuous if I try to summarize the immediate requirements of "psycho-neurology" as I see them.

Neuro-Dynamic Patterns

It is time that we should cease to overlook the absolute transparency of the principle of neurographic registration. It has remained obscure because we lack terms to describe its simplicity. The unquestionable truth is that the brain and nervous system

[17] The canalization concept has a long history and an honorable one dating essentially from the time of DesCartes who constructed, for human automatism, a scheme in analogy to the waterworks of French chateaux and their parks: Claparède has recently reminded us that this is still the most descriptive plan of how the nervous system acts as a combining mechanism for coördinating nervous impulses, and even a physiologist like Sir Michael Foster took the same view.

McDougall's theory of *inhibition by drainage* is a noteworthy extension of the canalization concept.

are burdened with the neurographic record in the same definite manner as a half-tone plate is burdened with its photographic record. In the printing press, the half-tone plate transfers the picture into ink-impulses. In a similar sense, the neurogram transmits an impression upon the pattern of muscle-behavior and upon the quality of gland-behavior and upon the course (not to say behavior) of consciousness. There is a patterned transfer of neurodynamic impulses from the neurogrammic web to these three effectors (if I may be allowed to so call them) and the question that remains is: "How shall we depict the nerve-tactics back of all this?"

The value of any analogy is that it makes it possible to think of something that is not yet clear, in terms of something that is already clear. Now, any printer will tell you that the half-tone plate is a photographic impression *carried on a system of dots* of different sizes and shapes and of correspondingly different capacities to convey flecks of ink to a sheet of paper. Similarly, we may say that the neurogram is an impress or picture of experience originally received onto and carried upon a system of meshes having the nature of a net. It is especially like a distorted hair-net with streamers, possessing varied connections with the effector termini—in spider-web fashion. All the strands, although connected, have differing capacities of conduction, both in amount and direction, so that they have a different permeability for conducting neurodynamic impulses to effector terminals like muscle and gland. These correspond, in final analysis, to the printed sheet where the end-result shows itself as the effector-pattern.

Unless psychologists are willing to make themselves familiar with the operation of this time-space mechanism of neurones to the degree that printers, in their daily labors, make themselves familiar with the mechanism of the half-tone imprint, we can hardly hope for a group of men to spring up who will be at home with the neurographic conception. New technical developments require, as William James points out, the creation of new terms; and from this standpoint, Prince's terminology is still somewhat difficult in view of the demonstrated need of familiarity with his views. Therefore, I take the liberty of somewhat overloading his conception with terms needed to do justice to its nuances.

Necessary Distinctions in Neurographic Concept

In the first place, is it not well to remember that registration, conservation and reproduction are viewed by Prince as distinct processes, however much they may intermingle? Why should not this be capable of sharper denotation in neurographic terms?

Let us call the network that carries the neurogram by the name *neurarkus*[18]—meaning, in Greek roots, a hair-net made of neurones. This analogy is exactly what the neurogram must conform to in its spatial aspect, with the proviso that the netting is *underneath* the brain coverings and that elongated meshes, extending for considerable distances, go into other parts of the nervous system. This neurarkus is the system of nerve-meshes that bears the neurogram. But in what phase—is it registered, conserved or reproduced? The answer is: "We cannot say unless we use distinctive terms." Let us grant that the neurarkus is a foundation for special dispositions affecting behavior and memory, provisionally viewing it as nothing more than the blank plate, or unmodified physical substrate. But let us broadly call the organized pattern or system of traces upon the neurarkus by the name of *neurarchy*. This means the portions of the nerve-net (neurarkus) that are so situated or so impressed or so charged that they govern or lead or control the way that stimuli travel. This must imply a form of neuro-electric conduction from receptor terminals to centers and again outwardly to effectors. Such is the principle of neurarchy, or of "governing disposition" in the neurarkus, regardless of the phase—whether of registered, conserved or reproduced *neurarchic* dispositions. These dispositions, at one time or another, must represent channels for re-conduction or at least for momentary reception of stimuli.

"It would be a gross exaggeration to say, on the basis of the evidence at our disposal, that all life's experiences persist as potential memories, or even that this is true of the greater number. It is, however, undoubtedly true that of the great mass of experiences which have passed out of all voluntary recollection, an almost incredible, even if relatively small, number still lie dormant, and, under favoring conditions, many can be brought within the field of conscious memory." ("*The Unconscious,*" page 84.)

Now, according to Prince, some neurarchic dispositions may fail to be conserved. This must mean that dispositions are sometimes registered although not conserved. We need a name, then, for that particular process which is *only* registration. What is more natural than to speak of an outline or graph? A *neurograph*, then, is a neurarchic disposition laid as it were magnetically upon a neurarkus

[18]This term is not euphonious but is employed here to give precision to the anatomical picture of brain-paths,

in such a manner that it composes some actual pattern, however temporary and however ready to be effaced or marred. While it lasts, it will lead or govern the propagation of impulses through some particular portion of a neurarkus. Elementary neurology will provide us with innumerable models of such patterns. Such neurographs can be diagrammed in three dimensions, provided we take heed of known localizations of brain functions and spend a few minutes bending wires to represent the canalizations involved in, say, a coördinated reflex. Now, how about the neurarchic dispositions that are conserved? It is obvious that they are best described by the term *neuroglyph* which implies a more deep-seated trace, or carved channel. It is understandable that it may take several neurographs passing over a neurarkus to effect that permanency that is implied by conservation, and thus carve a neuroglyph in the sense of a reliable neurodynamic track or web. But I ought not to overlook the fact here that there must be a great many neuroglyphs composed of channels which have never been "graphed," but which are deep tracks provided by organic inherited form. The original growth-tendency of the neurones, not registration, is responsible for such conservation. For instance, it requires no neurographic process to develop an eye-winking reflex path. That is a fixed neuroglyph which represents what is fancifully called ancestral memory or race memory. Consequently, it is well not to overlook the fact that probably very few neurographs are impressed upon any really blank neurarkus. That is, if there are any blank neurarkuses, they are probably extensions into the forebrain of networks already well-started as innate conduction channels in other parts of the neurarchic system. In fact, it is this situation which justifies McDougall's insistence upon the tremendous concatenation of purposive influences in organisms.

Neural Side of Purpose and Meaning

This brings us to the fact that Prince, McDougall and possibly Janet and Shand, have been ahead of their colleagues in insisting that the phase of reproduction of experience is not a mere copy of some experience, not a mere echo, but tinged, colored or tinctured with an instinctive or organic self-interest that brings into prominence the Law of the Whole Organism in the simplest of acts.[19] For my part, I have great sympathy with this view, although I have registered a middle position between Woodworth and McDougall

[19] "The Unconscious," page 118; see italics in footnote.

as regards the question of the origin of "drives."[20] This is relevant to the phase of reproduction of experiential records or, in other words, to the *neurogram*.

This hint of the *"neurogrammic* use of experiential traces" should, of course, point to the fact that I wish to speak of *neurograms* as the neurarchic disposition in its phase of reproduction. *Grammic* is the proper word to distinguish the reproduction from the master record which begins as a neurograph and continues as a neuroglyph. These three terms (neurograph, neuroglyph and neurogram) give us resourcefulness in explaining what really goes on in memory as a process, and the distinction permits me, at least for the present, to make clear what I think is the great contribution of the neurographic conception. The contribution lies in the possibility that it opens up of improving the art of *graphing* memories, of following the laws of conservation (cf. neuroglyphs) and of uncovering the rules of the neurogrammic process. The study of purpose or teleology is made more approachable. To what extent are acts insignificant and mere echoes; and to what extent can psychologists and educators and parents follow the MEANING back of neurogrammic operations?

In most discussions, meaning is thought of vaguely as essentially conscious; but Prince has indicated his position that consciousness of meaning is but a small part of the total state of mentality. Like an iceberg, a large portion of its bulk is beneath the surface. Under Prince's neurographic scheme, as I see it, meaning is a highly organized complex, in the formation and reproduction of which neurarchic dispositions in all three phases are compounded with a variable degree of consciousness. In other words, avoiding the term "complex" now popularly accepted in its narrow sense, we may say that meaning is a neurarchic matrix or mould-of-associations which has been built up in a manner to determine the cast of thought that shall form around the idea or stimulus called meaningful. In this matrix, many built-up canalizations guide the conduction of stimuli to their eventual outcome in muscular, glandular or conscious patterns of action.

On my own responsibility, I have come to regard consciousness (or, at any rate, its hypothetical substrate once called "psychoplasm") as a sort of third effector entitled to rank with the already accepted ones—muscle and gland substances.[21]

[20] "What Drives the Dream Mechanism?", Jour. Abn. Psych., October, 1920.
[21] See W. James, "Principles. . ." Vol. I, top of page 581.

As a corrective to the neglect of the "meaning of *meaning*" so marked up to 1914, Prince has made use of the analogy of a clock, the hands of which represent conscious equivalents; while meaning is represented by quite different "wheels within wheels" that remain out of sight. Prince's idea of Association Neuroses, covering the phenomena called Association of Ideas by Locke, imply a vast inter-relation of cogs and wheels that determine how emotions and other drives shall eventuate, with the distinctness of a watch-escapement. It is this definiteness and delicacy that I have attempted to translate into appropriate "neuro" language.

Need of Technique in Complex-Building

Lest I should seem to be speaking in the air, let me say that the principal inspiration for my work, for many years, in studying psychology in America has been the appalling realization that the large proportion of American parents and educators have not an adequate conception of the significance of the motions and the gestures and the acts of young people. It is this situation that inspired Henry James in many passages of "Daisy Miller." This story reveals by subtle characterization the fact that American behavior is apt to be denuded of an infinite variety of expressions, of modes, moods and modulations needed for effective social contact. In French-speaking countries generally, and in England among some classes, it is a custom that children, from their earliest years, should be implicitly instructed in the interpretation of slight changes of behavior as an index of character and motive, and as deeply significant of courtesy, or the reverse, in the daily affairs of life. It is, therefore, not surprising that, for many years before psychotherapy penetrated into America, the French vocabulary was stocked with terms that implied *psychological understanding.* It is an understanding which, in fact, probably accounts for many of the qualities of the French nation. This understanding is hardly dawning in America; hence, it has to be introduced to us now clumsily by the medium of "applied psychology" of the subconscious, of the unconscious and the like. Since it is not possible, in this melting pot of America, to gain the needed knowledge of behavior by the tuition of folk-ways and manners as developed through the racial consolidation that has gone on in France, is it not important that we should be reminded at this point, of the educational promise in the contribution of Morton Prince? His own words describe the goal of his work when he says:

"*And, above all, the formation of complexes* is the foundation stone of psycho-therapeutics."

"*The methods of* education and therapeutic suggestion *are variants of this mode of organizing mental processes. Both, in principle, are substantially the same, differing only in detail. They depend for their effect upon the implantation in the mind of ideational complexes organized by repetition, or by the impulsive force of their affective tones, or both. Every form of education necessarily involves the artificial formation of such complexes, whether in a pedagogical, religious, ethical, scientific, social, or professional field. So in psychotherapy by artfully directed suggestion, or education in the narrower sense, complexes may be similarly formed and organized. New points of view and "sentiments" may be inculcated, useful emotions and feelings excited, and the personality correspondingly modified. Roughly speaking, this is accomplished by suggesting ideas that will form* settings (*associations) that give new and desired meanings to previously harmful ideas; and these ideas, as well as any others we desire to implant in the mind, are organized by suggestion with emotions (instincts) of a useful, pleasurable, and exalting kind to form desirable sentiments, and to carry the ideas to fulfilment. Thus sentiments of right, or of ambition, or of sympathy, or of altruism, or of disinterestedness in self are awakened; and, with all this, opposing emotions are aroused to conflict with and repress the distressing ones, and the whole welded into a complex which becomes conserved neurographically and thereby a part of the personality.*

"*Under ordinary conditions of every-day mental life* social suggestion *acts like therapeutic suggestion. But the suggestions of every-day life are so subtle and insidious that they are scarcely consciously recognized.*"   ("*The Unconscious*," page 288.)

Prince has been "neurographically" interested in certain views of Shand and McDougall to the effect that a sentiment is a highly involved organization of neurarchic dispositions, and especially that it functions integratedly as a whole striving to fulfill its own end. We are now reminded of Aristotle and his concept of *entelechy*, this self-contained program within a system which works "in the direction of the goal." But couched in Aristotle's terms, man's *endeavor* was not understandable, whereas in neurographic terms, it can be understood by psychologists, parents and educators; what is more, strivings can be traced back to the experiential sources of good and bad social adjustment and neurarchic patterns can be visualized in a way to show us how to modify accurately and, as the French say, *en connaissance de cause,* those experiential records which have been badly made.

Now let me again keep my feet on the ground by stamping a heel into the fact that, all over America, there is going on a most insidiously false inculcation of impressions upon children by their parents, teachers and casual acquaintances; all of which can be diagrammed convincingly as *bad complex-building technique.* This is going on constantly among well-meaning people without arousing any notice or intelligent insight upon the part of those who are making the mistakes. Nor is there any scientific propaganda adequate for the training of parents in "better complex-building." It is for this reason that I have been interested in the historical position of Prince's neurographic theory; and not because it merely gratifies the scientific craving to visualize the neurarkus as a repository for the registration, conservation, and reproduction of experiences.

A Contribution to Mind-Training

What then, is the ultimate contribution of the neurogram? You can find it actually in Prince's own words and you will see in reading them that Prince has enriched by his canalization theory of complex-building the same program of mind-training and emotion-study that was placed on the agenda of the Cartesian System, back in 1637. Since then, it has been neglected by all but a few thinkers. At present, the existing non-neurographic formulations only touch the surface and are liable to unwise application because the mechanistic background is not understood—witness the abuse of *laissez faire* under the Play School method. The Principian psychology compels our interest because of its tendency to organize definitely the work of psychology for education and for social life by affording the nearest thing to a fool-proof explanation and visualization of what we are doing when we train the mind.

Of that sort, it seems to me, is the contribution of Morton Prince. It offers to the generation of psychologists who will make use of it, the "thread of Ariadne" long needed for a successful penetration into the secrets of the labyrinth we call Mind.

EE

BIBLIOGRAPHY OF DR PRINCE'S WRITINGS

BOOKS

Nature of Mind and Human Automatism. 1885.
The Dissociation of a Personality. 1906.
The Unconscious. 1913. Second Edition, 1919.
The Psychology of the Kaiser. 1915.
The Creed of Deutschtum. 1918.
Clinical and Experimental Studies in Personality. (*Collected Essays*). 1928.

COLLABORATIONS

Wood's *Reference Handbook to the Medical Sciences.* 1882
International System of Electro-Therapeutics. 1894
Diseases of the Nervous System. By American Authors. 1895
American System of Practical Medicine. 1898
Psychotherapeutics. 1913
Subconscious Phenomena. 1915
Harvard's "*H*" *Book* (*History of Football*.) 1923

I—GENERAL MEDICINE

Date of Publication	Article	Publication
1882	Is Acute Follicular Tonsillitis a Constitutional Disease ?	*Boston Med. & Surg. Jour.*, Vol. CVI, No. 5.
,,	Pancreatic Apoplexy ; With a Report of Two Cases.	*Boston Med. & Surg. Jour.*, Vol. CVII, Nos. 2 & 3.
,,	Unusual or Accidental Results of Vaccination.	*Boston Med. & Surg. Jour.*, Vol. CVI, No. 17.
1883	The Dangers from the Domestic Use of Polluted Waters	*City of Boston San. Records*, Vol. X, p. 308.
,,	Some Typhoid Epidemics of the Past Decade and the Necessity of Compulsory Disinfection.	*Boston Med. & Surg. Jour.*, Vol. CVIII, No. 9.
1889	The Occurrence and Mechanism of Physiological Heart Murmurs (Endocardial) in Healthy Individuals	*Medical Record*, Vol. 35, No. 16.
,,	Electrolysis : Proper and Improper Methods of Using it in Removal of Hair and other Kindred Operations	*Amer. Jour. of the Med. Sciences*, May, 1889.

Date of Publication	Article	Publication
1890	The True Position of Electricity as a Therapeutic Agent in Medicine	*Boston Med. & Surg. Jour.*, Vol. CXXIII, No. 14
1892	An Improved Method of Removing Vascular Growths of the Skin by Electrolysis	*Boston Med. & Surg. Jour.*, Vol. CXXVII, No. 4.
1895	What Number of Cases is necessary to Eliminate the Effect of Chance in Mortality Statistics, Especially those of Typhoid Fever : a Statistical Study	*Boston Med. & Surg. Jour.*, Oct., 1895.
,,	Hay Fever, Due to Nervous Influences, occurring in Five Members of the Same Family	*Annals of Gynæcology and Pædiatry*, 1895
1898	Health Board as a Part of the Army Medical Corps, distinct from the Hospital Service	*Medical Record*, Sept. 3, 1898
1901	Physiological Dilatation and the Mitral Sphincter as Factors in Functional and Organic Disturbances of the Heart	*American Jour. of the Medical Sciences*, Feb., 1901
1902	Osteitis Deformans and Hyperostosis Cranii ; a Contribution to their Pathology, with a Report of Cases	*American Jour. of the Medical Sciences*, Nov., 1903

FORENSIC MEDICINE

1887	A Case of Chronic Arsenical Poisoning of Supposed Criminal Nature, with Especial References to the Medico-Legal Aspect	*Boston Med. & Surg. Jour.*, Vol. CXVI, No. 18
1890	The Present Method of Giving Expert Testimony in Medico-Legal Cases, as Illustrated by one in which Large Damages were Awarded : Based on Contradictory Medical Evidence	*Boston Med. & Surg. Jour.*, Vol. CXXII, No. 4
1907	The Criminal Responsibility of Insane Persons	*Jour. of the A.M.A.*, Nov. 16, 1907, Vol. XLIX

II—NEUROLOGY

1885	How a Lesion of the Brain Results in that Disturbance of Consciousness known as Sensory Aphasia	*Jour. of Nervous and Mental Diseases*, Vol. XII, No. 3

Date of
Publication Article Publication

1886 Tenderness of the Spine in Health and Disease, and the Therapeutic Effects of Blistering over the Fourth and Fifth Dorsal Vertebrae *Boston Med. & Surg. Jour.*, Vol. CXV, No. 15

1889 Four Cases of " Westphal's Paradoxical Contraction " ; with Remarks on Its Mechanism *Boston Med. & Surg. Jour.*, Vol. CXX, No. 17

,, Two Cases of Pseudo-Locomotor Ataxia Following Diphtheria *Boston Med. & Surg. Jour.*, Vol. CXX, No. 24

,, Traumatic Neuroses *Boston Med. & Surg. Jour.*, Vol. CXX, No. 22

,, The somewhat Frequent Occurrence of Degenerative Disease of the Nervous System (Tabes Dorsalis and Disseminated Sclerosis) in Persons Suffering from Malaria *Journal of Nervous and Mental Diseases*, Oct., 1889

1891 Association Neuroses : a Study of the Pathology of Hysterical Joint Affections, Neurasthenia and Allied Forms of Neuro-Mimesis *Journal of Nervous and Mental Diseases*, May, 1891

1892 A Case of Functional Monoplegia in a Man due to Traumatism : Recovery *Boston Med. & Surg. Jour.*, Vol. CXXVI, No. 1

,, Two Fatal Cases of Cerebral Diseases (one of Confusional Insanity, the other of Doubtful Nature) following Grippe *Boston Med. & Surg. Jour.*, Vol. CXXVI, No. 10

,, Post-Hemiplegic Tumor of Paralysis Agitans *Boston Med. & Surg. Jour.*, Vol. CXXVI, No. 14

,, A Case of Cerebellar Tumor with Autopsy *Boston Med. & Surg. Jour.*, Vol. CXXVI, No. 21

,, Three Cases of Traumatic Hysterical Paralysis, of Twenty-nine, Twenty-eight and Twenty-nine Years' Duration respectively, in Males *American Journal of the Medical Sciences*, July, 1892

1894 Neuroses—Mode of Action of Electricity in Neuroses *International System of Electro-Therapeutics*

1895 Traumatism as a Cause of Locomotor Ataxia *Jour. of Nerv. & Ment. Diseases*, Feb., 1895

,, Diseases of the Spinal Cord *Diseases of the Nervous System.* By American Authors

Date of Publication	Article	Publication
1896	Remarks on the Probable Effect of Expert Testimony in Prolonging the Duration of Traumatic Neuroses	*Boston Med. & Surg. Jour.*, Vol. CXXXIV, No. 18
,,	A Case of Ideational Sadism (Sexual Perversion)	*Boston Med. & Surg. Jour.*, Vol. CXXXV, No. 8
1897	Hysterical Monocular Amplyopia Co-existing with Normal Binocular Vision	*Amer. Jour. of Med. Sciences*, Feb., 1897
,,	Idiopathic Internal Hydrocephalus (Serous Meningitis) in the Adult ; with Reports of Three Cases (two with Autopsies)	*Jour. of Nerv. & Ment. Diseases*, Aug., 1897
1898	Accident Neuroses and Football Playing	*Boston Med. & Surg. Jour.*,Vol. CXXXVIII, No. 17
,,	The Pathology, Genesis, and Development of some of the More Important Symptoms in Traumatic Hysteria and Neurasthenia	*Boston Med. & Surg. Jour.*, Vol. CXXXVIII, Nos. 22, 23, 24
,,	Habit-Neuroses as True Functional Diseases	*Boston Med. & Surg. Jour.*, Vol. CXXXIX, No. 24
,,	Fear-Neurosis	*Boston Med. & Surg. Jour.*, Dec. 22, 1898
,,	The Educational Treatment of Neurasthenia and Certain Hysterical States	*Boston Med. & Surg. Jour.*, Oct., 1898
,,	Hysterical Neurasthenia	*Boston Med. & Surg. Jour.*, Dec. 29, 1898
,,	Traumatic Neuroses	*American System of Practical Medicine*, 1898
1901	Section of the Posterior Spinal Roots for the Relief of Pain in a Case of Neuritis of the Branchial Plexus ; Cessation of Pain in the Affected Area ; Later Development of Brown-Séquard's Paralysis as a Result of Laminectomy ; Unusual Distribution of Root Anæsthesia ; Later Partial Return of Sensibility	*Brain*, Part XCIII, Spring Number, 1901

Date of Publication	Article	Publication
1901	The Great Toe (Babinski) Phenomenon: a Contribution to the Study of the Normal Plantar Reflex Based on the Observation of One Hundred and Fifty-six Healthy Individuals	*Boston Med. & Surg. Jour.*, Jan. 24, 1901
1905	The Course of the Sensory Fibres in the Spinal Cord and some Points in Spinal Localisation: Based on a Case of Section of the Cord	*Jour. of Nervous and Mental Diseases*, Feb., 1905
1907	A Study in Tactual Localisation in a Case Presenting Asteriognosis and Asymbolia due to injury to the Cortex of the Brain	*Jour. of Nervous and Mental Diseases*, Vol. XXXV, No. I
1908	Tactile Stereognosis and Symbolia : Have they Localisation in the Cerebral Cortex ?	*Jour. of Nervous and Mental Diseases*, Vol. XXXV, No. I
1910	Cerebral Localisation from the Point of View of Function and Symptoms	*Jour. of Nervous and Mental Diseases*, June, 1910
1917	The Prevention of so-called " Shell-Shock "	*Jour. of the American Med. Assn.*, Sept. 1
1919	Babinski's Theory of Hysteria	*Jour. Abnormal Psychology*, Vol. XIV, No. V

III—PSYCHOLOGY—PSYCHOPATHOLOGY— PSYCHIATRY

1882	Thought Transference or Telepathy	Wood's *Reference Handbook of the Medical Sciences*
1887	Thought Transference: a *Résumé* of the Evidence	*Boston Med. & Surg. Jour.*, Feb., 1887
1890	Some of the Revelations of Hypnotism, Post-Hypnotic Suggestion, Automatic Writing, and Double Personality	*Boston Med. & Surg. Jour.*, Vol. CXXII, Nos. 20 and 21
,,	Remarks on Hypnotism as a Therapeutic Agent in Medicine	*Boston Med. & Surg. Jour.*, Vol. CXXII, No. 14
1897	A Case of " Imperative Idea " or " Homicidal Impulse " in a Neurasthenic without Hereditary Taint	*Boston Med. & Surg. Jour.*, Vol. CXXXVI, No. 3
1898	Sexual Perversion or Vice ? : a Pathological and Therapeutic Inquiry	*Jour. of Nervous and Mental Diseases*, April, 1898

Date of Publication	Article	Publication
1898	A Contribution to the Study of Hysteria and Hypnosis ; being some Experiments on Two Cases of Hysteria and Physio-logico-Anatomical Theory of the Nature of these Neuroses	*Proceedings of Society for Psychical Research,* Part XXXIV, Dec., 1898
,,	An Experimental Study of Visions	*Brain,* Part LXXXIV, Winter Number, 1898
,,	Sexual Psychoses	*American System of Practical Medicine*
,,	The Development and Genea-logy of the Misses Beauchamp	*Proceedings of Society for Psychical Research,* Part XL, Feb., 1901
1905	Some of the Present Problems of Abnormal Psychology	Congress of Arts and Sciences (St Louis), 1904, Vol. V, p. 754 ; also *Psychological Review,* Vol. XII, Nos. 2–3
1905	Do Subconscious States Habitu-ally Exist Normally, or are they always either Artifacts or Abnormal Phenomena ?	*Psychological Review,* March–May, 1905
1906	The Psychology of Sudden Re-ligious Conversion	*Jour. of Abnormal Psy-chology,* Vol I, No. 1
1906	Hysteria from the Point of View of Dissociated Personality	*Boston Med. & Surg. Jour.,* Vol. CLV, Nos. 12 and 14
1907	Cases Illustrating the Educa-tional Treatment of the Psy-choneuroses	*Jour. of Abnormal Psychology,* Oct.–Nov., 1907
,,	A Symposium on the Subcon-scious (Janet and Prince)	*Jour. of Abnormal Psy-chology,* Vol. II, No. 1
1908	The Desirability of Instruction in Psychopathology in Our Medical Schools and its Intro-duction at Tufts	*Boston Med. & Surg. Jour.,* Vol. CLIX, No. 16
,,	Experiments in Psycho-Galvanic Reactions from Co-conscious (Subconscious) Ideas in a Case of Multiple Personality (Mor-ton Prince and Frederick Petersen)	*Jour. Abnormal Psy-chology,* Vol. III, No. 2
,,	Experiments to Determine Co-conscious (Subconscious) Ideation	*Jour. Abnormal Psy-chology,* Vol. III, No. 1
,,	The Unconscious	*Jour. Abnormal Psy-chology,* Vol. III, Nos. 4, 5, 6 ; Vol. IV, No. 1

Date of Publication	Article	Publication
1909	The Psychological Principles and Field of Psychotherapy	*Jour. Abnormal Psychology*, Vol. IV, No. 2 ; also *Psychotherapeutics*. Badger, Boston
„	The Subconscious	*Comptes Rendus*; International Congress of Psychologists, Geneva
1910	The Mechanism and Interpretation of Dreams	*Jour. Abnormal Psychology*, Vol. V, No. 2
„	The Mechanism and Interpretation of Dreams : a Reply to Dr Ernest Jones	*Jour. Abnormal Psychology*, Vol. V, No. 5
1911	The Mechanism of Recurrent Psychopathic States with Special Reference to Anxiety States—Presidential Address	*Jour. Abnormal Psychology*, Vol. VI, No. 2
1912	The Meaning of Ideas as Determined by Unconscious Settings	*Jour. Abnormal Psychology*, Vol. VII, No. 4
„	A Clinical Study of a Case of Phobia—A Symposium (Prince & Putnam)	*Jour. Abnormal Psychology*, Vol. VII, No. 4
1913	The Psychopathology of a Case of Phobia	*Jour. Abnormal Psychology*, Vol. VIII, No. 4
1916	The Subconscious Setting of Ideas in Relation to the Pathology of the Psychoneuroses	*Jour. Abnormal Psychology*, Vol. XI, No. 1
„	A World Consciousness and Future Peace	*Jour. Abnormal Psychology*, Vol. XI, No. 4
1917	Co-conscious Images	*Jour. Abnormal Psychology*, Vol. XII, No. 5
1919	Babinski's Theory of Hysteria	*Jour. of Abnormal Psychology*, Vol. XIV, No. 5
1919	The Psychogenesis of Multiple Personality	*Jour. Abnormal Psychology*, Vol. XIV, No. 4
1920	Miss Beauchamp: the Theory of the Psychogenesis of Multiple Personality	*Jour. of Abnormal Psychology*, Vol. XVI, No. 1, 1920
1921	The Structure and Dynamic Elements of Human Personality	*Jour. of Abnormal Psychology*, Vol. XVI, No. 6, 1920–21
1921	A Critique of Psychoanalysis	*Archives of Neurology and Psychiatry*, Vol. VI, p. 610

Date of Publication	Article	Publication
1922	An Experimental Study of the Mechanism of Hallucinations	*British Jour. of Psychology, Medical Section,* Vol. II, Part 3
1923	A Case of Complete Loss of all Sensory Functions, &c.	*Jour. of Abnormal Psychology,* 1923, Vol. XVIII
1923	Awareness, Consciousness, Co-consciousness and Animal Intelligence from the point of view of the Data of Abnormal Psychology—A Biological Theory of Consciousness	*Proceedings*: International Congress of Psychologists, Oxford
1924	The Problem of Human Personality	Read at Meeting of British Association for the Advancement of Science, Toronto (to be published)

IV—PHILOSOPHY

1885	The Question of a Vital Principle. A Reply to Professor Dwight	*Boston Med. & Surg. Jour.,* Vol. CXIII, Nos. 11–14
1891	Hughlings-Jackson on the Connection between the Mind and the Brain	*Brain,* Summer Number, 1891
1903	Professor Strong on the Relation between the Mind and the Body	*Psychological Review,* Vol. X, No. 6
1904	The Identification of Mind and Matter	*Philosophical Review,* Vol. XIII, No. 4
1908	Discussion of Professor Pierce's Version of the late " Symposium on the Subconscious "	*Psychology and Scientific Methods,* Vol. V, No. 3

V—BOOKS ABOUT DR. PRINCE

Morton Prince and Abnormal Psychology	*Prof. W. B. Taylor*

INDEX

A

Abraham, 381
Ach, 43, 84
Adler, A., 106, 107
Amblyopia:
  Hysterical, 234
Amnesia, 57, 59, 149, 193, 194, 235, 355
Amnesic apraxia, 222
Amsden, 67
Anæsthesia:
  Functional, 235
Analgesia, 56
Anger, 56, 57, 58, 60, 132, 133, 280
  Emotional movements in, 54, 55
Animal magnetism, 236
Animism, 168
Apraxia, 219, 222, 223
  Perseveration in, 222
Aristotle, 391-3
Army, 276
Art:
  Conflict and adjustment in, 373-383
  Ultimate function of, 374
Auto-suggestion, 307-310

B

Babinski, 237, 306
Bahnsen, Julius, 98
Bailey, T. J., 84
Bain, A., 84, 89, 90, 95
Balfour, Gerald, 198, 199
Baudouin, 305, 307
Beard, G. M., 182
Bergson, 42, 334
Berman, L., 111
Bernheim, 236, 305
Binet, 20
Bjerre, 321
Bleuler, E., 70, 71, 72, 73, 334
Boas, 137
Boven, 108
Brain:
  Development of, 5
  Human, evolution of, 4
Breuer, 322
Brown, William :
  " **Suggestion and Personality,**" 303-310
Bucard, 207
Bullough, 379
Burr, G. L., 173

C

Calef, 173
Campbell, C. Macfie :
  " **On Recent Contributions to the Study of the Personality,**" 63-75
Cannon, 47, 59, 111, 340
Carlson, 111
Carpenter, 317
Catalepsy, 224
Catch-phrases :
  Thraldom of, 8-11
Cerebellar disease, 221
Character:
  and inhibition, 77-138
  Classification of, 89-105
  Concept of, 110
  connection with sex impulses, 105
  Consolidation of, 92
  Definition of, 91
  from the angle of *Struktur* and *Gestalt* psychology, 113
  Historical, 83
  in children, 85, 137
  Index of, 122
  Inhibition as basis of, 115-122
  Investigation of, 105
  Moral, 82
  Psychological source of the regulative principles, 130
  Relation of intellect to, 127
  suggestions from psychiatry, 108
  Thought and, 127
Characterlessness of women, 123
Charcot, 233, 305
Chieftains:
  Mana in, 282
Children:
  Association of psycho-neurosis with mental deficiency in, 257-266
  Character in, 85, 137
  Curiosity of, 259, 261
  Fear in, 265
  " Sexual " feeling in, 265
Chorea, 221, 224
Christ, 276
  Equal love of, 276
Church, 276
  and witchcraft, 168
  Antagonism to magic of, 170
Claparède, Ed. :
  " **Does the Will Express the Entire Personality ?** " 37-43
Clear thinking :
  Evasion of, 9

Clinical psychology, 15-25
  Characteristics of, 16
  Relation to social psychology of, 21
Co-conscious personality, 194, 195, 198
Co-consciousness, 52, 191-203, 245-253, 329, 333
Conscience, 270
Conscious thought, 365
Consciousness, 196, 343
  Dissociation of, 235-237
  Double, 191
  Splitting of, 191
  What is, 315
Constitution:
  Concept of, 110
Convulsions, 224
Coriat, I. H., 176, 223
Coué, 237, 305, 309
Crile, 111
Crowd, 271, 278, 280, 343
  Defects and ferocities of, 271
  Emotional contagion in, 272, 273, 277, 284
Curiosity:
  Children's, 259, 261

D

Dana, Charles L. :
  " The Handwriting in Nervous Diseases, with Special Reference to the Signatures of William Shakespeare," 205-215
Danger:
  Dissociation during, 48, 51
  Emotional condition during, 53
  Experience during, 47-51
  Recollections of, 48
Dart, Raymond A., 7
Delusion of marital infidelity, 163
Dementia præcox, 68, 156, 338, 366, 367
  Stereotyped movements in, 225
Depression, 141, 142, 143, 147
  dreams, 355-364
Devotion, 276
Dianic cult, 171, 172
Downey, J. E., 124
Drake, 178
Dread:
  in group, 277, 279
  of society, 270
Dream(s), 325, 344
  Analogy of delusions to, 354
  Analysis, Freud's theory, 325
  Day, 327
  Depression, 356-364, 367
  Elation, 367
  Explanation of, 353
  images, 198
  Infantile sexual, 368
  Memory of, 355
  Metamorphosis of, 353-369
  Relation to waking stimulus, 368

Dream(s) *(cont.)* :
  Sexual, 368
  Symbolism of, 327, 328, 355
  thoughts, 198
  thoughts, change to waking thoughts, 366
  thoughts, mechanism by which they pass into waking activities, 354
Drever, J., 240
Dunlap, Knight, 314
" Subconscious, the Unconscious and the Co-conscious," 243-253
Dysdiadokokinesis, 221
Dysmetria, 221
Dyssynergia, 221

E

Ego, 43, 196, 197, 279, 283, 291
  Analysis of, 269
  Disintegration of, 203
Ego-ideal, 279, 283, 309
Ego-instincts, 276
Elation dreams, 367
Elliot, Hugh, 93
Emotion(s) :
  Asthenic, 47
  Cognitive effect of, 59
  connection with instincts, 47
  contagion in groups, 272, 273, 277, 284
  Effect on memory, 57
  Function of, 61
  Motor connection of, 47
  Primary, relation to instincts, 272
  Relation of endocrine glands to, 323
  Sthenic, 47, 54, 56, 61
  Wider functions of, 47
Emotional:
  movements, 54
  ties, 276, 277, 279, 282
Empathy, 32-33, 379, 380
  Bibliography of, 35
Encephalitis lethargica:
  Effect on handwriting of, 209
Endocrine glands :
  derangement in secretion produced by hysteria, 324
  relation to emotions, 323
Envy, 281, 285
Erlenmeyer, 207
Ethology, 83, 84
Excitement, 56, 60
  Emotional movements in, 55
Extraverts, 295, 296, 298
Extraversion, 302

F

Father:
  Christ, 276
  Equal love of, 282
  Primal, 282, 283, 285
  Surrogate, 276

Fear, 56, 57, 58, 60, 143
  Collective, 277
  Emotional movements in, 54, 55
Feeling, 297, 298
Ferenczi, S., 31
Fernald, G. G., 81, 82
Fiske, John, 173, 178
Flechsig, 316
Foreconscious, 329
Forel, 362
Fouillée, A., 42, 95, 96
Fraser, J. G., 169
Freud, S., 10, 11, 19, 20, 21, 23, 31, 43,
  65, 119, 200, 202, 236, 238, 239,
  241, 245, 269-285, 308, 313, 314,
  316, 322, 323, 324, 325, 326, 327,
  344, 353, 358, 375, 381, 390
Friedmann, R., 89
Friendship, 276

G

Galton, 85
Gestalt school, 407-8
Ginsberg, 245
God, 42
Goddard, Henry Herbert :
  " The Unconscious in Psycho-
  analysis. A Criticism," 311-329
Gregarious instinct, 22
Group, 280
  Dread in, 277, 279
  Emotional contagion in, 272, 273,
  277, 284
  ideal, 283
  leader, 276, 277, 280
  Leaderless, 279, 284
  mind, 271, 278
  Organisation in, 271
  Organised, 276
  Primitive, 271
  psychology, 269-285
  Religious, 278
  spirit, 281
Guiteau case, 160, 162

H

Habit, 247
Handwriting in nervous diseases, 205,
  215
Hart, Bernard :
  " The Development of Psycho-
  pathology as a Branch of
  Science," 229-241
Hartmann, 313
Head, Henry, 7
Herbart, 313
Herd instinct, 22, 275, 281
Hetero-suggestion, 307, 309
Heymans, G., 103
Hoch, 67, 354

Holt, E. B., 20, 126
Homosexuality, 357
Hoop, van der, 107
Horde Primal, 281, 282, 283, 285
  Father of the, 282, 285
  Leader of the, 284
Horton, L. H. :
  Prince's " Neurogram " Concept,
  385-419
Hose, 10, 137
Hunt, J. Ramsey :
  " The Static and Kinetic Represen-
  tations of the Efferent Nervous
  System in the Psycho-motor
  Sphere," 217, 227
Hunter, John I., 5, 7
Hutchinson, 177
Hypermnesia, retroactive, 58, 59
Hypnosis, 280, 282, 305
  Deep, 306
  Definition of, 306
  Relation of suggestion to, 305
Hypnotic somnambulism, 193, 235
Hypnotic state, relation of suggestion,
  31
Hypnotism, 192, 194, 200, 283, 306
Hypnotist, 282
Hysteria, 167, 192, 233, 236, 237, 307,
  338
  Derangement in secretion of endo-
  crine glands by, 324
  Psychokinetic and psychostatic
  manifestations of, 224
  Psychopathological conception of,
  233
Hysterical amblyopia, 234
Hysterical somnambulisms, 192, 193

I

Ideas, 251
Identification, 203, 279
Imitation, 274
Inhibition, 145, 280
  as basis of character, 115, 122
  Character and, 79-138
  of instinctive tendencies, 130
  of sexual instinct, 122
Insanity:
  Criteria of, 161
  Delusion of marital infidelity in, 163
Insanity cases :
  How verdicts are obtained in, 153
  Mental attitude of judges in, 159
  Partial responsibility for criminal
  acts in, 161
  Question of allowing medical wit-
  nesses to hear all testimony in
  (U.S.) Admiralty, 157
  trial to determine mental condition
  before trial for homicide, 160
  Writ of habeas corpus in, 154

Instinct(s), 20, 22, 117, 118, 136, 247
  Connections of emotions with, 47
  Ego-, 276
  Gregarious, 22
  Herd, 22, 275, 281
  Inhibition, 131
  Laughter, 273
  Love, 276
  Parental, 280
  Relation of primary emotions to, 272
  Self-preservative, 281
  Sexual, 80, 123, 270, 280, 281
  Sexual, inhibition, 122
  Sexual, obstruction, 280
  Social, 22, 269
  Unconscious, 319
Intelligence, evolution of, 3-8
Intention tremor, 221
Introjection, 33
Introverts, 295, 296, 298, 300
Introversion, 302
Intuition, 297, 298

J

James, William, 40, 47, 112, 147, 249
Janet, Pierre, 20, 42, 65, 192, 199, 200, 234, 235, 236, 240, 305, 313, 395, 396
  " Memories Which are Too Real," 139-150
Jastrow, J., 86, 87, 97, 109, 314
Jelliffe, Smith Ely:
  " Unconscious Dynamics and Human Behaviour: a Glimpse at Some Inter-Relationships of Structure and Function," 331-350
Jones, Ernest, 105, 309, 354, 368, 381
  " Abnormal Psychology and Social Psychology," 13-25
Jones, Tudor, 7
Jove, 251
Joy, 56
  Emotional movements in, 54, 55
Jung, C. G., 73, 74, 105, 106, 203, 241, 313, 390, 406, 407
  " Psychological Types," 287-302

K

Kahlbaum, 67
Kahn, 70, 71
Kant, 85
Kempf, 107
Kings, Mana in, 282
Kittredge, G. L., 173, 182, 188
Klages, 102
Koehler, 114, 407-8
Koffka, K., 114, 408
Kollarits, Jenö, 110
Kraepelin, 70, 74, 225
Kretschmer, Ernst, 68, 69, 71, 109, 110
Kroll, 223
Küppers, E., 335

L

Langfeld, Herbert Sidney :
  " Conflict and Adjustment in Art," 371-383
Laughter, 273
Laughter instinct, 273
Leader, 124, 276, 277, 280, 281, 284
  Death of, 278
  Equal love of, 276, 279, 282
  Prestige of, 274
Le Bon, 21, 270, 271, 273, 274, 283
Leftwich, R. W., 214
Leibnitz, 198
Lévy, 97
Lévy-Bruhl, 137
Libidinal ties, 277-279
Libido, 119, 201, 276, 277, 284, 336
  Sexual, 280, 285
Liepmann, 223
Lipps, 379
Locke, 394-5, 399
Lotze, 198
Love, 56, 58, 276, 279, 280
  Being in, 279, 280
  Christ's, 276, 279
  Emotional movements in, 54, 55
  Equal, 276, 279, 282
  for humanity, 276
  Parental, 276, 280
  Self-, *see* Narcissism
  Sexual, 280.
Lucka, E., 101, 102
Lunacy :
  Criminal, 160
  Criminal, partial responsibility, 161
  trials, how verdicts are obtained, 153
  trials, mental attitude of judges, 159
  trials, question of allowing medical witnesses to hear all testimony in (U.S.) Admiralty cases, 157
  trials, writ of *habeas corpus*, 154

M

McCharles, Stella B., 58
MacCurdy, John T. :
  " The Metamorphosis of Dreams," 351-369
McDougall, William, 10, 21, 47, 87, 92, 93, 117, 132, 137, 197, 198, 199, 271, 274, 277, 278, 306, 412
  " Professor Freud's Group Psychology and his Theory of Suggestion," 267-285
Magic, Antagonism of Church to, 170
Malapert, 96
Malebranche, 272
Mana, 282
Martin, 271

Medicine :
  Bad thinking in, 33
  Bad thinking in, bibliography, 36
Medico-legal experiences, 153-164
Memory :
  Effect of emotion on, 57
  Too real, 141-150
  Unreal, 145
Mental deficiency, association with psycho-neurosis, 257-266
Mental dissociation, 191-193
Mesmer, 236
Meumann, E., 98, 99, 100, 101
Meyer, Adolf, 68
Michotte, 43
Mill, J. S., 83, 84
Mills, Charles K. ;
  " Some Medico-Legal Experiences, with Comments and Reflections," 151-164
Mitchell, T. W. :
  "The Self and Co-consciousness," 189-203
Moore, G. H., 173
Motility, 219, 220, 221
  Hysterical disorders of, 224
Motor apraxia, 222, 223
  Perseveration in, 222
  Purposive, 219, 222
  Stereotyped, 219
  Stereotyped, in dementia præcox, 225
Münsterberg, 87, 313
Murray, Margaret A., 171, 176, 187
Myers, Charles S. ;
  " The Association of Psycho-Neurosis with Mental Deficiency," 255-266
Myers, Frederic, 192, 389
Myoclonus, 224
Myotonia, 221, 224

N

Narcissism, 278, 309
Nervous system :
  Efferent, new conception, 219
  Efferent, static and kinetic representations in psycho-motor sphere, 219-227
Neurogram concept, 387-419
Neurosis, 23, 307

P

Panic, 60, 277, 278
Parker, 8
Parmelee, 42
Paralysis :
  Functional, 235
Paralysis agitans, 221
  Effect on handwriting of, 209

Paramyoclonus multiplex, 221
Paresis, Effect on handwriting of, 210
Pathopsychology, 15
Paulhan, 42, 94, 95
Paulsson, 376
Pérez, 93
Perseveration, 219
  Intentional, 223
  Kinetic and static, 222-224
Personality :
  Co-conscious, 194, 195, 198
  Double, 48, 51, 191, 192, 194, 200, 235, 382
  Multiple, 149, 191, 192, 193, 198, 200, 203
  Secondary, 193, 194, 202
  Secondary, of trance mediumship, 199
  Study of, recent contributions, 65-75
  Suggestion and, 305-310
Petit mal, Effect on handwriting of, 212
Pfister, 107
Pick, 223
Prestige, 274
Prince, Morton, 3, 15, 20, 29, 43, 52, 65, 67, 150, 192, 195, 196, 197, 199, 201, 235, 245, 246, 247, 248, 305, 313, 314, 317, 326, 333, 382, 387-419
  bibliography of writings, 420-427
Prüm, 43
Psychic unity, 10
Psychoanalysis, 22, 200, 202, 203, 239, 320, 321, 324, 325, 344, 348, 353, 355-362
  Unconscious in, 313-329
Psychological scars, 147
Psychological types, 289-302
Psychology :
  Abnormal, 15-25
  Clinical, 15-25
  Clinical, characteristics, 16
  Clinical, relation to social psychology, 21
  Concepts of, construction, 231-242
  Faulty reasoning in, 34
  Group, 269-285
  Plea for elimination of evasive terms and phrases in, 11
  Social, 15-25
  Social, relation to clinical psychology, 21
Psycho-neurosis :
  association with mental deficiency, 257-266
Psychopathology, 15, 23
  development as branch of science, 231-242
  Use of catchwords in, 31
Psychoses, 233
Psycho-therapeutics, 320

R

Reciprocal innervation, 220
Regression, 284, 366, 368
Religion, 24
Repression, 43, 71, 200, 201, 202, 322, 324
Ribéry, 98
Ribot, 97
Rivers, 10, 241
Roback, A. A. :
"**Character and Inhibition,**" 77-138
Rosanoff, A. J., 109
Rugg, H., 124

S

Saltpêtrière, 306
Sanity :
  False criteria of, 161
Schallmeyer, 271
Schopenhauer, A., 128, 129
Self :
  Divisions of, 191
  love, see Narcissism
  preservation, 281
  sacrifice, 284
Senile tremor :
  Effect on handwriting of, 211
Sensation, 297, 298
Sense :
  of sight, 4
  of touch, 5
Sensuality, 276, 280
Sex theories, 238
Sexual :
  attraction, 276
  dreams, 368
  dreams, infantile, 368
  impulses, 285, 365
  impulses, connection with character, 105
  impulses, inhibited, 280, 282
  instinct, 80, 123, 270, 280, 281
  instinct, inhibition, 122
  instinct, obstruction, 280
  jealousy, 282, 285
  libido, 280, 285
  love, 280
  lust, 276, 280
  relationships, 24
  repression, 71
  tendencies, 280, 282
Shand, A. F., 47, 84, 90, 92, 415
Shellshear, Joseph, 7
Sighele, 271
Sight :
  Sense of, 4
Smith, G. Elliot :
  "**The Evolution of Intelligence and the Thraldom of Catch-Phrases,**" 1-11

Social :
  instinct, 22, 269
  psychology, 15-25
  psychology, relation to clinical psychology, 21
Society :
  Dread of, 270
Somnambulism, 235
  Hypnotic, 193, 235
  Hysterical, 192, 193
Sorrow, 58
  Emotional movements in, 55
Specht, Wilhelm, 15
Speech, 7
Spranger, 114, 115
Stärcke, 336
Stekel, 107
Stern, Erich, 114
Stern, William, 114
Stout, G. F., 310
Stratton, George M. :
  "**An Experience during Danger and the Wider Functions of Emotion,**" 45-62
Subconscious, 149, 192, 245-253, 313
Suggestion, 30-1, 236, 237, 273, 274, 281
  abuse of term, 30, 31
  and personality, 305-310
  Auto-, 307, 308, 309, 310
  Bibliography of, 35
  Hetero- 307, 309
  Hypnotic, 192
  Mutual, 274
  Post-hypnotic, 31
  relation to hypnosis, 31, 305
  relation to waking state, 31
  Theory of, 274, 276, 285
  Theory of, Freud's, 269, 285
Superman, 282
Symbols :
  Typical, 10
Sympathy, 133

T

Tabes, dorsalis, effect on handwriting, 211
Taboo, 282
Tarde, 274
Taylor, E. W. :
  "**Some Medical Aspects of Witchcraft,**" 165-188
Temperament, 84, 85, 89, 90, 98-110, 292
  Concept of, 110
  Differentiation of, 289
Tenderness, 280
Tertullian, 187
Thinking, 297, 298
Thought and character, 127.
Thoughts, 251
Totemism, 282

Touch, Sense of, 5
Tremor, 224
Trotter, Wilfred, 22, 271, 272, 275, 281
Types, 289-302

U

Unconscious, 202, 238, 240, 245-253, 313, 333, 334, 337, 343, 365
   cerebration, 317
   Concepts of, 313
   dynamics and human behaviour, 333-350
   in psychoanalysis, 313-329
   instinct, 319
   Term, 315
Upham, C. W., 174, 175, 177, 188

V

Van der Hoop ;
   see Hoop, van der
Vision, foundation of man's mental powers, 4
Volition, 39, 40, 42, 43, 310

W

Waking state, Relation of suggestion to, 31
Waking thoughts, 354

Walshe, 223.
Warren, 42
Webb, E., 123
Weininger, Otto, 85
Wells, F. L., 67
Wendell, B., 182
Wertheimer, 114
Westermarck, 137
White, William, A., 107
   " **Notes on Suggestion, Empathy, and Bad Thinking in Medicine,**" 27-36
Wiersma, E., 103
Will, 92
   Definition of, 39
   does it express the entire personality ? 39-43
Wilson, 223
Winsor, Justin, 173
Wishes, 251
Witchcraft :
   in America, 173-188
   Medical aspects of, 167-188
   Salem cases, 28, 33-48, 168, 173-188
   Suppression of, 172
   Term, origin and development, 168
Women, Characterlessness, 123
Wundt, W., 21, 87, 98, 99

Owing to the order of the contributions to this volume having been changed at the last minute, the necessary alterations in the INDEX were overlooked, and the references as printed are therefore incorrect. The following KEY INDEX will remedy this defect.

For 1–11	. . .	*read* 1–11
13–23	. . . . .	217–227
25–48	. . . . .	165–188
49–61	. . . . .	13–25
63–74	. . . . .	255–266
75–88	. . . . .	229–241
89–106	. . . . .	45–62
109–122	. . . . .	287–302
123–132	. . . . .	27–36
133–151	. . . . .	351–369
153–171	. . . . .	311–329
173–186	. . . . .	151–164
187–206	. . . . .	331–350
207–221	. . . . .	189–203
223–233	. . . . .	243–253
235–246	. . . . .	139–150
247–257	. . . . .	205–215
259–271	. . . . .	371–383
273–291	. . . . .	267–285
293–299	. . . . .	37–43
301–362	. . . . .	77–138
363–375	. . . . .	63–75
377–384	. . . . .	303–310
385–419	. . . . .	385–419